Health Issues

MAGILL'S CHOICE

Health Issues

Volume 1

Abortion – Hypertension

edited by
The Editors of Salem Press

project editor
Tracy Irons-Georges

SALEM PRESS, INC.
Pasadena, California
Hackensack, New Jersey

The essays in *Magill's Choice: Health Issues* were adapted from *Women's Issues* (1997), *Encyclopedia of Family Life* (1998), *Children's Health* (1999), *Encyclopedia of Environmental Issues* (1999), *Aging* (2000), *Magill's Choice: Psychology and Mental Health* (2000), and *Magill's Medical Guide, Second Revised Edition* (2002). All bibliographies have been updated, and formats have been changed.

∞ The paper used in these volumes conforms to the American National Standard for Permanence of Paper for Printed Library Materials, Z39.48-1992 (R1997).

Library of Congress Cataloging-in-Publication Data
Health issues / edited by the editors of Salem Press ; project editor, Tracy Irons-Georges
    p.   cm. — (Magill's choice)
Includes bibliographical references and index.
ISBN 0-89356-042-1 (set). — ISBN 0-89356-048-0 (v. 1). — ISBN 0-89356-049-9 (v. 2)
    1. Public health. 2. Social medicine. I. Irons-Georges, Tracy. II. Salem Press.
III. Series

RA425.H39 2001
362.1—dc21

200102087

First Printing

PRINTED IN THE UNITED STATES OF AMERICA

Table of Contents

Publisher's Note

The maintenance of health has always been a crucial concern both for individuals and for societies. *Health Issues* focuses on important topics in public health such as epidemic, occupational, and environmental diseases, as well as on such social issues as ethical debates and the financial and sociological impact of particular diseases.

This set offers 251 articles adapted from other Salem Press products: *Women's Issues* (1997), the *Encyclopedia of Family Life* (1998), *Children's Health* (1999), the *Encyclopedia of Environmental Issues* (1999), *Aging* (2000), *Magill's Choice: Psychology and Mental Health* (2000), and *Magill's Medical Guide, Second Revised Edition* (2002). All essays have been updated with the latest information and bibliographical sources.

Examined here are preventive measures such as exercise, vitamin supplements, and prenatal care. The myriad ramifications of diseases such as AIDS, Alzheimer's disease, and cancer are discussed, as well as traditional and alternative treatments, including gene therapy, biofeedback, and acupuncture. Emerging, or reemerging, public health threats receiving coverage include sick building syndrome, tuberculosis, and Lyme disease. Social trends that put health at risk are addressed, such as eating disorders, steroid abuse, smoking, and domestic violence. Some medical or industry practices that have aroused controversy are considered, such as circumcision, hysterectomy, cosmetic surgery, pesticide use, and the genetic engineering of foods. Issues pertaining to vulnerable groups—children, teenagers, and the elderly—are highlighted.

Each article begins with information about type of health issue and a brief definition of the topic. The text of the essay follows, divided into helpful subheadings that guide the reader through the discussion. An author byline, a bibliography, and cross-references to other entries in the encyclopedia conclude every entry. At the back of volume 2 can be found a full Alphabetical List of Entries and a Category List by type of issue: children's health, economic issues, elder health, environmental health, epidemics, ethics, industrial practices, medical procedures, men's health, mental health, occupational health, prevention, public health, social trends, treatment, and women's health. Volume 2 also features a Glossary of relevant medical terms and a comprehensive subject Index.

Health Issues is made possible by the work of many physicians, academicians, and other scholars. We would like to extend our gratitude to them. A list of their names and affiliations appears in the front of volume 1.

Contributor List

Richard Adler
University of Michigan, Dearborn

E. Victor Adlin, M.D.
Temple University School of Medicine

Patricia A. Ainsa, M.P.H.
University of Texas at El Paso

Bruce Ambuel
Medical College of Wisconsin

P. Michele Arduengo
Morningside College

Iona C. Baldridge
Lubbock Christian University

Lawrence W. Bassett, M.D.
Iris Cantor Professor of Radiology
University of California, Los Angeles,
*   School of Medicine*

Paul F. Bell
The Medical Center, Beaver, Pennsylvania

Alvin K. Benson
Brigham Young University

Cynthia Beres
Independent Scholar

Carol D. Berkowitz, M.D.
Harbor-UCLA Medical Center

Matthew Berria
Weber State University

Robert W. Block, M.D.
University of Oklahoma

Paul R. Boehlke
Dr. Martin Luther College

Barbara Brennessel
Wheaton College

Peter N. Bretan, M.D.
University of California Medical Center,
*   San Francisco*

Mitzie L. Bryant
St. Louis Board of Education

Edmund C. Burke, M.D.
University of California Medical Center,
*   San Francisco*

Louis A. Cancellaro, M.D.
Veterans Affairs Medical Center, Mountain
*   Home, Tennessee*

Byron D. Cannon
University of Utah

Jack Carter
University of New Orleans

Sonya H. Cashdan
East Tennessee State University

Karen Chapman-Novakofski
University of Illinois

Paul J. Chara, Jr.
Loras College

Francis P. Chinard
New Jersey Medical School

Arlene R. Courtney
Western Oregon State College

Maureen C. Creegan
Dominican College of Blauvelt

Margaret Cruikshank
University of Maine

Roy L. DeHart, M.D., M.P.H.
University of Oklahoma

Patrick J. DeLuca
Mt. St. Mary College

Shawkat Dhanani
West Los Angeles VAMC

M. Casey Diana
University of Illinois

Kristen L. Easton
Valparaiso University

C. Richard Falcon
Roberts and Raymond Associates,
Philadelphia

L. Fleming Fallon, Jr., M.D., M.P.H.
Jameson Hospital, New Castle,
Pennsylvania

Frank Fedel
Henry Ford Hospital, Detroit

Mary C. Fields
Collin County Community College

K. Thomas Finley
State University of New York, Brockport

Bonnie Flaig
Kalamazoo Valley Community College

Kimberly Y. Z. Forrest
Slippery Rock University

Ronald B. France
LDS Hospital, Salt Lake City, Utah

Katherine B. Frederich
Eastern Nazarene College

C. George Fry
Lutheran College of Health Professions

Keith Garebian
Independent Scholar

Soraya Ghayourmanesh
City University of New York

Wallace A. Gleason, Jr., M.D.
University of Texas, Houston

D. R. Gossett
Louisiana State University—Shreveport

Karen Gould
Independent Scholar

Daniel G. Graetzer
University of Montana

Hans G. Graetzer
South Dakota State University

L. Kevin Hamberger
Medical College of Wisconsin

Ronald C. Hamdy, M.D.
James H. Quillen College of Medicine

Linda Hart
Independent Scholar

H. Bradford Hawley, M.D.
Wright State University

Robert M. Hawthorne, Jr.
Independent Scholar

Celia Ray Hayhoe
University of Kentucky

Diane Andrews Henningfeld
Adrian College

Martha M. Henze, R.D.
Boulder Community Hospital, Colorado

Mary Ann Holbein-Jenny
Slippery Rock University

David Wason Hollar, Jr.
Rockingham Community College

Betsy B. Holli
Dominican University

Carol A. Holloway
Independent Scholar

Robert M. Hordon
Rutgers University

Howard L. Hosick
Washington State University

Jennifer J. Hostutler
University of Akron

Katherine H. Houp
Midway College

Shih-Wen Huang, M.D.
University of Florida

Larry Hudgins, M.D.
Veterans Affairs Medical Center, Mountain
Home, Tennessee

Diane White Husic
East Stroundsburg University

Vicki J. Isola
Independent Scholar

Albert C. Jensen
Central Florida Community College

Michelle L. Jones
Muskingum College

Karen N. Kähler
Independent Scholar

Karen E. Kalumuck
Cañada College

Armand M. Karow
Xytex Corporation

Robert Kastenbaum
Arizona State University

Laurence M. Katz
University of North Carolina at Chapel Hill

Mara Kelly-Zukowski
Felician College

Cassandra Kircher
Elon College

Hillar Klandorf
West Virginia University

Sharon L. Larson
University of Nebraska-Lincoln

Shirley A. Leckie
University of Central Florida

Gary J. Lindquester
Rhodes College

Stan Liu, M.D.
*University of California, Los Angeles,
School of Medicine*

Joe E. Lunceford
Georgetown College

Fai Ma
University of California, Berkeley

John Arthur McClung, M.D.
New York Medical College

Maxine M. McCue
College of Eastern Utah-San Juan Campus

Nancy E. Macdonald
University of South Carolina at Sumter

Wayne R. McKinny, M.D.
University of Hawaii School of Medicine

Scott Magnuson-Martinson
South Dakota State University

Louise Magoon
Independent Scholar

Nancy Farm Manniko
Michigan Technological University

Bonita L. Marks
University of North Carolina at Chapel Hill

Charles C. Marsh, Pharm.D.
University of Arkansas for Medical Sciences

Linda Mealey
University of Queensland

Randall L. Milstein
Oregon State University

Paul Moglia
*St. Joseph's Medical Center, Yonkers,
New York*

John Monopoli
Slippery Rock University

Sharon Moore, M.D.
*Veterans Affairs Medical Center, Mountain
Home, Tennessee*

Rodney C. Mowbray
University of Wisconsin, LaCrosse

Trina Nahm-Mijo
*University of Hawaii-Hawaii Community
College*

Donald J. Nash
Colorado State University

Cherilyn Nelson
Eastern Kentucky University

Anthony J. Nicastro
West Chester University

Jane Cross Norman
Tennessee State University

Kathleen O'Boyle
Wayne State University

Janet Rose Osuch, M.D.
Michigan State University

Oliver Oyama
*Duke/Fayetteville Area Health Education
Center*

Maria Pacheco
Buffalo State College

Cheryl Pawlowski
University of Northern Colorado

Kate L. Peirce
Southwestern Texas State University

Joseph G. Pelliccia
Bates College

Leslie Pendleton
Independent Scholar

Thomas W. Pierce
Radford University

Nancy A. Piotrowski
University of California, Berkeley

George R. Plitnik
Frostburg State University

Lillian M. Range
University of Southern Mississippi

Wendy E. S. Repovich
Eastern Washington University

Kris Riddlesperger
Texas Christian University

Connie Rizzo, M.D.
Pace University

Larry M. Roberts
Independent Scholar

Gene D. Robinson
James Madison University

John Alan Ross
Eastern Washington University

John G. Ryan, Dr.P.H.
University of Texas, Houston

William J. Ryan
Slippery Rock University

Virginia L. Salmon
Northeast State Technical Community College

Robert Sandlin
San Diego State University

Steven A. Schonefeld
Tri-State University

John Richard Schrock
Emporia State University

Rebecca Lovell Scott
College of Health Sciences

Rose Secrest
Independent Scholar

Kevin S. Seybold
Grove City College

Martha Sherwood-Pike
University of Oregon

R. Baird Shuman
University of Illinois, Urbana-Champaign

Bobbie Siler
Medical College of Ohio

Sanford S. Singer
University of Dayton

Virginia Slaughter
University of Queensland

Genevieve Slomski
Independent Scholar

Roger Smith
Linfield College

Lisa Levin Sobczak, R.N.C.
Independent Scholar

Diane Stanitski-Martin
Shippensburg University

Sharon W. Stark
Monmouth University

Irene Struthers
Independent Scholar

Wendy L. Stuhldreher, R.D.
Slippery Rock University

Billie M. Taylor
Independent Scholar

John M. Theilmann
Converse College

Nicholas C. Thomas
Auburn University at Montgomery

Roberta Tierney
Indiana University and Purdue University

Leslie V. Tischauser
Prairie State College

CONTRIBUTORS

James T. Trent
Middle Tennessee State University

Mary S. Tyler
University of Maine

Maxine Urton
Xavier University

Kimberly A. Wallet
Lamar University

Annita Marie Ward
Salem-Teikyo University

Marcia Watson-Whitmyre
University of Delaware

David J. Wells, Jr.
University of South Alabama Medical Center

Diane E. Wille
Indiana University Southeast

Lee Williams
Independent scholar

Bradley R. A. Wilson
University of Cincinnati

Virginia M. Witt, M.D.
St. Joseph's Hospital and Medical Center

Jay R. Yett
Orange Coast College

Kathleen M. Zanolli
Kansas University

Chester J. Zelasko
Buffalo State College

Health Issues

✧ ABORTION

Type of issue: Ethics, medical procedures, social trends, women's health
Definition: The induced termination of pregnancy, which is usually legal only before the fetus is viable.

Abortion is the deliberate ending of a pregnancy before the fetus is viable, or capable of surviving outside the woman's body. It has been practiced in every culture since the beginning of civilization. It has also been controversial.

ABORTION IN THE UNITED STATES

In the United States, abortion before quickening was legal until the 1840's. By 1841, ten states declared abortion to be a criminal act, but punishments were weak and the laws frequently ignored. The movement against abortion was led by the American Medical Association (AMA), founded in 1847. Doctors were becoming increasingly aware that the "first sign of life" took place well before the fetus actually moved. By this time, scientists had established that fetal development actually began with the union of sperm and egg. In 1859, the AMA passed a resolution condemning abortion as a criminal act. Within a few years, every state declared abortion a felony. Not until 1950 did the AMA reverse its position, when it began a new campaign to liberalize abortion laws. Many doctors were concerned about the thousands of women suffering from complications and even death from illegal abortions. In 1973, the Supreme Court of the United States ruled in *Roe v. Wade* that abortions were generally legal. That ruling made abortions in the United States available on the request of pregnant women.

In the nineteenth century, it is believed that there was one abortion for every four live births, a rate only a bit lower than that in the latter part of the twentieth century. The number of abortions in any year varied from 500,000 to 1 million, most of them illegal. In 1969, the Centers for Disease Control (CDC), a branch of the U.S. Department of Health and Human Services, began an annual abortion count. Legal abortions in 1970 numbered about 200,000. The number of illegal abortions is unknown. Ten years later, legal abortions reached 1,200,000 and by 1990 had increased to 1,600,000; they have remained at that level fairly consistently since then. The CDC estimated that there were about 325 abortions for every 1,000 live births in the 1980's, a number consistent with findings for the 1990's. The number of abortions in any year rarely fluctuated by more or less than 3 percent from these figures.

In *Roe v. Wade*, the Supreme Court ruled that abortions were legal under certain conditions. Those conditions included the welfare of the woman and the viability of the fetus. During the first three months of pregnancy, according to the Court, the government had no legitimate interest in regulating abortions. The only exception was that states could require that abortions be performed by a licensed physician in a "medical setting." Otherwise, the decision to abort was strictly that of the pregnant woman as a constitutional right of privacy. During the second trimester, abortions were more restricted. They would be legal only if the woman's health needed to be protected and would require the consent of a doctor. The interest of the fetus would be protected during the third trimester, when it became able to survive on its own outside of the woman's body, with or without artificial life support. States, at this point, could grant abortions only to women for whom, according to medical opinion, the continued pregnancy would be life-threatening. The determination of viability would be made by doctors, not by legal authorities. This ruling effectively struck down all antiabortion laws across the United States.

In the aftermath of *Roe v. Wade*, abortion became an intensely emotional political issue in the United States. The Hyde Amendment of 1976 eliminated federal funding for abortions, and other legislation blocked foreign aid to programs such as family planning that members of Congress who were opposed to abortion saw as "pro-abortion." In *Webster v. Reproductive Health Services* (1989), the Supreme Court upheld its ruling in *Roe v. Wade*, but it also sustained a rule forbidding the use of public facilities or public employees for carrying out abortions. The Court also supported a requirement that a test for viability be done before any late abortion and said states could ban funding for abortion counseling. The issue continued to divide Americans, with opponents arguing that abortion at any point in the process of birth was murder.

Reasons for Seeking an Abortion

A 1987 survey done by the Alan Guttmacher Institute of 1,900 women who had abortions revealed the most common reasons for making that decision. Ninety-three percent of the respondents gave more than one reason, but these reasons could usually be reduced to four basic notions. The most common was that having a baby would interfere with work or going to school. Next came not being able to afford a child. Third was a concern about relationship problems with the father. The last was that the potential mother did not want to be a single parent.

A study done by the CDC of what types of women wanted to have an abortion revealed that almost 60 percent were experiencing their first pregnancy. Women beneath the poverty level, regardless of race, religion, or ethnic background, were more likely to have an abortion than middle-class women. African American and Hispanic women had higher rates of abortion than did white women. The largest number of abortions were performed on white, single women, eighteen to twenty-five years of age. This same group, however, also had the highest number of live births.

Religion appeared to make little difference: The percentage of Catholic women having abortions was actually a bit higher than the percentage of Protestant women. The lowest percentage of abortions was found among Evangelical, "born-again" Christians. Teenagers under fifteen and women over forty had the highest rates of abortion of any age groups. The study showed that the reasons for late abortions, defined as those sixteen weeks or later after conception, differed somewhat from those given by women who had their abortions during the first trimester. Two key factors were involved in late abortions. Seventy-one percent of the women interviewed said that they had waited so long because they had not realized they were pregnant or did not know soon enough how long they had been pregnant. Fifty percent said that they had taken so long because they had problems raising enough money to pay for an abortion. Thus, poverty appears to be a leading cause of late abortions. Many in this latter group also reported that they had to leave their home states to obtain legal abortions because there were no facilities in these states. Almost 90 percent of counties in the United States do not have facilities or doctors who will perform abortions. Death rates for women who have abortions after sixteen weeks are thirty times higher than the rate at eight weeks.

ABORTION PROCEDURES

A variety of techniques can be used to perform abortions. They vary according to the length of the pregnancy, which is usually measured by the number of weeks since the last menstrual period (LMP). Instrumental techniques are usually used very early in a pregnancy. They include a procedure called menstrual extraction, in which the entire contents of the uterus are removed. It can be done as early as fourteen days after the expected onset of a period. A major problem with this method is a high risk of error; the human embryo may still be so small at this age that it can be missed. It is also true that a high proportion of women undergoing this procedure turn out not to have been pregnant. Nevertheless, this method is easy to do and very safe. Death rates from this technique average less than 1 out of 100,000.

About 96 percent of all abortions in the United States are done by a procedure known as vacuum aspiration, or suction curettage. This technique can be used up to about fourteen weeks after the LMP. It can be performed with local anesthesia and follows these steps. First, the cervix is expanded with metal rods that are inserted into it one at a time, with each rod being slightly larger than the previous one. When the cervix is expanded to the right size, a transparent, hollow tube called the vacuum cannula is placed into the uterine cavity. This instrument is attached to a suction device, which looks something like a drinking straw. An electric or hand-operated vacuum pump then empties the uterus of its contents. Finally, a spoon-shaped device called a curette is used to check for any leftover tissue in the uterus. The entire procedure takes less than five minutes. This method, first used in China in 1958, is among the safest procedures in medicine. There are about six times more maternal deaths during regular birth than during vacuum aspiration.

An older method, dilation and curettage (D & C), was common up to the 1970's, but it has largely been replaced by vacuum aspiration. In a D & C, the cervix was expanded or dilated, and a curette was used to scrape out the contents of the uterus. The biggest difference was the use of general anesthesia during the process. Since most abortion-related deaths result from complications from anesthesia, a method that requires only local anesthesia, such as aspiration, greatly reduces the dangers of the procedure.

For the period from thirteen to twenty weeks, a method called dilation and evacuation (D & E) is usually preferred. The cervix is expanded with tubes of laminaria (a type of seaweed), and the fetus is removed with the placenta, the part of the uterus by which the fetus is nourished. Forceps, suction, or a sharp curette is sometimes used. The procedure is usually safe, but sometimes a large fetus must be crushed and dismembered in order to remove it through the cervix. This process can be upsetting for the doctor and the patient and is more dangerous than procedures done earlier in the pregnancy. Generally, the later abortions are performed, the more dangerous they are for women.

Physicians can also use "medical induction" techniques when required. Amnioinfusion is an old example of this method that was used on fetuses from sixteen to twenty weeks old. This process has largely been replaced by D & E, which has proved far less dangerous. Amnioinfusion usually required hospitalization, local anesthesia, and the insertion of a large needle into the uterus. Between 100 and 200 milliliters of fluid were withdrawn and a similar amount of hypertonic saline solution was infused into the uterine cavity. Within ninety minutes, the fetal heart would stop. The woman would go into labor and deliver a dead fetus within twenty-four to seventy-two hours. These kinds of abortions generally had much higher risks of complications than did D & E. On rare occasions, a fetus was born alive, but the main risks were infection, hemorrhage, and cervical injuries to the woman. The psychological difficulties associated with such long labor are very upsetting, especially the knowledge that the fetus delivered will be dead.

Another method used prostaglandins, naturally occurring hormones that cause uterine contractions and expulsion of the fetus, rather than a saline solution. The hormones could be given to the patient in several different ways: intravenously, intramuscularly, through vaginal suppositories, or directly into the amniotic sac. Prostaglandins are used for inducing second trimester abortions and are as safe as saline solutions. Their major advantage is to reduce the time for the abortion, but they also have severe side effects.

They cause intense stomach cramps and other gastrointestinal discomfort, and about 7 percent of the fetuses expelled show some sign of life.

Surgical techniques for abortion are very rare, although sometimes they prove necessary in special cases. Hysterotomy resembles a Cesarean section. An incision is made in the abdomen, and the fetus is removed. Hysterotomy is usually used in the second trimester, but only in cases where other methods have failed. The risk of death is much higher in this procedure than in most others. Even more rare is a hysterectomy, the removal of the uterus. This is done only in cases in which a malignant tumor threatens the life of the pregnant woman.

In the late 1980's, the French "abortion pill," RU-486, was approved for use in many parts of Europe. By the mid-1990's, it had been used in more than fifty thousand abortions. Progesterone is a hormone that tells the uterus to develop a lining that can be used to house a fertilized egg. If the egg is not fertilized, the production of progesterone stops, and the uterine lining is discarded during menstruation. RU-486 contains an antiprogesterone, which means that it prevents the production of progesterone. The pill has proved to be effective about 90 percent of the time if used in early pregnancy.

A few serious side effects sometimes occur with RU-486, the major one being sustained bleeding. About one out of a thousand users bleeds so much that a transfusion is required. Cramps and nausea are also reported in a number of cases. There is apparently no effect on subsequent pregnancies. The drug must be taken under medical supervision and requires, under French law, at least three visits to a doctor's office. The first visit is for testing and counseling. On the second visit, the patient is given the drug. On the third, she receives an injection of prostaglandin. In late 2000, RU-486 was approved for use in the United States.

RELATIVE RISKS OF LEGAL VS. ILLEGAL ABORTIONS

Abortion is the most frequently performed surgical procedure in the United States. As long as women have unwanted pregnancies, that will continue to be true. Abortion is a very safe procedure, although there can be some complications. Generally, however, the earlier the procedure is performed, the less the risk. The lowest chance of medical complications occurs during the first eight weeks of pregnancy. After eight weeks, the risk of complications increases by 30 percent for each week of delay. Nevertheless, the death rate per case is very low, about half that for tonsillectomy. These statistics apply only to those areas of the world where abortion is legal, since women in those places tend to have earlier abortions.

In the United States, deaths declined when abortions became legal in 1973. Before the *Roe v. Wade* decision, it was estimated that anywhere from a few hundred to several thousand American women died every year from the procedure. The best estimate was that in the 1960's, about 290 women died every year as a result of complications from abortions. In the 1980's, the average was twelve per year, mostly from anesthesia complications. More than 90 percent of abortions in the United States take place during the first twelve weeks of pregnancy.

—Leslie V. Tischauser

See also Abortion among teenagers; Birth control and family planning; Birth defects; Condoms; Ethics; Fetal tissue transplantation; Genetic counseling; Hippocratic oath; Law and medicine; Miscarriage; Morning-after pill; Pregnancy among teenagers; Sterilization; Women's health issues.

FOR FURTHER INFORMATION:
Githens, Marianne, and Dorothy McBride Stetson, eds. *Abortion Politics: Public Policy in Cross-Cultural Perspective.* New York: Routledge, 1996. The essays in this collection provide some insight on the contentious nature of this issue. Includes bibliographical references and an index.
Paul, Maureen, et al., eds. *A Clinician's Guide to Medical and Surgical Abortion.* New York: Churchill Livingstone, 1999. Includes a historical review and an analysis of the epidemiological and public health aspects of abortion. Discusses preprocedure assessment and management, abortion techniques and procedures, postabortion management, and abortion service delivery.
Sciarra, John J., et al. *Gynecology and Obstetrics.* Rev. ed. Vol. 6. Philadelphia: Harper & Row, 1996. A textbook that discusses methods, demographics, health concerns, and the psychological and medical consequences of abortions.
Sloan, Irving J. *The Law Governing Abortion, Contraception, and Sterilization.* Legal Almanac Series. London: Oceana, 1996. Covers historical and modern legislation relating to abortions, contraception, and the rights of minors to these services. Appendixes include selected state and federal laws.
Solinger, Rickie, ed. *Abortion Wars: A Half Century of Struggle, 1950-2000.* Berkeley: University of California Press, 1998. Solinger is a noted historian of reproductive behavior and its social and cultural meanings. Here she brings together activists, providers, attorneys, and academics for this collection of essays, which takes a strong pro-rights stance and examines abortion as it figures in the United States and countries around the world.

✧ ABORTION AMONG TEENAGERS

Type of issue: Children's health, ethics, medical procedures, social trends, women's health

Definition: The medical termination of a pregnancy by a teenage girl.

Each year, according to the Alan Guttmacher Institute, a leading provider of information on abortion, more than one million teenagers in the United States become pregnant. Almost nine out of ten of these pregnancies are unintended. As a consequence, about one-third (35 percent) of teenage girls who become pregnant decide to have an abortion. This means that there are more than 350,000 teenage abortions every year in the United States.

THE SOCIETAL CONTEXTS OF TEENAGE PREGNANCY

The United States has far more abortions than any other wealthy, developed country. For example, in the Netherlands where teenage sexual activity occurs at about the same rate as it does in the United States, only about one out of ten teenage girls becomes pregnant. Experts believe that this difference is accounted for by the easier availability of contraception and family planning services in the Netherlands and by the fact that Dutch teenagers receive much more sex education than do Americans. American teenagers, both male and female, have limited knowledge about ways of preventing pregnancy, even though four out of five report having had intercourse by the time they reach eighteen years of age. This sexual activity is not always voluntary, especially for very young women. Of those girls under fifteen who reported having sexual relations, more than 60 percent said that the sex was forced upon them by older males.

Teenagers with unplanned pregnancies generally face difficult, lonely choices, especially if they are poor or if they are living in broken families. Teenage girls who give birth and keep their babies are likely to drop out of school, go on public assistance, develop health problems (both mother and child), and live in single-parent households. Teenage marriages are much more likely to end in divorce than are later marriages. The younger the mother, the more likely the child will suffer from medical, psychological, economic, and educational disadvantages.

By 1998, twenty-eight of the fifty U.S. states had enacted laws restricting access to abortion for girls under eighteen by requiring involvement of one or both parents in the abortion decision. These laws required medical personnel to notify a girl's parents if she requests an abortion. Only two states—Connecticut and Maine—and the District of Columbia allowed teenage girls the right to obtain abortions on their own.

The U.S. Supreme Court ruled that a state cannot give parents the absolute right to deny abortion to their daughter. In some states, girls who do not want their parents notified can seek a judicial bypass, which requires authorization from a judge before an abortion can be performed. The judge is required to give the authorization unless he or she decides that the girl is too immature to make the decision by herself.

If any woman, regardless of age, is going to have an abortion, it is best to have the procedure done as early as possible in the pregnancy. Thus, laws that make teenagers wait before an abortion is performed also increase the risk of complications. According to the best evidence, about 1 in every 100,000 legal abortions results in the death of the pregnant woman. If an abortion takes place before the eighth week of pregnancy, then the death rate is only about 2 out of 1 million. The rate increases after the twelfth week of pregnancy, however, to about 12.7 deaths per 100,000 abortions. The death rate for illegal abortions in all age groups is about four times higher. Early abortion lessens the risk to the health of the teenager, and abortions are among the safest of any type of medical procedure.

THE ABORTION DEBATE

The major debate over abortion is one of ethics: Is it right to end a pregnancy deliberately before the fetus is capable of living outside the uterus? The Supreme Court's decision in *Roe v. Wade* (1973) made the right to an abortion, at least during the first twelve weeks of pregnancy, legal in the United States. The question concerning teenage pregnancy is whether girls under the age of eighteen are ready to make the decision to abort an unwanted pregnancy on their own or whether they should be required to notify their parents or guardians first.

U.S. states justify parental involvement laws by arguing that the decision to end a pregnancy is not simply a medical choice but one that can have a significant long-term impact on a teenager's psychological and emotional health and that teenagers are not ready to make such difficult decisions by themselves. Critics of parental consent point out, however, that several states allow teenagers to marry without parental consent, while others even allow teenagers to drop out of school without parental involvement. Even more striking is the fact that, in 1998, forty-five states allowed a teenage mother to place her baby for adoption without consulting an adult. It can be argued that difficult decisions such as these are just as important in a young person's life as is the choice to have an abortion. If teenagers can make these choices on their own, should they also have the right to end a pregnancy?

The debate over abortion is based on ethics. New abortion techniques have largely eliminated any major medical complications for the teenager or adult woman undergoing this procedure. Factors involved in the choice of whether to have an abortion vary from individual to individual. Restrictive laws create problems of their own. If a parent or judge makes the decision and a young woman is forced to have a baby against her will, the consequences can be devastating. She may decide to run away from home and have an illegal abortion, which is dangerous and unsafe. Restrictions can rob a young woman of the power to take control of her own life and may force her to raise her baby in poverty and isolation.

—*Leslie V. Tischauser*

See also Abortion; Birth control and family planning; Condoms; Ethics; Pregnancy among teenagers; Women's health issues.

FOR FURTHER INFORMATION:

Baird, Robert M., and Stuart E. Rosenbaum, eds. *The Ethics of Abortion: Pro-Life vs. Pro-Choice.* Rev. ed. Buffalo, N.Y.: Prometheus Books, 1993. Covers a wide range of opinions.

Feinberg, Joel, and Susan Dwyer, eds. *The Problem of Abortion.* 3d ed. Belmont, Calif.: Wadsworth, 1997. An excellent selection of articles.

Gordon, Mary. *Good Boys and Dead Girls and Other Essays.* New York: Viking Press, 1991. Has several interesting essays on abortion as well as the accounts of several women recalling abortions from their teenage years.

Solinger, Rickie, ed. *Abortion Wars: A Half Century of Struggle, 1950-2000.* Berkeley: University of California Press, 1998. Solinger is a noted historian of reproductive behavior and its social and cultural meanings. Here she brings together activists, providers, attorneys, and academics for this collection of essays, which takes a strong pro-rights stance and examines abortion as it figures in the United States and countries around the world.

✧ ACUPUNCTURE

Type of issue: Medical procedures, treatment

Definition: An ancient therapy developed in China in which designated points on the skin are stimulated by the insertion of needles, the application of heat, massage, or a combination of these techniques in order to treat impaired body functions or induce anesthesia.

The theory and practice of acupuncture is rooted in the Chinese concept of life—the Ch'i (pronounced "chee")—which, according to ancient writings, is the beginning and the end, life and death. The belief, which has been handed down for thousands of years, is that all things animate and inanimate have an internal source of energy. This energy stabilizes the chemical composition of matter, and when this matter is broken down, energy is released. The Chinese view differs from the Western view of life in its adherence to the belief that human beings are all one with the cosmos, obeying the rhythms of the natural order. This oneness with the entire universe is represented by two forces: Yin and Yang.

Yang, the positive force in human beings and nature, is exemplified by powerful elements such as heat, energy, vitality, the lush growing period of summer, and the sun. Yin, on the other hand, is the passive, almost negative force that is most obvious during winter, when plant growth almost comes to a standstill and certain animals hibernate. The Yin force is believed to be at work nightly in humans when they sleep. People who suffer from rheumatic pains frequently claim that they can forecast a change in the weather by noting the onset of those pains, and many people respond emotionally to the flow of energy in their bodies. They can feel either full of life or deeply depressed for no apparent reason.

THE FLOW OF CH'I

According to the ancient Chinese system of medicine, there are two categories of organs associated with the Ch'i: the Tsang and the Fou. The Fou is the group of organs that absorb food, digest it, and expel waste products. They are all hollow organs such as the stomach, the large and small intestines, the bladder, and the gallbladder, and all are Yang by nature. Tsang organs are all associated with the blood—the heart, which circulates the blood around the body; the lungs, which oxygenate the blood; the spleen, which controls the red corpuscles; and the liver and the kidneys. These organs are Yin by nature. For the flow of energy to remain steady, it must pass unimpeded from one organ to another. If the organ is weak, the resultant energy that is passed on to the next organ is weakened. Acupuncture stimulates specifically designated points on the body (called "meridians") and corrects the problem.

According to the Chinese, the human "circuit" of energy is made up of twelve meridians, which stretch along the limbs from the toes and the fingers to the face and chest. There are six meridians in the upper limbs and six in the lower. Ten meridians are connected to a main organ by branches from the sympathetic nervous system, and each of these meridians contains the Ch'i, which varies in strength and is governed by the nerve impulses arising from the organs. The meridians and their attendant vessels contain the flow of energy that enables the body to function efficiently.

The meridian points that proved to be effective for certain ailments were organized, and specific names were given to each. Later, the meridian line concept was hypothesized in order to explain the effectiveness of the points. These meridian points were selected by observing the effects of stimulation on particular signs and symptoms.

According to modern medical concepts, some of these points are thought to be relating points at which the autonomic nervous system is stimulated by a specific visceral disorder. Anatomically, some of the meridian points appear to correspond to areas where a nerve appears to surface from a muscle or areas where vessels and nerves are relatively superficially located, such as areas between a muscle and a bone or between a bone and a joint. These areas are generally composed of connective tissue.

Tapping the Flow

The meridians are stimulated by the insertion of needles. The needles that are commonly used range in size from the diameter of a hair to that of a sewing needle. In China, round and cutting needles are commonly used. The lengths of the needles range from approximately 0.14 millimeter to approximately 0.34 millimeter. In Europe, the needles are slightly shorter and slightly wider in diameter.

The needles are made of gold, silver, iron, platinum, or stainless steel. Stainless steel needles are most commonly used. Infection caused by needle puncture is said to be extremely rare. This may be the case because the minor injury created by the needle is controlled by biological reaction. It is routine to wipe the skin with alcohol before inserting the sterilized needle. The needle itself may be wiped with alcohol sponges before each insertion on the same patient. Needles are discarded after being used in patients with a history of jaundice or hepatitis.

Insertion of a needle requires great skill and much practice. There are three different angles of penetration into the skin: perpendicular, oblique, and horizontal. These angles correspond to 90 degrees, 45 degrees, and a minimum angle, respectively. The angles may be chosen on the basis of the thickness of the skin and the proximity to muscle or bone at the desired puncture point. The depth of penetration will vary, with an average of 10, 30, and 40 millimeters in the head, shoulder, and back regions, respectively.

Tapping (the tube method) is one method of insertion: When the diameter of the needle is small, this method is extremely effective. The needle is placed into the tube from either direction, and the tube is shorter than the needle by 5 millimeters or more. Gentle tapping of the needle handle with the right index finger introduces the needle easily. The tapping finger must be removed from the needle head immediately; otherwise, it causes pain. The tube is removed gently with the right index finger and thumb.

In the twirling method (the freehand method), the left thumb and index finger make contact at the acupuncture point. The left hand is called the pushing hand. Next, the skin is cut with the needle tip, after which the needle is inserted by pushing and twirling it with the right hand.

Needle Manipulation

The objective of the advancement of the needle and the needle motion is to create a needle feeling in the patient. This is a dull, aching, paralyzing, or compressing feeling or a combination of these sensations that radiates to a distal or proximal portion of the body. When the patient notices the needle feeling, the operator increases the feeling by using various needle motions. Numerous motions are available, such as the single-stick, twirling, vibration, intermittent, and retention motions.

The amount of stimulation equals the strength of stimulation multiplied by the number of treatments; this is dependent on the sensitivity of the patient. Gradual increases of stimulation are essential. In general, for acute disease, treatment is usually given once a day for ten days and then terminated for three to seven days. For chronic ailments, treatment is administered once every two to three days for ten treatments and then terminated for seven days. The patient is placed in a supine, sitting, prone, or side position—the position that is most convenient for the patient and physician. A special position, however, may be needed in order to relax the painful area.

Western Uses for Acupuncture

The basic approach of modern medicine involves removing the causal factor of disease. In this approach, the pain associated with disease or with a surgical procedure may not be eradicated instantaneously, however, and the management of pain becomes an issue until the disease is cured or until the surgery and recuperation are complete. Controlling chemical receptors and reducing the sensitivity of those receptors is one way of treating pain. Intensive studies of the stimulation that causes pain have indicated that intrinsic chemical substances (polypeptides) such as histamine and serotonin, which stimulate the receptors, are essential for pain. Therefore, an antagonistic drug for these chemicals is often effective in controlling pain. Although acupuncture is used to treat conditions as diverse as allergies, circulatory disorders, dermatologic disorders, gastrointestinal disorders, genital disorders, musculoskeletal disorders, neurologic disorders, and psychiatric and emotional disorders, the use of acupuncture for pain control (analgesia) can be described as the most basic level of treatment.

The popularity of acupuncture, like that of most techniques and discoveries, has waxed and waned throughout the years; for the most part, however, the Chinese have remained faithful to the five-thousand-year-old practice. The laws and method of acupuncture have endured, although these methods have been increasingly combined with Western medical techniques.

—Genevieve Slomski

See also Addiction; Alternative medicine; Biofeedback; Holistic medicine; Homeopathy; Pain management; Stress; Yoga.

FOR FURTHER INFORMATION:

Ernst, Edzard, and Adrian White, eds. *Acupuncture: A Scientific Appraisal.* London: Butterworth Heinemann Medical Publishers, 1999. Examines acupuncture's possible mechanisms of action. Contains chapters on both Eastern and Western approaches. Reviews the evidence for the effectiveness of acupuncture and provides in-depth coverage of safety aspects.

Manaka, Yoshio, Kazuko Itaya, and Stephen Birch. *Chasing the Dragon's Tail: The Theory and Practice of Acupuncture in the Work of Yoshio Manaka.* Brookline, Mass.: Paradigm, 1997. The definitive text by Manaka, one of the most famous acupuncturists of the twentieth century. Explains his treatment approach and his research in and understanding of acupuncture.

Mann, Felix. *Acupuncture: Cure of Many Diseases.* 2d ed. London: Butterworth Heinemann Medical Publishers, 1992. Written by a practicing acupuncture therapist. A beginning book on the theory and practice of acupuncture.

Stux, Gabriel, and Bruce Pomeranz. *Basics of Acupuncture.* 4th ed. New York: Springer-Verlag, 1998. An updated reference on acupuncture that provides details about the procedure. Also examines the history of acupuncture treatment.

Tan, Leong T., et al. *Acupuncture Therapy.* 2d rev. ed. Philadelphia: Temple University Press, 1976. A useful introduction to the theory and practice of acupuncture. The authors state that acupuncture, as a simple, efficient, and effective means of medical therapy, has successfully withstood the tests of time and scrutiny, earning acceptance in the United States. Numerous charts and illustrations. Bibliography.

✧ ADDICTION

Type of issue: Mental health, social trends

Definition: A psychological and sometimes physiological process whereby an organism comes to depend on a substance; defined by a persistent need to use the substance and to increase the dosage used as a result of tolerance, as well as the experience of withdrawal symptoms when the substance is withheld or use is reduced.

Addiction is a disorder that can affect any animal and may result from the use of a variety of psychoactive substances. Typically, it involves both psychological and physiological dependence. Psychological dependence is marked by compulsions to use a substance of abuse because of its reinforcing qualities. Physiological dependence results when the body responds to the presence of the addictive substance. Tolerance, withdrawal, and significant decreases in psychological, social, and occupational dysfunction characterize physiological dependence.

THE DEVELOPMENT OF TOLERANCE

Tolerance involves pharmacokinetics, pharmacodynamics, and environmental or behavioral conditioning. Pharmacokinetics refers to the way in which a biological system, such as a human body, processes a drug. Substances are subject to absorption into the bloodstream, distribution to different organs (such as the brain and liver), metabolization by these organs, and then elimination. Over time, the processes of distribution and metabolism may change, such that the body eliminates the substance more efficiently. Thus, the substance has less opportunity to affect the system than it did initially, reducing any desired effects. As a result, dose increases are needed to achieve the initial or desired effect.

Pharmacodynamics refers to changes in the body as a result of a pharmacologic agent being present. Tissue within the body responds differently to the substance at the primary sites of action. For example, changes in sensitivity may occur at specific sites within the brain, directly or indirectly impacting the primary action site. Direct changes at the primary sites of action denote tissue sensitivity. An example might be an increase in the number of receptors in the brain for that particular substance. Indirect changes in tissue remote from the primary action sites denote tissue tolerance, or functional tolerance. In functional tolerance, physiologic systems that oppose the action of the drug compensate by increasing their effect. Once either type of tolerance develops, the only way for the desired effect to be achieved is for the dose of the substance to be increased.

Finally, environmental or behavioral conditioning is involved in the development of tolerance. Organisms associate the reinforcing properties of substances with the contexts in which the drugs are experienced. Such contexts may be physical environments, such as places, or emotional contexts, such as when the individual is depressed or anxious. Over the course of repeated administrations in the same context, the tolerance that develops is associated with that specific context. Thus, an organism may experience tolerance to a drug in one situation, but not another. Greater doses of the reinforcing substance would be needed to achieve the same effect in the former situation, but not in the latter.

VARIATIONS IN TOLERANCE DEVELOPMENT

Tolerance develops differently depending on the type of substance taken, the dose ingested, and the routes of administration used. Larger doses may contribute to quicker development of tolerance. Similarly, routes of administration that produce more rapid and efficient absorption of a substance into the bloodstream tend to increase the likelihood of an escalating pattern of substance abuse leading to dependence. For many drugs, injection and inhalation are two of the fastest routes of administration, while oral ingestion is one of the slowest. Other routes include intranasal, transdermal, rectal, sublingual, and intraocular administration.

For some substances, the development of tolerance also depends on the pattern of substance use. For example, even though two individuals might use the same amount of alcohol, it is possible for tolerance to develop more quickly in one person than in the other. Two individuals might each drink fourteen drinks per week, but they would develop tolerance at different rates if one consumes two drinks each of seven nights and the other consumes seven drinks each of two nights in a week. Because of their patterns of use, the first drinker would develop tolerance much more slowly than the second, all other things being equal.

WITHDRAWAL

Withdrawal occurs when use of the substance significantly decreases. Withdrawal varies by the substance of abuse and ranges from being minor or nonexistent with some drugs (such as hallucinogens) to quite pronounced with other drugs (such as alcohol). Mild symptoms include anxiety, tension, restlessness, insomnia, impaired attention, and irritability. Severe symptoms include convulsions, perceptual distortions, irregular tremors, high blood pressure, and rapid heartbeat. Typically, withdrawal symptoms can be alleviated or extinguished by readministration of the substance of abuse. Thus, a compounding problem is that the addicted individual often learns to resume drug use in order to avoid the withdrawal symptoms.

Addiction occurs with both legal and illegal drugs. Alcohol and nicotine are two of the most widely abused legal addictive drugs. Over-the-counter drugs, such as sleeping aids, and prescription drugs, such as tranquilizers (for example, sedative-hypnotics) and antianxiety agents, also have addiction potential. Common illegal addictive drugs include cocaine, marijuana, hallucinogens, heroin, and methamphetamine.

Not everyone who uses these substances will automatically become addicted. In the United States, for example, surveys have shown that approximately 65 percent of adults drink alcohol each year. In contrast, less than 13 percent of the population goes on to develop alcohol problems serious enough to warrant a medical diagnosis of alcohol abuse or dependence. Similarly, despite the fact that large numbers of individuals are prescribed opiates or sedative-hypnotics for pain while hospitalized, roughly 0.7 percent of the adult population is addicted to opiates and 1.1 percent is addicted to sedative-hypnotics or antianxiety drugs. Thus, the development of addiction often requires repeated substance administration, as well as other biological and environmental factors.

CONSEQUENCES OF ADDICTION

When addiction is present, the consequences are multiple and complex. While substance abuse involves deteriorated functioning in psychological, social, occupational, or physical functioning, substance dependence usually involves more severe problems in each of these areas for significantly longer amounts of time. Psychologically, problems with depression, anxiety, the ability to think clearly or remember information, motivation, judgment, and one's sense of self may result. Socially, one can become isolated from friends and family, or even unable to deal with the stresses and demands of normal, everyday relationships. Finally, occupational disruptions can result from the inability to plan, to manage one's feelings and thoughts, and to deal with social interactions.

In terms of health, there are many acute and chronic effects of addiction. With cocaine, for example, acute cardiac functioning may be affected, such that the risk of heart attacks is increased. Similarly, individuals addicted to opiates, alcohol, and sedative-hypnotics must contend with such risks as falling into a coma or experiencing depressed respiratory functioning. Finally, the acute effects of any of these drugs can impair judgment and contribute to careless behavior. As a result, accidents, severe trauma, and habitually dangerous behavior, such as risky sexual behavior, may be associated with addiction.

Chronic health consequences are common. Smoking is associated with cancers of the mouth, throat, and lungs, as well as premature deterioration of the skin. Alcohol is associated with cancers of the mouth, throat, and stomach, as well as ulcers and liver problems. General malnutrition is a risk for heroin and alcohol users, since they often fail to eat properly. Injected drugs such as heroin and cocaine are associated with problems such as hepatitis and acquired immunodeficiency syndrome (AIDS), since shared needles may transmit blood-borne diseases. Finally, addiction contributes to health problems in the unborn children of addicted individuals. Problems such as low birth weight in the children of smokers, fetal alcohol syndrome in the children of female drinkers, and withdrawal difficulties in the children born to other types of addicts are well documented.

PSYCHOLOGICAL TREATMENT

Because of the combination of psychological and physiological dependence, addiction is a disorder that often demands both psychological and pharmacological treatments. Typically, interventions focus on decreasing or stopping the substance use and reestablishing normal psychological, social, occupational, and physical functioning in the addicted individual. Though the length and type of treatments may vary with the particular addictive drug and the duration of the addiction problem, similar principles are involved in the treatment of all addictions.

Psychological treatments focus primarily on extinguishing psychological dependence, as well as on facilitating more effective functioning by the addicted individual in other areas of life. Attempts to change the behavior and thinking of the addicted individual usually involve some combination of individual, group, and family therapy. Adjunctive training in new occupational skills and healthier lifestyle habits are also common.

In general, treatment focuses on understanding how the addictive behavior developed, how it was maintained, and how it can be removed from the person's daily life. Assessments of the situations in which the drug was used, the needs for which the drug was used, and alternative means of addressing those needs are primary to this understanding. Once these issues are identified, a therapist then works with the client to break habitual behavior patterns that were contributing to the addiction (for example, driving through neighborhoods where drugs might be sold, going to business meetings at restaurants that serve alcohol, or maintaining relationships with drug-using friends). Concurrently, the therapist helps the client design new behavior patterns that will decrease the odds of continued problems with addiction. Problems related to the drug use would then be addressed in some combination of individual, family, or group therapy.

The therapy or therapies selected depend on the problems related to drug use. For example, family therapy might be more appropriate in cases in which family conflicts are related to drug use. In contrast, individual therapy might be more appropriate for someone whose drug use is linked to thinking distortions or mood problems. Similarly, group therapy might be most appropriate for individuals lacking social support to deal with stress, or whose social interactions are contributing to their drug use. Regardless of the type of therapy, however, the basic goal remains: facilitating the client's solving of his or her specific problems. Additionally, the development of new ways of coping with intractable problems, rather than relying on drug use as a means of coping, would be critical.

Cognitive and behavioral therapies have been quite useful for breaking the conditioned effects of addiction. Some psychological dependence, for example, is based on placebo effects. A placebo effect occurs as a result of what people believe a drug is doing for them, rather than from anything that the drug actually has the power to accomplish. In addition, the practice of using addictive drugs within certain contexts is associated with drug tolerance, such that certain situations trigger compulsions leading to drug use. In this way, cognitive therapy can be used to challenge any faulty thinking associations that individuals have made about what the drugs do for them in different situations. This may involve increasing patients' awareness of the negative consequences of their drug use and challenging what they perceive to be its positive consequences. As a complement, such therapies correct distorted thinking that is related to coping with stressful situations or situations in which drug use might be especially tempting. In such situations, individuals might actually have the skill to handle the stress or temptation without using drugs. Without the confidence that they can successfully manage these situations, however, they may not even try, instead reverting to drug use. As such, therapy facilitating realistic thinking about stress and coping abilities can be quite beneficial.

Similarly, behavioral therapies are used to break down conditioned associations between situations and drug use. For example, smokers are sometimes made to smoke not in accordance with their desire to smoke, but according to a schedule over which they have no control. As a result, they are made to smoke at times or in situations where it is inconvenient, leading to an association between unpleasant feelings and smoking. While such assigned drug use would not be used with illegal drugs, the basic principles of increasing negative or unpleasant feelings with drug use in specific situations can be used. Rewarding abstinence has also been a successful approach to treatment. In this way, positive reinforcement is associated with abstinence and may contribute to behaviors related to abstinence being more common than behaviors related to drug use.

PHARMACOLOGICAL TREATMENT

Pharmacological treatments concentrate on decreasing physical dependence on the substance of abuse. They rely on behavioral principles and on five primary strategies. The first strategy, based on positive reinforcement, is pharmacological replacement. Prescribed drugs with effects at the sites of action similar to those of the addictive drug are used. These prescribed drugs, however, usually fail to have reinforcing properties as powerful as the addictive drug and focus mainly on preventing the occurrence of withdrawal symptoms. Nicotine patches for smokers and methadone for heroin users are examples of replacement therapies.

A second strategy involves the use of both reinforcement and extinction, the behavioral process of decreasing and eventually extinguishing the drug-taking behavior. Partially reinforcing and partially antagonistic drugs are prescribed. The net effect is that the prescribed drug staves off withdrawal symptoms, but yields less reinforcement than drug replacement therapy, serving to facilitate the process of extinction for the drug taking.

Antagonists, or drugs that completely block the receptors responsible for the reinforcing effects of the drug action, are prescribed alone as a third strategy. With this strategy, extinction is the primary behavioral principle in effect. The prescribed drug blocks the primary receptor sites and does not yield positively reinforcing drug effects. Even if the addictive drug is taken in addition to the antagonist, no positively reinforcing effects are experienced. Thus, without reinforcement, drug-taking behavior should eventually cease. Naltrexone, typically used for opiate addiction, is a good example of this strategy.

Punishment is another behavioral principle used in pharmacological therapy. Metabolic inhibitors, or drugs that make the effects of the addictive substance more toxic, are often used to discourage drug use. Antabuse, a drug often given for problems with alcohol, is such a substance. When metabolic inhibitors are prescribed, individuals using these drugs in combination with their substance of abuse experience toxic and unpleasant effects. Thus, they begin to associate use of the addictive substance with very noxious results and are discouraged from continuing their drug use.

Symptomatic treatment of withdrawal effects is used as a fifth strategy. Based on reinforcement, this strategy simply encourages the use of drugs likely to reduce withdrawal effects. Unfortunately, these drugs may also have abuse potential. For example, when benzodiazepines are given to individuals with alcohol or opiate dependence, one dependency may be traded for another. As such, symptomatic treatment is helpful but is not a treatment of choice by itself. In fact, none of these pharmacological treatments is recommended for use in isolation; they are recommended for use with complementary psychological treatments.

SOCIETAL ATTITUDES TOWARD SUBSTANCE USE AND ABUSE

The use of substances to alter the mind or bodily experiences is a practice that has been a part of human cultures for centuries. Time and again, even through legislated acts such as Prohibition, drug and alcohol use have persisted. The continued use of drugs for recreational and medicinal practices seems virtually inevitable, and it is unlikely that substance abuse and dependence will disappear from the world's societies. Consequently, an understanding of substance use, how it leads to addiction, ways to minimize the development of addiction problems, and strategies for improving addiction treatments will be critical.

At different times in history, addiction has been viewed as strictly a moral, medical, spiritual, or behavioral problem. As the science of understanding and treating addiction has progressed, the variety of ways in which these aspects of addiction combine has been noted. Modern treatments and theories no longer view addiction from one strict point of view, but instead recognize the heterogeneity of paths leading to addiction. Such an approach has been helpful not only in treating addiction but also in preventing it. Efforts to curb the biological, social, and environmental forces contributing to addiction have become increasingly important.

Addiction remains a disorder with no completely effective treatment. Of individuals seeking treatment across all addictive disorders, fewer than

20 percent succeed the first time that they attempt to achieve long-term abstinence. As a result, individuals suffering from addiction often undergo multiple treatments over several occasions, with some individuals experiencing significant problems throughout their lives. Even though treatments for physiological and psychological dependence offer some improvement, much work remains to be done. In this context, the challenge ahead is not to prevent all substance use, but rather to decrease the odds that a person will become addicted. Improving the pharmacological and psychological treatments currently available will be important. Discoveries of new ways of tailoring treatment for addiction to the needs and backgrounds of the different individuals affected will be one critical task for health professionals. Continued exploration of new pharmacological treatments to combat withdrawal and facilitate abstinence is necessary.

—*Nancy A. Piotrowski*

See also Alcoholism; Alcoholism among teenagers; Alcoholism among the elderly; Drug abuse by teenagers; Eating disorders; Recovery programs; Smoking; Steroid abuse; Stress; Tobacco use by teenagers.

FOR FURTHER INFORMATION:
Dupont, Robert L. *The Selfish Brain: Learning from Addiction.* Washington, D.C.: American Psychiatric Association, 1997. Discusses the commonalities across different types of addiction in an easy-to-understand manner.
Julien, Robert M. *A Primer of Drug Action.* 9th ed. New York: W. H. Freeman, 2000. A nontechnical guide to drugs written by a medical professional. Describes the different classes of drugs, their actions in the body, their uses, and their side effects. Basic pharmacologic principles, classifications, and terms are defined and discussed.
Miller, William R., and Nick Heather, eds. *Treating Addictive Behaviors: Processes of Change.* 2d ed. New York: Plenum Press, 1998. This book, written by medical and psychological scientists, is an overview of treatment strategies for problems ranging from nicotine to opiate addiction. Psychological, behavioral, interpersonal, familial, and medical approaches are outlined and discussed.
Schlaadt, Richard G., and Peter T. Shannon. *Drugs: Use, Misuse, and Abuse.* 4th ed. Englewood Cliffs, N.J.: Prentice Hall, 1994. A good introduction to the complex issues surrounding addiction and drug use. Describes different drugs of abuse, individual differences in drug use, legal and social issues, and continuing controversies. Also included is an overview of the differences between illegal and legal drugs, as well as drug myths and facts.
Weil, Andrew, and Winifred Rosen. *From Chocolate to Morphine: Everything You Need to Know About Mind-Altering Drugs.* Rev. ed. Boston: Houghton Mifflin, 1998. This book on psychoactive substances provides basic informa-

tion to the general reader. Psychoactive substances are identified and defined. Also outlines the relationships between different types of drugs, the motivations to use drugs, and associated problems. As the title suggests, the discussion ranges from legal, caffeinated substances to illegal and prescription drugs.

❖ AGING

Type of issue: Elder health, mental health, social trends
Definition: The manifestation of biological, psychological, and sociocultural events occurring in a human being over the passage of time.

Gerontologists, those people who study aging, make two important distinctions regarding the aging process. First, chronological aging, which occurs with the passage of time from birth or conception, is distinguished from functional aging, measured by how well people function over that passage of time. Second, longevity, the average number of years people can expect to live, is distinguished from life span, the theoretical upper limit on how long a person can live. These distinctions provide a necessary context for understanding the course of the biological, psychological, and sociocultural facets of aging.

THE EXPANDING HUMAN LIFE SPAN

Advances in medicine and health care, especially in the eradication of many childhood diseases, greatly increased the longevity of humans in the twentieth century. To illustrate, only 4 percent of Americans were age sixty-five and older at the beginning of the twentieth century. By the close of that century, that percentage had more than tripled to approximately 13 percent, with life expectancy reaching the high seventies. This optimistic picture, however, needs to be qualified in two regards. First, longevity varies greatly across culture and era. For example, Moses, living in the thirteenth century B.C.E., wrote in the Ninetieth Psalm of the Bible that the life expectancy of his contemporaries was between seventy and eighty years. Furthermore, extrapolations from Leonard Hayflick's work on cell division begun in the 1950's strongly suggest that there is an upper limit to how long a person can live: approximately 120 years, the same number that is told to Noah in Genesis 6:3.

Great variation is also found between the genders within most species of animals. The general rule is that females experience greater longevity than males. Among humans, female life expectancy is approximately seven years longer.

PROGRAMMED EVENTS AND RANDOM OCCURRENCES

Why are there consistent differences in the course of aging among the sexes and species? An obvious inference is that all animals are biologically determined to live a particular number of years and then die. Three main theories interpret aging as the consequence of purposeful, predetermined events.

The cellular clock theory is based on Hayflick's work with cell cultures derived from embryonic tissue. A 1990 study by Hayflick demonstrated that human cells placed in a dish and fed nutrients grow, divide, and multiply rapidly at first. The rate of division then slows down, and the cells die somewhere between forty and sixty divisions, with male cells ceasing their doubling before female cells. Hayflick's explanation is that an intracellular clock determines an end to each cell's life.

The genetic design theory, proposed by Charles Minot in 1908, contends that the deoxyribonucleic acid (DNA) of every cell determines the course of aging in that cell. In other words, aging is designed into the "blueprint" of each organism at the time of conception. Consistency of aging in a species is therefore seen to be the consequence of similar DNA.

Extracellular mechanisms are the focus of the neuroendocrine theory. Many declines in vitality are induced by drops of particular hormones. For example, dehydroepiandrosterone (DHEA) diminishes with age, and some research indicates that supplements of DHEA in older adults restore many youthful characteristics. According to this theory, aging is predetermined by changes in endocrine gland functioning that reduce levels of various hormones.

Theories of aging based on random events can be roughly categorized into three types. The wear-and-tear approach to aging assumes that people and all other biological organisms simply wear out like machines. Aging is seen to be an erosion process, and the greater the stress on the body, the greater the acceleration of aging. For example, the more skin is exposed to the sun, the more rapidly it ages.

Error theories of aging focus on something going wrong with physiological functioning. Many sorts of errors are implicated in aging. Some of these errors may be intracellular, such as flaws in the transcription process involving ribonucleic acid (RNA) that lead to the loss of DNA or flaws in enzymes that impair the production of proteins. Other errors may be extracellular, such as the immune system attacking and weakening the host body or failures to maintain proper homeostatic balances such as temperature or blood sugar level.

A third random event approach to aging emphasizes the accumulation of harmful substances which then interfere with the smooth functioning of the body. Some of the accumulated substances are produced within the body, such as waste products, genetic mutations, cross linkages (interconnections that reduce pliability in bodily tissues), and caramelization (coating of proteins by excess sugars). Some harmful substances come from outside the body. Free radicals—molecules with one or more unpaired electrons—are highly reactive and can initiate chemical changes in the wrong place and at the wrong time. Oxygen is a major source of free radicals, and breathing ensures a constant influx of these damaging substances. While free radicals are also produced in the body and play roles in digestion and immunological responses, their accumulation, if not checked by antioxidants and free radical scavengers such as melatonin, inevitably leads to physiological damage. Various pollutants and drugs can also add and subtract from the vigors of youth. For example, smokers show excessive and accelerated wrinkling of the skin as compared to nonsmokers.

No one theory of aging, whether based on random or programmed events, offers a complete explanation of the aging process. That is why many gerontologists adopt an eclectic perspective that views aging as a consequence of numerous events, designed and undesigned.

External Aging

Normal aging involves bone loss that is more severe in women (30 percent) than in men (17 percent). Two main consequences follow when the bones lose calcium. First, osteoporosis, in which bone loss leads to a stooping posture and a high risk of fractures, increases in incidence. Second, height decreases with aging. Lifetime average losses in height are greater for women (2.0 inches) than for men (1.25 inches), with the rate of loss increasing with age. Tooth loss is primarily a result of periodontal disease, the swelling and shrinking of infected gums, not calcium loss.

While height declines with age, the pattern is different for weight. Most studies show increases of weight until the mid-sixties and then declining weight through late adulthood. Because excess weight is a risk factor for premature death, late adulthood averages are lower, in part, because of the smaller representation of heavier individuals. Other dimensions of human stature also change with aging. The nose and ears elongate. The chest and head increase in circumference. The trunk becomes thicker, and the legs and arms become thinner, although arm span shows only a slight decrease through the years. Muscle mass, particularly the percentage of lean muscle tissue, decreases with age and further alters physical appearance.

The aging of the skin is a consequence of both preventable and unpreventable factors. What is unpreventable is the inevitable loss of elastin and collagen proteins that help the skin retain its suppleness. What is preventable are two lifestyle choices that dramatically impact the rate and severity of wrinkling. Smoking, which accelerates the loss of collagen, leads to excessive wrinkling. In the case of heavy smokers, the wrinkling is several times more severe than in nonsmokers. Time spent in the sun also greatly influences wrinkling: The greater the exposure to the sun, the earlier and more excessive the wrinkling and the greater the risk of skin cancer.

A slowing in the growth rate of hair and fingernails (but not toenails) is observed with aging. The slowing of the growth rate in hair is more rapid in men than in women and can lead to baldness. High levels of certain androgen hormones, which men have more of, appear to play the key role in this process. Graying is caused by decreases of melanin, a pigment that gives hair its color. Body hairs also become less numerous during the aging process; an exception is that hair on the upper lip of women, particularly after the menopause, often increases.

Physical strength and capacity for exercise begin to show declines in the thirties and are related primarily to decreases in muscle tissue. In general, people who maintain good and consistent exercise patterns throughout their lives exhibit considerably smaller declines than those whose lifestyles are sedentary.

The Senses

Several changes occur with aging that impair the ability of the eyes to convey the physical world. Changes in the lens of the eye that affect vision are usually first noticed by people in their forties. The lens becomes thicker and harder through the years, which begins to interfere with the ability to see things close to the eyes. The result is presbyopia, or farsightedness, which is why middle-aged adults usually need reading glasses. The lens also begins to cloud with aging, a condition called cataracts, further obscuring vision in most elderly people. The opening permitting light to reach the lens is called the pupil, and its ability to dilate decreases with age. This results in less light being allowed to enter the eye and can cause night blindness. Directly in front of the pupil is a chamber containing a fluid called aqueous humor. A decrease in the amount of aqueous humor leaving this chamber can result in a buildup of pressure called glaucoma that, if unchecked, can lead to blindness. Two other notable changes in vision are linked with aging. First, peripheral vision usually begins to decrease in the late fifties to sixties. Second, there is often a decrease in the ability to perceive blues and greens.

Hearing losses with age occur in ability to detect both pitches and loudness. By the mid-thirties, people begin a progressive loss of the ability to hear higher-pitched sounds, a condition called presbycusis. Furthermore, because the pitch range of male hearing is lower than female hearing, hearing loss enters the range of normal human conversation sooner in men than in women. There is also a diminishment in loudness perception, which is measured in decibels. Both long exposures to dangerous decibel levels (over 90 decibels) and shorter exposures to extremely high decibel levels will damage hearing cells and increase hearing deficits.

Age-related deficits in taste are the result of degenerative changes in the taste buds that reduce the perception of bitterness and saltiness more than sourness or sweetness. Thirst tends to slacken with age, increasing the risk of dehydration, especially in the elderly.

Several studies have also recorded drops in the sense of smell. This drop in the ability to detect odors includes a diminished ability to detect faint odors and a lesser ability to judge the magnitude of strong odors. The decline is steeper and more rapid for men than women.

The sense of touch is actually at least three senses, each mediated by different sense organs: skin contact and movement, temperature, and pain. Research indicates some decline in all three tactile abilities. The vestibular sense, or sense of balance, begins to decline in the fifties. Impairment of this sense combined with bone loss greatly increases the risk of broken bones as people grow older.

INTERNAL SYSTEMS

Changes in both the quality and quantity of sleep occur with age. Rapid eye movement (REM) sleep, which facilitates learning and is characterized by a high prevalence of dreaming, gradually declines from birth to death. The amount of sleep also declines from birth to late adulthood: from about sixteen hours to a little under seven hours. As people move into middle age, they typically wake up more frequently from their sleeping (maintenance insomnia) and end their sleeping periods sooner (termination insomnia).

Diseases of the cardiovascular system became the leading causes of death in most industrialized countries during the course of the twentieth century. Great variability in the rates of heart attacks, atherosclerosis (thickening and hardening of the arteries), and other cardiovascular problems among different nations demonstrates the importance of environmental factors, particularly diet, in addition to normal aging. What is normal is that both the heart and the blood vessels become less flexible. A combination of these changes and lifestyle dynamics makes several diseases more prevalent with aging. Systolic blood pressure increases and can result in hypertension (high blood pressure); diastolic blood pressure does not increase with aging. Decreased oxygen to the heart can lead to chest pains called angina or, in the case of a complete blockage, a stroke. Decreased heart output and increased blood pressure lead to increased fluid around the heart, a condition called congestive heart failure, a leading reason for hospitalization in the elderly.

Declines in the functioning of the organs of the digestive system associated with aging are generally not severe enough to cause major health problems. There are decreases in several digestive enzymes, particularly the protein enzyme hydrochloric acid, secreted by the stomach. On the other hand, bile, which is stored in the gallbladder and helps to break down fats, can increase in concentration and lead to gallstones. The liver, which produces bile and plays the major role in regulating blood contents, shows

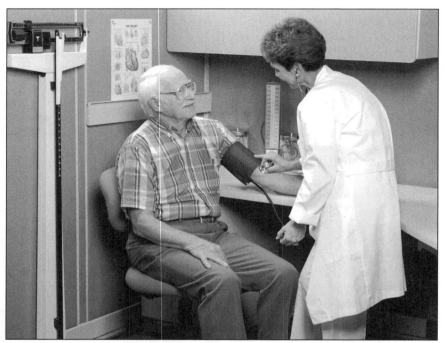

Periodic monitoring of blood pressure is recommended to detect hypertension in older adults. (Digital Stock)

some shrinkage with age. Hardening of the liver, termed cirrhosis, is more attributable to alcohol consumption than to normal aging.

The general rule regarding the aging of the endocrine system, the cells and tissues that produce hormones, is that lesser amounts of various hormones are produced and cells become less responsive to the hormones. Drops in melatonin lead to sleep problems; in thyroxin, to decreases in metabolism; in insulin and glucagon, to greater difficulty regulating the blood sugar level; and in androgens and estrogens, to declining reproductive ability and deficits in muscles and bones.

Systemic Slowdown

Healing capacity is reduced in two ways as people age. Wound repair is slower in older people, and the strength of the repairs is diminished. Once the healing process is completed, however, the repairs are basically as good in older people as in younger individuals. Inflammatory response to irritants is reduced with increasing age, as is immune system responsiveness. Skin with greater exposure to the sun heals slower than skin that is infrequently exposed to the sun.

The body's main defense against attacking microorganisms and foreign materials is the immune system. To function effectively, the immune system must maintain a balance between the extremes of too much activity, in which immune cells attack other cells of the body as foreign, and too little activity, in which foreign invaders to the body are not repulsed. As people grow older, there is an increased tendency for the immune system to lose that necessary balance. Thus, cancers become more likely as a result of immunological underreactiveness and, conversely, overreactiveness leads to autoimmune disorders such as certain kinds of arthritis. The most significant observable change in the immune system occurs in the thymus gland, which shrinks after puberty and loses over 90 percent of its original size by the age of fifty. The effectiveness of white blood cells, such as the lymphocytes and neutrophils, also decreases with the increase in years.

One of the reasons that people typically put on excess weight during middle age is a decrease in the basal metabolic rate (BMR). Declines in the BMR mean that less food is "burned" as fuel and more food is turned into fat stores. The good news about a lowered BMR is that it is linked with greater longevity: Mammals with lower BMRs generally outlive mammals with higher BMRs, which is also one reason that females (with lower BMRs) outlive males.

Age-related changes in the nervous system have a significant impact on the physiological, psychological, and social aspects of aging. As people age, there are two primary changes observed in their nervous systems. First, the speed of messages to and from nerve cells (neurons) slows down about 10 percent. This slowing is partly responsible for increases in reaction time and a general decrease in the speed at which older people do activities. The second major change in the nervous system is a shrinkage in size. For example, measures of the size of the human brain reveal average decreases of approximately 10 percent from young adulthood to late adulthood. This decrease is partly attributable to losses of neurons and partly the consequence of shrinkage of the neurons themselves.

There are significant age-related differences in declining reproductive ability (called the climacteric) between females and males. By around the age of fifty, a decline in the number of a woman's eggs and an associated decline in estrogen levels result in irregular menstrual periods and eventually the cessation of the menstrual cycle (the menopause), ending her ability to reproduce naturally. Furthermore, by middle age a woman's remaining eggs begin to deteriorate in quality, diminishing her likelihood of becoming pregnant. Shrinkage in the size of the uterus, vagina, and breasts is also typical in postmenopausal women.

There is no naturally induced end to a male's reproductive capability. Declining hormone levels do, however, lead to a decline in the number of sperm produced as a man ages. The most problematic change associated with this gradual climacteric is the enlargement of the prostate gland and an increased risk of prostate cancer in elderly men. As men age, obtaining an erection becomes more difficult but maintaining it becomes easier.

The most significant change in the respiratory system is a drop of over 50 percent in vital capacity (the amount of air volume that can be inspired) from young to late adulthood. Calcification of air passages, increased rigidity of the rib cage, reductions of elastin and collagen in the lungs (reducing their flexibility), and decreases in muscle strength all play a role in this decline.

The ability to control body temperature is reduced as people grow older due to a reduction in sweat glands, subcutical skin (which controls the loss of body heat), and the density of the circulatory system of the skin. These changes put the elderly at greater risk in extremes of both cold and hot temperatures.

Problems with the urinary tract can be a major source of embarrassment for the elderly. Approximately half of all people over the age of sixty-five have some problems with bladder control. The functioning of the kidneys also declines about 50 percent from young to late adulthood.

Slowing Aging

Three primary factors will help a person to live long and well: good genes, a good environment, and a good lifestyle. Because the first two factors are largely the result of other people's decisions, gerontologists have usually emphasized lifestyle choices for people who want to do something about how they age. Lifestyle decisions have the greatest impact on functional aging. Consistent and moderate exercise, a diet high in fruits and vegetables, lower exposure to harsh environments, maintenance of proper weight, and intellectual stimulation have all been demonstrated to improve the quality of life in the later years. Of particular interest in this regard has been work with a group of nuns in Mankato, Minnesota, who are being studied because of their mental sharpness in their elderly years and their great longevity. The nuns lead very stimulating intellectual lives, and autopsies of their brains have revealed fewer signs of aging than in comparable groups. The implication from this research is that intellectual activity slows the ravages of aging.

The search for the proverbial fountain of youth and immortality has been the preoccupation of scholar and nonscholar alike throughout the centuries. Many of the supposed "wonder cures" for aging have had consequences worse than the natural progression of aging itself. Research, however, has provided some hope of increasing the life span. Studies with a variety of mammalian species have found that significant drops in caloric intake translate into significant increases in both functional and chronological aging. Nevertheless, limits remain to the beneficial effects of caloric restriction.

—*Paul J. Chara, Jr.*

See also Alcoholism among the elderly; Alzheimer's disease; Arthritis; Breast cancer; Broken bones in the elderly; Cancer; Canes and walkers; Cardiac rehabilitation; Colon cancer; Cosmetic surgery and aging; Death and dying; Dementia; Dental problems in the elderly; Depression in the elderly; Diabetes mellitus; Elder abuse; Emphysema; Euthanasia; Exercise and the elderly; Falls among the elderly; Foot disorders; Hair loss and baldness; Health insurance; Hearing aids; Hearing loss; Heart attacks; Heart disease; Heart disease and women; Hormone replacement therapy; Hospitalization of the elderly; Illnesses among the elderly; Immunizations for the elderly; Incontinence; Infertility in men; Infertility in women; Influenza; Injuries among the elderly; Living wills; Lung cancer; Macular degeneration; Malnutrition among the elderly; Mammograms; Mastectomy; Medications and the elderly; Memory loss; Menopause; Mobility problems in the elderly; Muscle loss with aging; Nursing and convalescent homes; Nutrition and aging; Obesity and aging; Osteoporosis; Overmedication; Pain management; Parkinson's disease; Preventive medicine; Prostate cancer; Prostate enlargement; Reaction time and aging; Safety issues for the elderly; Screening; Sexual dysfunction; Skin disorders with aging; Sleep changes with aging; Strokes; Suicide among the elderly; Temperature regulation and aging; Terminal illnesses; Vision problems with aging; Weight changes with aging; Wheelchair use among the elderly.

FOR FURTHER INFORMATION:

Erikson, Erik H., and Joan M. Erikson. *The Life Cycle Completed.* Extended version. New York: W. W. Norton, 1997. This final work of a noted developmental psychologist, with additional material by his wife, presents an eloquent affirmation of what elderly people can become.

Evans, William, J., Jacqueline Thompson, and Irwin H. Rosenberg. *Biomarkers: The Ten Keys to Prolonging Vitality.* New York: Simon & Schuster, 1992. Guidelines for how diet and exercise can improve the aging process are described.

Hayflick, Leonard. *How and Why We Age.* New York: Ballantine Books, 1994. A preeminent scientist offers a comprehensive examination of the aging process.

Levinson, Daniel J., et al. *The Seasons of a Man's Life.* New York: Ballantine Books, 1978. Examines the issues with which individuals grapple as they age in the book that popularized the concept of midlife crisis.

Weiss, Rick, and Karen Kasmauski. "Aging: New Answers to Old Questions." *National Geographic* 192, no. 5 (November, 1997). Presents an excellent overview on aging and the techniques used to slow it down.

✧ AIDS

Type of issue: Epidemics
Definition: A disorder that develops when the human immunodeficiency virus (HIV) attacks the body's T cells, eventually destroying them in sufficient numbers to render victims of the disease unable to fight opportunistic infections that, in cases of full-blown AIDS, lead to their deaths.

No one really knows how long ago AIDS first afflicted human populations, but it received its first official recognition in the United States in 1981. The disease probably took lives for at least a decade prior to its being recognized and diagnosed. AIDS was characterized by a wasting away of those who fell ill with it.

SYMPTOMS AND SYSTEMIC EFFECTS

A first symptom was often the appearance of black, purple, or pink spots on the extremities that were diagnosed as a rather rare condition called Kaposi's sarcoma. This was once thought to be a form of cancer of the walls of blood and lymphatic vessels, although it is no longer classified as cancer in the conventional sense.

Other frequent precursors of AIDS are persistent flu-like symptoms, a general loss of weight, diarrhea, continued nausea, and, in some patients, dementia. These symptoms may be accompanied or followed by *Pneumocystis carinii* pneumonia (PCP), which is the most common cause of death in AIDS patients, who are also particularly vulnerable to tuberculosis. Both PCP and tuberculosis attack the lungs, causing severe respiratory problems in those afflicted with these diseases.

It is perhaps imprecise to say that people die of AIDS. It is more accurate to say that people suffering from AIDS are left with an immune system so weakened that it cannot serve its normal purpose, that of warding off infection. The cells that attack disease in the body, having been consumed by the HIV, are rendered useless. As T cell counts drop, usually to below five hundred, patients lack defenses against the opportunistic diseases that they contract and that generally kill them.

The immune system functions in such a way that cells attacked by viruses typically respond by releasing chemicals that summon white blood cells, the body's chief defense against disease. Some of these white cells, called macrophages, consume offending germs before they are able to cause an infection. Other such cells, called lymphocytes, produce antibodies in the form of proteins that attach themselves to parts of virus proteins, preventing them from attacking the cells they seek to destroy or weakening them, thus clearing the path for macrophages to destroy them.

The lymphocytes called killer T cells destroy infected cells and cancer cells. Another type of T cell, called a helper T cell, causes lymphocytes designated B cells, to propagate and produce antibodies bent on attacking cells infected by viruses. In AIDS victims, the T cells are so diminished that the body's natural defenses virtually disappear.

SLOW RECOGNITION OF THE AIDS EPIDEMIC

In its earliest manifestations, AIDS baffled medical researchers. The virus that causes it, while so fragile that it dies almost immediately on exposure to air, is capable of endlessly changing its shape and characteristics so that those devising ways to fight it have to find ways to fight a multiplicity of related viruses.

HIV is particularly insidious because it can lurk undetected for long periods—some AIDS researchers say for more than ten years—in the bloodstreams, lymph nodes, and livers of those who have been infected. The infected person may display no symptoms of the disease. The presence of HIV can be detected through a relatively simple blood test, but those who are asymptomatic often see no reason to be tested. False negatives can be recorded if one is tested shortly after exposure. Tests given three or more months after exposure produce the most reliable results.

AIDS was first thought to be a disease that mostly afflicted homosexual males who contracted it through the exchange of body fluids during sex, particularly anal sex, in which the passive partner (bottom) was more susceptible to contracting the disease than the active partner (top). Because of the stigma attached to the gay lifestyle, government agencies and the medical profession responded to the growing AIDS epidemic more slowly than they characteristically respond to health emergencies and potential epidemics.

Although the Centers for Disease Control (CDC) issued warnings about the disease as early as 1981, President Ronald Reagan never publicly acknowledged its existence until 1987, a lapse for which he made a public apology in 1990. United States Surgeon General C. Everett Koop recognized the threat and urged the establishment of national sex education programs, but with a public either apathetic about the disease or openly hostile toward those who had it, the lag time between its discovery and concerted efforts to control it was shockingly long.

Ultimately, it was the AIDS deaths of such prominent people as actor Rock Hudson, tennis star Arthur Ashe, and child activist Ryan White that heightened public awareness of the AIDS dilemma. It soon became apparent that AIDS was not wholly a gay disease but one that could afflict other groups of people, including children born to parents who carried the virus and heterosexual men and women who engaged in unprotected sex. Prostitutes, both male and female, were particularly vulnerable.

People at Risk for Contracting HIV

People who received blood transfusions in the early days of the epidemic, as was the case with Ryan White, a hemophiliac who required regular transfusions, had little protection against receiving tainted blood. This problem has diminished in recent years. Another high-risk group was intravenous drug users who often injected themselves with needles that had been used previously by other addicts whose blood, clinging to the shared needle, carried the virus.

Medical personnel began to exercise extreme caution to avoid sticking themselves with needles they had used for injecting patients. New protocols were developed for the disposal of such needles and of other materials used with HIV-positive patients. As people became more cognizant of the causes of AIDS, physicians, nurses, dentists, and oral hygienists began routinely to wear latex gloves and masks in all their contacts with patients.

When the disease was first brought to public attention, the public was extremely fearful that it might be spread through touching, sharing food, and kissing. Although such fears were groundless, some medical personnel, including physicians and dentists, refused to treat those suffering from AIDS. Parents rebelled against school districts that integrated HIV-positive children into the general school population. Some such prejudices continue to exist, although the more enlightened members of society realize that the possibility of infection exists only where bodily fluids have been exchanged intravenously or through sexual contact.

The best defenses against AIDS are sexual abstinence and the use of measures to prevent infection. Sexual encounters should involve the use of condoms unless one is absolutely certain that his or her partner is not infected. Complete honesty about sexual matters is essential for married people or for those in committed relationships. Members of such relationships who have unprotected sex with one other person are at risk not only from the person with whom they have an encounter but from every person with whom that person has had previous unprotected encounters. It is essential in any casual sexual encounter that body fluids not be exchanged.

Treatment Options

Although AIDS has been an acknowledged health problem since 1981, no cure for the disease has emerged nor have vaccines been developed to prevent infection. The CDC and other government agencies have engaged in considerable research to find both a cure and a preventive vaccine, but progress has been slow, often hampered by lack of funding and by the stigma that still makes AIDS a politically uncomfortable topic for public discussion.

Scientists have found HIV particularly challenging to combat because it is such a complex virus and because it has the ability to change itself, virtually to reinvent itself, almost at will. Vaccines that have controlled or eliminated such diseases as polio, smallpox, and measles are effective because they are aimed at viruses that, although complex, remain relatively stable. HIV is part of a different category of viruses altogether.

Despite the challenges that HIV offers, considerable headway has been achieved in making the presence of this virus in HIV-positive people manageable for considerable periods of time. There was a 19 percent decrease in AIDS-related deaths from the first nine months of 1995 to the first nine months of the following year, with 37,900 such deaths recorded in the United States in 1995 and 30,700 recorded in 1996.

When AIDS was first recognized in 1981, a diagnosis was equivalent to a death sentence. It was not until 1986 that the CDC revealed that a new drug, azidothymidine, commonly called AZT, first developed in 1964 as a cancer drug and sold under the brand name Retrovir, was proving effective in combating retroviruses, of which HIV was one. CDC's tests showed that those on a course of AZT showed a weight gain within four weeks, whereas those on the placebo lost weight. After six months, just 1 of the AIDS patients on AZT had died, whereas 19 of the 137 patients in the group receiving the placebo had succumbed.

So dramatic were the initial results that the United States Food and Drug Administration approved of the CDC's halting the study and granted approval to distribute AZT in 1987. The drug worked by blocking the ability of an enzyme necessary for the early stage of HIV reproduction to function. Not only were the lives of AIDS sufferers being extended, but they were also less subject to the opportunistic infections that had plagued them in the past. The drug also appeared to inhibit the growth of the virus in the brain, thereby reducing substantially the dementia that earlier AIDS victims had often endured. AZT treatment of HIV-positive pregnant women reduced by two-thirds the risk that the disease would be transmitted from mother to baby.

Even though AZT quickly became the major drug for treating AIDS, it was not without its hazards. A very toxic drug, AZT was first given in large doses at frequent intervals. It took the medical profession some time to realize that smaller doses taken less frequently were beneficial. The drug, even when the dosage was reduced, caused such substantial side effects in many patients that an estimated 40 to 80 percent had to discontinue treatment because of acute anemia, diarrhea, nausea, and damage to the liver, bone marrow, and nerves. Even those with minimal side effects often were taken off the drug because they developed a resistance to it.

Physicians soon learned that it was more effective to treat HIV-positive and AIDS patients with several drugs rather than merely with AZT. When a single drug is used, any particles of the virus not killed by the drug may mutate, creating a new strain of HIV that becomes resistant to the drug. When three drugs are used simultaneously, the virus has to go through three mutations, which is much more difficult for it to do.

These drug cocktails, while effective in reducing substantially the amounts of virus present in the blood—sometimes to virtually undetectable levels—involve taking between fourteen and twenty pills and capsules a day and having one's life revolve around medicating at precise times twenty-four hours a day. To violate the strict routine imposed by such a course of medication is to invite failure, yet many people on this routine are destined to stay on it throughout their lives.

The most promising treatment for HIV was developed after researchers discovered the HIV protease in 1986. Protease is needed if HIV is to reproduce in the later stages of its life cycle. Protease inhibitors prevent such reproduction, but the early ones were so toxic in tests on humans and animals that they could not be used. Finally, however, less toxic versions of the protease inhibitors were developed and by 1994, they went beyond slowing viral reproduction as AZT had, seemingly eliminating it altogether.

It has been determined that in the first few weeks after infection, HIV occurs in the lymph nodes where standard blood tests do not detect it. Tests have shown that during this period, HIV makes billions of copies of itself every day. By the time HIV is detected in the bloodstream, the lymph nodes have probably been destroyed and the immune system is collapsing. Therefore, it is now thought that protease inhibitors should be used as soon after exposure as possible.

Cost has been an inhibiting factor in the treatment of HIV-positive and AIDS patients. Therapy with three protease inhibitors costs between twelve and sixteen thousand dollars a year. Many insurance companies balk at covering such expenses, and a number of states limit state-funded treatment to one protease inhibitor, whereas seventeen states provide none. In Third World countries, where AIDS is wiping out huge numbers of people, treatment is virtually unobtainable. Those who are HIV-positive simply wait for their devastated immune systems to collapse and give way to full-blown AIDS, which will quickly be followed by death from one or more opportunistic diseases.

THE SCOPE OF THE PROBLEM

In order to gain a perspective on the HIV/AIDS dilemma, it is necessary to realize the extent of it. No continent is exempt from AIDS, and the United States is less affected than some other parts of the world where the problem is intensified by both poverty and political infighting that make the care of AIDS victims severely substandard, indeed, virtually nonexistent except for what families can to do provide for stricken relatives.

The highest incident of AIDS is in sub-Saharan Africa, where well over 20 million people are afflicted. Nearly 6 million cases are reported in south and southeast Asia, a million and a half in Latin America. This compares with about 860,000 cases in North America. Statistics show that worldwide, just under 6 million people were newly infected in 1997 alone. Of these, just over 2 million were women and about 590,000 were children. The number of children orphaned by AIDS through the deaths of both parents is estimated at over 8 million, most of them in Third World countries.

In 1997, over 30 million people worldwide suffered from HIV/AIDS. In that year, some 2.3 million died of AIDS-related diseases, although in the same year there was a percentage decrease in AIDS deaths in the United States, partly because many people were avoiding risky sexual and drug encounters, but mostly because of the availability of protease inhibitors and other drugs that reduce AIDS from an unquestionably fatal disease to a manageable one that is often compared to diabetes, which is manageable through medications.

Half of all HIV-positive people develop AIDS within nine years of the onset of the infection, and 40 percent die within ten years. The only reasonable way to conquer this disease is through the development of one or more vaccines that will make people immune from it. If an HIV/AIDS vaccine is developed, the next major tasks facing agencies like the World Health Organization will be to find money to produce it for the whole world and to devise a means of inoculating entire populations in the Third World—Africa, Latin America, and Asia. But developing a vaccine for HIV/AIDS is much more complicated than developing one for many of the other diseases that have been brought under control.

To begin with, there are at least twelve identifiable strains of HIV, each unique, each diabolically tricky in reinventing itself. A vaccine that offers immunity to one strain of the virus may well leave one defenseless against other strains. A further complication is that most effective vaccines have been produced by using weakened or inactivated forms of the virus that the vaccine is being created to attack. HIV, however, changes form with such lightning speed that the danger of transmitting the virus to those being inoculated is quite real. Viruses against which successful vaccines have been devised, unlike HIV, do not attack and destroy the immune system. They trigger antibodies that combat the offending cells that cause the disease. With HIV, there is the danger that the virus will change form quickly enough that any antibodies produced will not recognize the characteristics of the viruses they are supposed to attack. This could result in the collapse of the immune system in a person who, before the immunization, was healthy.

Because of the risks involved, testing of HIV/AIDS vaccines in the United States has been carried out mostly on monkeys and chimpanzees, whose immune systems are much like those of humans. One genetically engineered vaccine was given to chimpanzees who were injected one year later with enough of the AIDS virus to infect about 250 animals. Subsequent tests revealed that these animals were completely free of the virus, although there is always the danger that some remnant of it might still lurk somewhere in the systems of the inoculated animals. This test has been sufficiently promising, however, that limited testing is being done on human subjects who are HIV-negative.

—R. Baird Shuman

See also AIDS and children; AIDS and women; Epidemics; Sexually transmitted diseases (STDs); Terminal illnesses.

FOR FURTHER INFORMATION:

Bellenir, Karen, ed. *AIDS Sourcebook.* 2d ed. Detroit: Omnigraphics, 1999. This book provides the most comprehensive coverage currently available on matters relating to AIDS. It is rich with statistical information. Its sections on the management of the disease and prevention are particularly notable.

Bartlett, John G., and Ann K. Finkbeiner. *The Guide to Living with HIV Infection.* 4th ed. Baltimore: The Johns Hopkins University Press, 1998. Developed at the AIDS clinic of the Johns Hopkins University Hospital; offers practical advice for dealing with HIV and AIDS on a day-to-day basis. Goes into such matters as making legal and financial decisions and preparing to die.

Check, William A. *AIDS.* Philadelphia: Chelsea House, 1999. This volume, part of *The Encyclopedia of Health,* is directed toward the adolescent audience. The presentation is crisp and direct; C. Everett Koop's introduction well organized and effective.

Houts, Peter S., ed. *Home Care Guide for HIV and AIDS: For Family and Friends Giving Care at Home.* Philadelphia: American College of Physicians, 1998. Well organized, as comprehensive as any book available on the practical aspects of managing HIV/AIDS treatment at home. Deals not only with the problems of the afflicted but also with the problems of those who care for them.

Shein, Lori. *AIDS.* San Diego: Lucent Books, 1998. Aimed at general and adolescent audiences. Strong chapter on prevention. Offers a list of AIDS organizations.

✧ AIDS AND CHILDREN

Type of issue: Children's health, epidemics
Definition: The effects of human immunodeficiency virus (HIV) on the children, who often acquired it from their mothers during childbirth.

As a segment of the growing AIDS epidemic, pediatric cases offer a unique set of issues pertaining to the transmission, physical health, and psychological care of children and their families.

Reported AIDS Cases Among Children and Teenagers in the United States

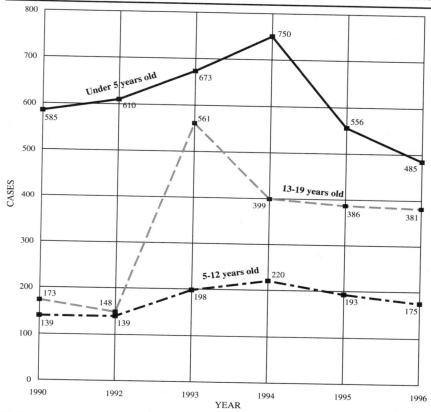

SOURCE: *Statistical Abstract of the United States 1997. Washington, D.C.: GPO, 1997.*

Awareness and detection of the disease known as acquired immunodeficiency syndrome, or AIDS, began in the 1980's, and the first cases of children with AIDS appeared in 1982. AIDS was diagnosed only after the struggle to determine the reason behind immunodeficiency and opportunistic infections that began to occur in children under the age of two. Such baffling cases had appeared in the late 1970's but were not yet linked with the AIDS disorder.

INCIDENCE AND SPREAD

The number of pediatric cases of AIDS reached 189 by the end of 1981. The number of cases increased during that decade, and by the middle of 1992 more than 4,000 cases of pediatric AIDS in the United States had been reported to the Centers for Disease Control (CDC). In comparison to the number of AIDS cases reported for individuals age thirteen and older, pediatric cases represented only 2 percent of all diagnoses. At the same time, however, AIDS continued to climb as one of the leading causes of death among children.

Cases of pediatric AIDS are distributed throughout the United States. The metropolitan areas and larger cities, such as New York, Miami, and Washington, D.C., have a greater proportion of pediatric AIDS cases. In addition, a greater number of pediatric AIDS cases are found among African American children. There are slightly more cases of AIDS among male children than among female children, a difference attributed to transfusions of tainted blood to male hemophilia patients.

TRANSMISSION OF THE VIRUS

Most children acquire AIDS through the transmission of human immunodeficiency virus (HIV) by their mothers. Known as "vertical transmission," this can occur during pregnancy through the placental tissue or amniotic fluid, during labor and delivery via blood or vaginal secretions, or postnatally through mothers' breast milk. Nevertheless, not all infants born to HIV-positive women acquire HIV. About half of all infected infants test positive for HIV soon after birth, indicating that the virus was transmitted during pregnancy. Some cases of HIV in fetuses have been detected as early as the first and second trimesters by testing fetal tissue. Evidence of infection, however, may not appear until a few days, months, or even years following birth.

HIV-infected children are thus often the result of HIV-infected mothers. Many such mothers are intravenous drug users. Most other women infected with HIV are believed to have acquired the virus by heterosexual contact with male intravenous drug users. Some of these women may also have exchanged sex for drugs, engaged in unprotected sex, or had sex with multiple partners.

Cases of pediatric AIDS can also be transmitted through the receipt of blood and blood products. The number of cases of HIV transmission linked to blood transfusions has drastically decreased since 1985 because of more stringent procedures for screening blood by medical personnel. While not generally acknowledged, it is also possible for children to acquire HIV through sexual abuse, child prostitution, or children's use of intravenous drugs.

PHYSICAL HEALTH EXPERIENCES

HIV affects the immune system, thus rendering infected children vulnerable to common infections and opportunistic infections. Children are more susceptible to infections than adults, because, unlike adults, they have not had time to develop a healthy immune system prior to becoming infected. Symptoms of the disease vary in number, duration, and severity from child to child. Children infected with HIV alternate between ill and healthy periods and are often asymptomatic in their early lives. The earlier children show symptoms of HIV, the more rapid the advancement of the disease and the progression toward death.

In 1987 the CDC designed a classification system specifically for children. This classification system lists many diagnoses as AIDS indicators and is arranged in such a way so that practitioners can track the progress of the disease. Although this system is very similar to that used for adults, two conditions are listed for children only: a chronic lung condition called lymphoid interstitial pneumonitis and recurrent serious bacterial infections.

Some of the more common symptoms in HIV-infected children include recurrent diarrhea, thrush, fever, malnutrition, and failure to thrive. Failure to thrive can include a lack of height and weight gain and a lack of growth of head circumference. HIV-infected children may also experience bacterial infections, such as sinusitis, meningitis, pneumonia, urinary tract infection, and anemia—an extremely common symptom.

The opportunistic infection *Pneumocystis carinii* pneumonia (PCP), considered to be the most common opportunistic infection for infants and children, affects about half of all children with AIDS. The signs of PCP include shortness of breath, fever, cough, and rapid breathing. Often the disease indicating the presence of HIV, it is most often diagnosed in the early months of life and is associated with a high rate of mortality.

Neurologic disease, another potential diagnosis, can cause developmental delay, loss of previously achieved milestones, and attention deficits. Children with neurologic disease may experience seizures, weakness, or even blindness. In the advanced stages of HIV infection, the virus can cause damage to the central nervous system, the heart, lungs, and kidneys.

EFFECTS ON FAMILIES

Children and other family members can be affected by pediatric AIDS in numerous ways. If children require hospitalization, they may be separated from their families for extended periods, thus necessitating their segregation from the family environment. In other circumstances, infants may be abandoned or relocated to other family members' homes, because caregivers are unable to care for their children's needs, as in the case of drug-addicted mothers. In addition, caregivers may also be infected with HIV, thus intensifying the impact of all aspects of the disease.

Families with HIV-infected children may also suffer financially. Physical care, equipment, visits by doctors and specialists, and the costs of hospitalization and medication are just some of the expenses that families with seriously ill members face. If families' resources are limited, provisions for basic needs may be inadequate. Proper nutrition, vital to attempting to maintain children's health, may have to be sacrificed in order to pay health costs. Caregivers' health may also be at risk, as they ignore their own needs while trying to meet those of their sick children.

Family members may find that they must take on new roles, as they become nurses or income providers. Siblings may report feeling neglected or may feel burdened by the added responsibilities placed on them. Grandparents or other extended family members may assume greater primary caregiving responsibilities. Married couples may experience stress because their time and energy often become focused on their ailing children. Such experiences can emotionally drain family members, especially those who do not have adequate coping skills. Taking time for other family members and expressing appreciation for their contributions can help to reduce the intensity of these difficulties.

Anticipatory grief, guilt, anxiety, and depression are some of the commonly faced emotional problems. These emotions can be triggered or heightened by social stigmatization, lack of social support, a reduction in the amount of time for socializing or being alone, and a sense of being overwhelmed by the physical and emotional burden of caring for terminally ill loved ones.

Other children may be discouraged from spending time with children who have pediatric AIDS because of the fear of transmission. However, this fear is often based on a lack of knowledge about the disease. On the other hand, in order to ease some of the burden on families with ill children, the community may provide them with support, such as child care while parents run errands or take required time for themselves. The medical community can potentially offer support and understanding, providing parents with referrals to community programs and personnel that may be of assistance. The reaction and assistance of family members and the community are key to the impact upon the family system.

—*Kimberly A. Wallet*

See also AIDS; AIDS and women; Children's health issues; Depression in children; Epidemics; Sexually transmitted diseases (STDs); Terminal illnesses.

FOR FURTHER INFORMATION:
Cohen, Felissa L., and Jerry D. Durham, eds. *Women, Children, and HIV/AIDS.* New York: Springer, 1993.
Kelly, Patricia, Susan Holman, Rosalie Rothenberg, and Stephen Paul Holzemer, eds. *Primary Care of Women and Children with HIV Infection: A Multidisciplinary Approach.* Boston: Jones and Bartlett, 1995.
Pizzo, Philip A., and Catherine M. Wilfert, eds. *Pediatric AIDS: The Challenge of HIV Infection in Infants, Children, and Adolescents.* 3d ed. Baltimore: Lippincott Williams & Wilkins, 1999.

Sherr, Lorraine, ed. *AIDS and Adolescents.* Amsterdam: Harwood Academic, 1997.

Zeichner, Steven L., and Jennifer S. Read, eds. *Handbook of Pediatric HIV Care.* Baltimore: Lippincott Williams & Wilkins, 1999.

❖ AIDS AND WOMEN

Type of issue: Epidemics, women's health

Definition: The effects of human immunodeficiency virus (HIV) on the female body.

Acquired immunodeficiency syndrome (AIDS), which is caused by HIV, presents a real and significant threat to women's health. By the early 1990's, HIV was spreading four times faster among women than among men, and it was the fifth leading cause of death of women aged fifteen to forty-four in the United States. Additionally, a disproportionate number of minority women had contracted HIV. While African American and Hispanic women constituted 21 percent of the general population, they made up 74 percent of all women with HIV. This trend seemed not to stem from racial issues but rather was representative of the socioeconomic statistics of the epidemic.

Prior to 1992, the majority of cases of HIV in women were caused by intravenous drug use. Since 1992, the majority of reported new transmissions have been from sexual activities. It is considerably more likely for a man to transmit the virus to a woman through intercourse than it is for a woman to transmit the virus to a man. There are two primary reasons for this finding: because semen is introduced into the vagina during ejaculation and because microscopic tears may occur in the vaginal tissue during intercourse, breaking the skin barrier and allowing the virus easy access to open tissue. Consequently, the use of a condom is considered helpful in reducing the risk of transmission, although it does not provide complete protection. Only by abstinence from intercourse can one be sure to avoid contracting HIV through sexual contact.

THE EFFECTS OF THE VIRUS

At one time it was believed that women had a significantly reduced survival time compared to men after becoming infected with HIV, but this trend is more accurately a reflection of the socioeconomic status of women with the virus. In women, the virus was first seen in those with a history of blood transfusion (a few cases) and in those who used drugs intravenously, women who traditionally represented a poor economic picture. In men, the virus made its first significant statement among white gay men, who as a group were more educated, had greater access to the health care system, and were in potentially better health in general than members of poorer populations. It is also true that until the 1990's, all major HIV studies of drugs, treatments, and diseases associated with AIDS were conducted on male subjects; there were no reliable data to determine the action of the virus in women. More recent research, however, indicates that women often have different health problems after contracting HIV but that their life span is equal to that of men if all other factors are equal.

THE NEEDS OF WOMEN WITH HIV

Areas of special consideration for women with HIV include physical, psychological, and social needs. Physically, women with HIV have a greater incidence of sexually transmitted diseases, including human papillomavirus (genital warts), chlamydia, candidiasis (yeast infections), and herpes than do women who are not HIV-positive. They also have a greatly increased incidence of uterine, ovarian, cervical, and breast cancers. Once any infection or cancer occurs in a woman with HIV, it may be very difficult to cure or slow the process of that disease because of the compromised condition of the patient's immune system. Along with such gender-specific diseases and sexually transmitted diseases, a woman with HIV also must cope with all the other diseases that affect a failing immune system, such as pneumonia and various cancers.

Another physical consideration for women is the possibility of conceiving or continuing a pregnancy once they have tested positive for HIV. If the drug zidovudine (formerly azidothymidine, or AZT) is used from the earliest point possible in pregnancy, the infant's chances of contracting HIV may be reduced to as low as 5 percent. Questions arise, however, regarding the advisability of maintaining a pregnancy if AZT was not started early. Such a dilemma might arise, for example, if the diagnosis of AIDS had not yet been made, if the mother is quite ill with HIV and the pregnancy may hasten the mother's death regardless of medication, or if the mother has no way to ensure support of a child after her own death. To resolve these issues, the woman may seek a therapeutic abortion, which may be available depending on the laws in her state.

In addition to the need to deal with the diagnosis of HIV, there are special psychological considerations depending on what stage of life the woman has recently entered. A woman with HIV may be facing adolescence, early adulthood, middle age, or elder years. It is important for an individual who is HIV-positive to accomplish the tasks of each stage of life, just as it is for uninfected women. In the 1990's, there was a new category of women entering adolescence, those who were born HIV-infected and had lived all their lives in that state.

The social needs of the HIV-positive woman are numerous and should be broadly defined because, as with psychological needs, each case differs.

Financial security is necessary through the progress of the virus, to cover not only health care and the payment of medical bills but also food, clothing, shelter, possibly the provision of the same for dependents, and transportation. The woman with HIV also needs support for her life and lifestyle, and privacy and security considerations accompany the seeking of such help. A woman who has kept her HIV status secret risks letting her family and friends know of the illness, and if there are children involved, she runs the risk of having her children removed from her care. If she is an intravenous drug user, she may be at legal risk if she seeks help. Social support also may be required in the notification of any past sexual partners who may have been exposed to the virus; such contact may be difficult, but it is necessary.

By the beginning of the twenty-first century, twenty years into the AIDS epidemic, women had not had a primary voice in research, treatment trials, or the allocation of funds. As the spread of HIV has led to a primarily heterosexual transmission of the virus, the special needs of women with the disease have begun to emerge. There is a distinct need for further study on the impact of HIV and AIDS on the female body.

—Kris Riddlesperger

See also Abortion; AIDS; AIDS and children; Alcoholism; Condoms; Epidemics; Hospice; Sexually transmitted diseases (STDs); Terminal illnesses; Women's health issues.

FOR FURTHER INFORMATION:

Cotton, Deborah J., and D. Heather Watts, eds. *The Medical Management of AIDS in Women.* New York: Wiley-Liss, 1997.

Fan, Hung, Ross F. Conner, and Luis P. Villarreal. *The Biology of AIDS.* 4th ed. Boston: Jones and Bartlett, 2000.

Stine, Gerald J. *Acquired Immune Deficiency Syndrome: Biological, Medical, Social, and Legal Issues.* 3d ed. Englewood Cliffs, N.J.: Prentice Hall, 1997.

_____. *AIDS Update 2001.* Upper Saddle River, N.J.: Prentice Hall, 2000.

White, Edith. *Breastfeeding and HIV/AIDS: The Research, the Politics, the Women's Responses.* Jefferson, N.C.: McFarland, 1999.

✧ ALCOHOLISM

Type of issue: Mental health, social trends
Definition: The compulsive drinking of and dependency on alcoholic beverages; viewed as psychological in origin, it can be arrested but not cured.

In 1992, it was estimated that nearly 70 percent of Americans used alcoholic beverages, that more than ten million such people were involved in the severe substance abuse of alcohol, and that about 250,000 alcohol-related deaths occur each year.

THE PHYSIOLOGY AND PSYCHOLOGY OF ALCOHOLISM

Some deaths attributable to alcohol occur as a result of alcohol poisoning, from excessive consumption in a short time period. The drug primarily depresses the action of the central nervous system, creating the desired euphoric effects of alcohol consumption. Given a drink or two, a drinker may become relaxed and uninhibited. A few more drinks, however, may increase blood alcohol levels above .10 and further depress the central nervous system, causing lack of coordination, slurred speech, and stuporous sleep. If just a little more alcohol is imbibed before stupor occurs and blood alcohol levels rise much above .25, further depression of the central nervous system stops breathing and kills.

People engaged in substance abuse of alcohol, alcoholics, carry out repeated, compulsive abuse that may make them unable to retain their jobs, to obtain an education, or to engage in responsible societal roles. Eventually, alcoholics damage their brains and other body tissues irreversibly. Often, they die of these afflictions or by suicide triggered by depression or terrifying hallucinations. They also engage in behavior that is dangerous to themselves and others, such as driving under the influence or violence.

Chronic alcoholism damages many body organs. Best known is liver disease, or cirrhosis of the liver. Another common affliction is organic brain damage. Mental disorders caused by injury to the cerebral hemispheres may include delirium tremens and Korsakoff's psychosis. Both delirium tremens, characterized by hallucination and other psychotic symptoms, and Korsakoff's psychosis, which is characterized by short-term memory loss and confabulation, or stories to cover this loss, may be accompanied by severe physical debility requiring hospitalization.

In addition, alcoholism damages the kidneys, the heart, and the pancreas. In fact, a large number of instances of diseases of other organs are thought to arise from alcohol abuse. Also, much evidence suggests that alcoholism greatly enhances the incidence of mouth and throat cancer resulting from smoking tobacco.

Severe effects in the liver occur because most ingested alcohol is metabolized there. In the presence of alcohol, most other substances normally metabolized by the liver—the factory bloc of the body—are not changed into useful and essential forms. One example has to do with fat, a major dietary source of energy. Decreased fat metabolism in the livers of alcoholics results in the fat accumulation—a fatty liver—that precedes cirrhosis of the liver. Cirrhosis results in the replacement of liver cells with nonfunctional fibrous tissue.

Another problem that results from excessive alcohol metabolism is that the liver no longer destroys the many other toxic chemicals that are eaten. This defect adds to problems seen in cirrhosis and leads to dissemination of such chemicals through the body, where they can damage other body parts. In addition, resistance to the flow of blood through the alcoholic liver develops, which can burst blood vessels and cause dangerous internal bleeding. As a consequence of these problems, alcoholic liver disease, or cirrhosis, has become a major, worldwide cause of death from disease.

POSSIBLE CAUSES FOR ALCOHOLISM

There is no one clear physical explanation for the development of alcoholism. Most often, it is viewed as the result of a biological predisposition to addiction and/or social problems and psychological stresses, especially in those socioeconomic groups in which consumption of alcoholic beverages is equated with manliness or sophistication. Other proposed causes of behaviors that lead to alcoholism include habitual drinking, other mental health problems, domineering parents, adolescent peer pressure, personal feelings of inadequacy, loneliness, job pressures, and marital discord.

The fact that 20 percent of children of alcoholics tend to develop the disease, compared to 4 percent of the children of nonalcoholics, has led to investigations of the genetic proclivity for alcoholism. The fact that 80 percent of the progeny of alcoholic parents escape alcoholism, however, diminishes support for such theories. On the other hand, there are clearer indications that genetic factors are important to distaste for alcohol, precluding the development of alcoholism in some ethnic and national groups.

Another disease attributable to alcoholism is fetal alcohol syndrome, which occurs in many children of mothers who drank heavily during pregnancy. Such children may be hyperactive, mentally retarded, and facially disfigured, and they may exhibit marked growth retardation. Fetal alcohol syndrome is becoming more frequent as alcohol consumption increases worldwide.

Commonly observed symptoms of alcoholism are physical dependence on alcohol consumption shown by tremors, shakes, other physical discomfort, and excitability reversed only by alcohol intake; blackout and accompanying memory loss; diminished cognitive ability, exhibited as an inability to understand verbal instructions or to memorize simple series of numbers; and relaxed social inhibitions. These symptoms are attributable to the destruction of tissues of the central nervous system. Diminished sexual activity and sexual desire may also result from excessive alcohol consumption. A high level of alcohol appears to cause diminished libido and impotence. In addition, alcohol may even increase the rate of destruction of existing testosterone in the body.

Treating Alcoholism

While no immediate cure for alcoholism is known, treatments for alcohol problems with demonstrated effectiveness do exist. Treatments involving a combined biological, psychological, and social approach, complete with follow-up, often appear most helpful. For most individuals, however, an important phase—or possibly even a permanent feature—of treatment involves total abstinence from alcoholic beverages, all medications that contain alcohol, and any other potential sources of alcohol in the diet.

Two well-known medical treatments for enforcing sobriety are the drugs disulfiram (Antabuse) and citrated calcium carbonate (Abstem). These drugs are given to alcoholics who wish to avoid all use of alcoholic beverages and who require a deterrent to drinking to achieve this goal. Neither drug should ever be given secretly by well-meaning family or friends because of the serious dangers that Antabuse and Abstem pose if an alcoholic back-slides and drinks alcohol.

These dangers are the result of the biochemistry of alcohol utilization via the two enzymes (biological protein catalysts) alcohol dehydrogenase and aldehyde dehydrogenase. Normally, alcohol dehydrogenase converts alcohol to the toxic chemical acetaldehyde, and aldehyde dehydrogenase quickly converts the acetaldehyde to acetic acid, the main biological fuel on which the body runs. Either Abstem or Antabuse will turn off aldehyde dehydrogenase and cause acetaldehyde levels to build up in the body when alcohol is consumed. The presence of acetaldehyde in the body then quickly leads to violent headache, great dizziness, heart palpitation, nausea, and vertigo. When the amount of alcohol found in a drink or two (or even the amount taken in cough medicine) is consumed in the presence of either drug, these symptoms can escalate to the extent that they become fatal.

As a result of the symptoms of alcohol withdrawal common during detoxification and the presence of other mental health disorders in nearly half of all individuals diagnosed with alcohol dependence, other therapeutic drugs are often used in treatment. Examples include lithium, tranquilizers, and sedative hypnotics. The function of these psychoactive drugs is to diminish the discomfort of alcohol withdrawal. Lithium treatment, which must be done with great care because it can become very toxic, appears to be effective only in the alcoholics who drink because of depression or bipolar disorder.

The use of tranquilizers and the related sedative hypnotics must also be done with great care, under close supervision of a physician. Many such drugs are addictive. In addition, some of these drugs have strong synergistic (additive) effects when mixed with alcohol, and such synergism can be fatal.

Alcoholics Anonymous and Other Group Therapies

It is believed that the advent of Alcoholics Anonymous in the 1930's has been crucial to the perception of alcoholism as a disease to be treated, rather than as immoral behavior to be condemned. This organization operates on the premise that abstinence is the best course of treatment for alcoholism—an incurable disease that can, however, be arrested by the cessation of all alcohol intake. The methodology of the organization is psychosocial. First, alcoholics are brought to the realization that they can never use alcoholic beverages without succumbing to alcoholism. Then, the need for help from a "higher power" is identified as crucial to abstinence. In addition, the organization develops a support group of people in the same situation.

Estimates of the membership of Alcoholics Anonymous in 1992 ranged between 1.5 and 4 million, meaning up to one-third of American alcoholics were affected by its tenets. These people, ranging widely in age, achieve results varying from periods of sobriety (lasting longer and longer as membership in the organization continues) to lifelong sobriety. A deficit of the sole utilization of Alcoholics Anonymous for alcoholism treatment—in the opinion of some experts—is lack of medical, psychiatric, and trained sociological counseling. The results of the operation, however, are viewed by most as beneficial to all parties who seek help from the organization.

Alcohol rehabilitation centers apply varied combinations of drug therapy, psychiatric counseling, and social counseling, depending on the treatment approach for the individual center. Group therapy, however, is the dominant mode of treatment in the United States. Counseling can identify the factors leading to alcohol abuse, explore and help to rectify the associated problems, provide emotional support, and refer patients to Alcoholics Anonymous and other long-term support efforts. The psychotherapist also has experience with managing clients who use or have used psychoactive drugs, understands behavioral modification techniques, and can determine whether an individual requires institutionalization.

Behavior modification is a cornerstone of alcoholism psychotherapy, and many choices are available to all alcoholics desiring psychosocial help. An interesting point is that autopsy and a variety of sophisticated medical techniques such as CT (computed tomography) and PET (positron emission tomography) scans identify the atrophy of the cerebral cortex of the brain in many alcoholics. This damage is viewed as participating in the inability of alcoholics to stop drinking, their loss of both cognitive and motor skills, and the eventual development of serious conditions such as Korsakoff's psychosis and delirium tremens.

—Sanford S. Singer; updated by Nancy A. Piotrowski

See also Addiction; Alcoholism among teenagers; Alcoholism among the elderly; Dementia; Fetal alcohol syndrome; Recovery programs.

FOR FURTHER INFORMATION:
Berkow, Robert, and Andrew J. Fletcher, eds. *The Merck Manual of Diagnosis and Therapy.* 17th ed. Rahway, N.J.: Merck Sharp & Dohme Research Labs,

1999. This book contains a compendium of data on the etiology, diagnosis, and treatment of alcoholism. Contains good cross-references to the psychopathology related to the disease, drug rehabilitation, and Alcoholics Anonymous. Designed for physicians, it is also valuable to the layman.

Collins, R. Lorraine, Kenneth E. Leonard, and John R. Searles, eds. *Alcohol and the Family*. New York: Guilford Press, 1990. This book is divided into segments on genetics, family processes, and family-oriented treatment. Genetic testing and markers are well covered, and adolescent drinking, children of alcoholics, and alcoholism's effect on a marriage are also discussed. Evaluates the ability of the family to cope with stresses of alcoholism and its treatment.

Cox, W. Miles, ed. *The Treatment and Prevention of Alcohol Problems: A Resource Manual*. Orlando, Fla.: Academic Press, 1987. This work contains much information on the psychiatric and behavioral aspects of alcoholism. It is also widely useful in many other related issues, including Alcoholics Anonymous, marital and family therapy, and alcoholism prevention.

Eskelson, Cleamond D. "Hereditary Predisposition for Alcoholism." In *Diagnosis of Alcohol Abuse*, edited by Ronald R. Watson. Boca Raton, Fla.: CRC Press, 1989. This article provides useful data on the genetic aspects of alcoholism, concentrating on metabolism, animal and human studies, teetotalism, familial alcoholism, and genetic markers. Sixty-five references are included.

Torr, James D. *Alcoholism*. San Diego, Calif.: Greenhaven Press, 2000. This well-balanced selection of primary source materials is designed for children in grades six through twelve. A lengthy bibliography and a list of organizations to contact are appended.

✧ Alcoholism among teenagers

Type of issue: Children's health, mental health, social trends
Definition: The consumption of alcoholic beverages (such as beer, wine, or liquors) despite the occurrence of repeated social, interpersonal, or legal problems occurring as a result of that use over the course of a year.

Alcohol abuse is a specific diagnosis given for alcohol problems, as described in the *Diagnostic and Statistical Manual of Mental Disorders* (4th ed., 1994, DSM-IV) by the American Psychiatric Association. It is characterized by repeated psychological, legal, and social problems occurring as a result of alcohol use over the course of a year. Alcohol abuse is distinct from alcohol dependence, which refers to physical and psychological reliance on alcohol despite the presence of problems associated with its use. Both conditions can be diagnosed in children, teenagers, and adults.

Symptoms of alcohol abuse might include repeated legal problems (such as public drunkenness, driving while under the influence, truancy, violence, and crimes related to drinking or other criminal offenses occurring when under the influence). They might also include arguments and violent or aggressive behavior in which drinking results in social problems with friends or family members. Other types of problems that might signal a diagnosis of alcohol abuse would be an adult or child repeatedly not fulfilling what is expected of him or her in daily life, such as not going to work, being late to work, or missing or skipping school because of drinking.

The abuse of alcohol as a public health problem has also been linked to binge drinking. Young drinkers are especially prone to binge drinking because alcohol is not as available to them as it is to older drinkers. It is illegal for minors to purchase alcohol in the United States, so having alcohol available to consume can affect how individuals drink. What often happens with teenagers is that they will drink as much as they can when alcohol is available to them, on weekends or at parties, and then abstain when not at such events. Unfortunately, this pattern is conducive to the development of some tolerance to alcohol. Additionally, it is often linked to poor judgment, which may lead to risky sexual behavior (such as unprotected sex), the operation of an automobile while under the influence, or the taking of other drugs. There is also the risk that young or inexperienced drinkers who binge—by thinking that they can drink as much as they want without suffering anything worsse than a hangover—inadvertently put themselves at risk for alcohol poisoning.

TEENS, FAMILIES, AND ALCOHOL

By the age of eighteen years, nearly 80 percent of children and teenagers in the United States will experiment with alcohol. Not all will go on to abuse alcohol or to develop more severe problems. Differences in genetics, the influence of family and friends, community norms and expectations, self-esteem, and career and academic interests make some children and teenagers more likely to develop problems than others. Young people who are more likely to develop problems such as alcohol abuse tend to be impulsive, to be less interested in school work, to have lower levels of achievement in school, to be more uninhibited, to experience less positive feelings, to be more tolerant of deviant behavior in others, and to have a greater sensitivity to the positive physical and emotional effects of alcohol. Additionally, children who perceive their friends and family to be accepting of alcohol use are more likely to use alcohol. Those who come from families in which there are alcohol problems are generally at greater risk for problems than those who do not. This is particularly true for teenage boys of fathers with alcohol problems.

Teenagers are also more likely to have problems with alcohol if they have problems with self-regulation, have poor self-esteem, or are more susceptible to peer pressure. Parents may recognize budding alcohol problems in children who drink heavily or talk about drinking heavily as acceptable behavior, have friends who drink heavily or talk about drinking heavily as acceptable behavior, glamorize alcohol use or collect promotional materials on drinking products, or begin to have significant negative changes in their relationship with their parents, school performance, moodiness, sleeping habits, choice of friends, or interests in the future.

In general, the earlier alcohol use starts in childhood, the more likely it is that this use will lead to heavier drinking in the teenage years. Alcohol problems in the teenage years do not necessarily mean that a person will go on to develop alcohol problems as an adult, but the possibility remains. Because young adults and teenagers are exposed to risks as a result of drinking, understanding their alcohol problems, exclusive of problems experienced by adults, is important. Accidents, loss of life, damaged academic performance, social relationship problems, exposure to sexually transmitted diseases, and other risky situations can result from alcohol misuse and abuse by teenagers and younger children.

Attempts by parents and other adults to delay when a child's experimentation with alcohol starts can be valuable. Some indication exists that children of parents who do not drink at all or who drink very little begin experimentation at later ages. Additionally, having parents who are effective at providing support, setting standards for behavior, and giving guidance lessens the risk for alcohol abuse in teenagers and children. Children of parents who act proactively (who try to prevent problems before they happen) also tend to begin experimentation at later ages. Finally, teenagers who are more involved in school and who are more aware of the potential harmful effects of alcohol delay their drinking experimentation.

Alcohol abuse can also show up in the lives of children as a result of drinking done by their parents. Fetal alcohol syndrome is one example. In this case, it is not the children who abuse alcohol but rather their mothers, who drink while pregnant. Fetal alcohol syndrome is a medical condition resulting directly from the effects on the fetus of the mother's drinking. In the worst cases, it can result in fetal death. In less severe cases, a child of a parent who drank during pregnancy can experience mild to severe facial and dental abnormalities, mental impairments, or problems related to the skeleton and the cardiovascular system. Problems with vision, hearing, and attention span are also common. These problems are thought to result from the alcohol interfering with embryonic development.

Children of alcoholic fathers also can have difficulties in learning, language, and temperament. The causes of such problems are multiple and need to be determined. They include the contribution of genetics and the effects of growing up in a home that may be less stable as a result of alcohol-related social, occupational, or psychological problems in the father.

ALCOHOL ABUSE EDUCATION AND TREATMENT

Treatment for alcohol abuse can take several different forms: primary, secondary, and tertiary prevention. In primary prevention, treatment is applied to the population as a whole. An example might be a campaign against driving while drunk that is advertized on television, such as those promoted by many major beverage companies and groups like Mothers Against Drunk Driving (MADD). Similarly, educational programs focused on educating women about the dangers of drinking while pregnant can be seen as primary prevention approaches. Another example might be educating store clerks and store owners about the laws and fines that may be applied to individuals who sell alcohol to minors. In each case, the effects of the treatment are on the community as a whole, and the attempt is made to avoid a problem before it happens.

In secondary prevention, treatment is applied to individuals who are at a higher-than-average risk. Examples of such groups would be children of parents with alcohol problems and children who might be anxious, prone to panic, or depressed and may drink to calm their feelings. Treatment might include giving these children health education information about why people use alcohol (such as social pressure, uncomfortable feelings, boredom) and then teaching them other ways to handle those kinds of problems. Having such children talk to psychological counselors or medical doctors to treat depression or anxiety might also be appropriate. They might also be taught the skills necessary to refuse alcohol in situations where it is tempting to use it. Similarly, since some alcohol use is generally considered socially acceptable, secondary intervention might also include teaching a drinker how to drink in a safer manner or in a manner that is not harmful. With teenagers and children, however, it is important to keep in mind that any alcohol use by minors is illegal in the United States and can have legal consequences if it is occurring outside the home or without responsible parental supervision.

In tertiary prevention, treatment is applied to individuals who already have developed alcohol dependence, including children, teenagers, and adults. People can try to quit drinking on their own; however, withdrawal from alcohol can be fatal. As such, it is important for individuals thinking about quitting alcohol consumption to talk to a doctor. For schoolchildren, talking to a health teacher, school nurse, or counselor may be the best way to start. Depending on how long the person has been drinking, different types of treatment might be suggested. If dependence is severe, then seeking a doctor may be necessary for detoxification, a process of being taken off of alcohol in a safe manner. If dependence is less severe, then nonmedical treatments may be sufficient. Such treatments might include counseling, group support, or learning new ways to handle problems that the person was trying to handle with alcohol. Learning what caused the drinking, finding other means of meeting personal needs, and behaving in new ways to break old habits can be as important as any medical interventions in learning how to quit.

It is important to realize that alcohol abuse in children and teenagers may involve different issues for girls and boys. Some studies have suggested that boys who have more severe problems with alcohol early on in life, particularly those who have fathers or other male relatives with alcohol problems, are more likely to have a biological propensity to alcohol. Similarly, girls who have alcohol problems as children or adolescents are more likely to have problems with mood, such as depression, mood swings, or anxiety, particularly if they have mothers or female relatives with similar problems. Treatment may need to take these issues into account. For some, this may mean that medication is a best first strategy. For others, it may mean that supportive counseling may be critical to the cessation of alcohol abuse. In each case, the gender and other background characteristics of the child or adolescent must be considered for the best match to treatment. Additionally, problems such as emotional, physical, or sexual abuse must be explored and ruled out in children abusing alcohol. Often, alcohol and other drugs may be used by a child as a coping strategy for dealing with difficult family situations. In such cases, addressing the underlying situation is of critical importance for the immediate and long-term well-being of the child or adolescent.

ALCOHOL USE VERSUS ABUSE

Alcohol use has been a common social practice for thousands of years. Done with care and under safe conditions, it may add to the enjoyment that most people experience in social situations. In excess, however, alcohol can contribute to social and health problems in children, teenagers, adults, and families as a whole. Understanding the difference between acceptable levels of alcohol use, as compared to alcohol abuse and alcohol dependence, is important.

In the United States, while the number of individuals who drink alcohol has remained fairly constant, average alcohol consumption, heavy drinking, and alcohol-related problems are increasing. Additionally, adolescents are currently drinking, drinking heavily, and experiencing alcohol-related problems at younger ages than they have in the past. Prevention and treatment efforts need to be targeted toward delaying alcohol use in early adolescence and using educational and community resources to promote safe drinking practices. This has been recognized by the alcoholic beverage industry, which is now promoting safer drinking campaigns, and will continue to be important in the future for the betterment of public health.

—*Nancy A. Piotrowski*

See also Addiction; Birth defects; Child abuse; Children's health issues; Depression in children; Drug abuse by teenagers; Fetal alcohol syndrome; Recovery programs; Smoking; Tobacco use by teenagers.

For Further Information:

Collins, R. Lorraine, Kenneth E. Leonard, and John R. Searles, eds. *Alcohol and the Family*. New York: Guilford Press, 1990. This book is divided into segments on genetics, family processes, and family-oriented treatment. Genetic testing and markers are well covered, and adolescent drinking, children of alcoholics, and alcoholism's effect on a marriage are also discussed. Evaluates the ability of the family to cope with stresses of alcoholism and its treatment.

Forrest, Gary G. *How to Cope with a Teenage Drinker: Changing Adolescent Alcohol Abuse*. Northvale, N.J.: Jason Aronson, 1997. This book is written for parents or friends who know a teenager who may have an alcohol problem. Guidelines for helping teenagers recognize such problems are given.

Julien, Robert M. *A Primer of Drug Action*. 8th ed. New York: W. H. Freeman, 1998. This is a nontechnical guide to mind-altering drugs: their effects, practical uses, and how they work.

Torr, James D. *Alcoholism*. San Diego, Calif.: Greenhaven Press, 2000. This well-balanced selection of primary source materials is designed for children in grades six through twelve. A lengthy bibliography and a list of organizations to contact are appended.

Weil, Andrew, and Winifred Rosen. *From Chocolate to Morphine: Everything You Need to Know About Mind-Altering Drugs*. Rev. ed. Boston: Houghton Mifflin, 1998. This book describes a variety of mind-altering substances. The history, methods, and pros and cons of the use of these substances are described.

✧ ALCOHOLISM AMONG THE ELDERLY

Type of issue: Elder health, mental health, social trends

Definition: A general set of problems associated with alcohol abuse (psychological, social, and legal problems related to alcohol use) and alcohol dependence (a physical and psychological reliance on alcohol despite repeated significant problems associated with its use).

"Alcoholism" is a vague clinical term that is sometimes used to describe the condition in which an individual is afflicted with severe physical, social, and psychological problems related to alcohol use. It is not a medical diagnostic term. Rather, it is a colloquial term used to describe the state of an individual experiencing a general set of problems associated with the more formal diagnostic conditions known as alcohol abuse and alcohol dependence. Alcohol abuse is a specific diagnosis given for alcohol problems in which physical dependence on alcohol is not indicated. In cases of alcohol abuse, repeated and significant psychological, legal, and social problems tend to occur over the course of a year. The diagnosis of alcohol abuse is distinct from that of alcohol dependence and is described in the fourth edition of the *Diagnostic and Statistical Manual of Mental Disorders* (1994, DSM-IV) by the American Psychiatric Association. Alcohol dependence refers to both physical and psychological reliance on alcohol, despite the presence of repeated significant problems associated with its use for a period of a year or more.

PREVALENCE AND SPECIAL PROBLEMS

Alcohol problems can be diagnosed in individuals of any age; alcoholism among the elderly is thus to be expected at about the same rate as it would be in other adult age groups. In the elderly, however, alcoholism can be related to more significant problems because of the physical, mental, psychological, social, and financial vulnerabilities that can accompany later life. Changes in resilience accompanying later life can magnify the impact of problems related to alcohol by making recovery from such problems more difficult. This is especially true for elderly women, as physiological differences between men and women appear to cause alcohol problems to escalate in severity more quickly in older adult women than in older adult men.

Problematic alcohol use in elders is especially complicated by the greater physiological effects of alcohol that result from changes in how alcohol is processed by the body. As the body ages, the liver and other organs are less able to process alcohol out of the body, thereby altering tolerance to alcohol. As a result, alcohol stays in the body longer and has a more pronounced effect. This slowing of the body's ability to process substances also affects the processing of other drugs, which may also stay in the body longer. This can create drug interaction problems in the elderly, as they are especially likely to take prescription and nonprescription drugs on a regular basis.

Alcohol can intensify the effects of certain drugs, and vice versa; such interactions are particularly hazardous in the elderly. Combined with sedatives, alcohol can cause severe respiratory problems and also worsen problems related to balance. For elders already having respiratory or balance problems, such intensified effects can be very dangerous, leading to increased risk for falls, other accidents, or even death. Similarly, alcohol taken in combination with diuretics can be particularly dangerous, as the combination may encourage dehydration and can affect kidney functioning and blood pressure in a dangerous manner.

TREATMENT AND INTERVENTION

Alcohol problems in the elderly can come in two important types. For some, problems with alcohol may merely represent a continuation of lifelong habits. In these cases, the problems are chronic and will most likely require intensive intervention and management. Chronic problems of this type may lead to premature aging, serious cardiovascular health problems, cancers, and death, as well as severe difficulties with memory and other mental problems such as organic brain syndromes, aphasias, and dementias.

For other elderly people, though, problems related to alcohol may be a new development. In some cases, such problems may be situational, resulting from a recent stressor such as a death or loss of a loved one. Alcohol may be being used as a means of managing grief or depression. In these cases, interventions from someone such as a psychologist or geriatric psychiatrist may be warranted. Such assistance can help to address the root problem and also decrease the chance that a secondary problem with alcohol might develop as a result of repeated use.

Similarly, short-term alcohol problems may result from a lack of knowledge about drug interactions with alcohol. In these cases, the dissemination of information from a pharmacist about the dangers of mixing drugs and alcohol can prevent the elder from using alcohol in dangerous ways. Similarly, education from a family physician about how alcohol interacts with certain health conditions, such as heart problems, blood pressure problems, diabetes, depression, anxiety, insomnia, and stomach problems can also be useful in decreasing misuse of alcohol.

Alcohol problems may be more difficult to diagnose in the elderly than in younger adults. Older adults often do not show obvious signs of intoxication and withdrawal; moreover, when such symptoms appear, they may be attributed to other problems related to aging. Additionally, confusion of alcohol problems with other age-related conditions such as tremors, forgetfulness, and disorientation may obscure an accurate diagnosis. Alcohol problems in the elderly may also be masked by other physical or psychological conditions. Such conditions may bring an elder in for treatment, but the alcohol problem may go undetected. Screening for alcohol problems and questioning by medical professionals about alcohol use are thus important, as missing such problems may predispose an elder to relapse and worsened problems in the future.

Signs of problem drinking among the elderly may include any of the following: unusual increases in falls or accidents, slurring of speech, anxiety, insomnia or other sleep disorders, irritability, social withdrawal, efforts to hide or lie about the use of alcohol or other drugs, increased consumption of alcohol following significant losses, drinking alone more often, gulping of drinks or drinking fast, loss of interest in food, or any social, medical, or financial problems that appear to be caused or exacerbated by drinking. Evidence of any of these conditions may suggest a need for further medical evaluation.

—*Nancy A. Piotrowski*

See also Addiction; Aging; Alcoholism; Alcoholism among teenagers; Depression in the elderly; Medications and the elderly; Overmedication; Suicide among the elderly.

FOR FURTHER INFORMATION:

American Psychiatric Association. *The Diagnostic and Statistical Manual of Mental Disorders: DSM-IV-TR*. Rev. 4th ed. Washington, D.C.: Author, 2000.

Fanning, Patrick, and John T. O'Neill. *The Addiction Workbook: A Step-by-Step Guide to Quitting Alcohol and Drugs*. Oakland, Calif.: New Harbinger Press, 1996.

Miller, William R., and Ricardo F. Munoz. *How to Control Your Drinking: A Practical Guide to Responsible Drinking*. Rev. ed. Albuquerque: University of New Mexico Press, 1990.

Roukema, Richard W. *What Every Patient, Family, Friend, and Caregiver Needs to Know About Psychiatry*. Washington, D.C.: American Psychiatric Press, 1998.

✧ ALLERGIES

Type of issue: Environmental health, occupational health, public health

Definition: Exaggerated immune reactions to materials that are intrinsically harmless; the body's release of certain chemicals during allergic reactions may result in discomfort, tissue damage, or even death.

Allergies represent inappropriate immune responses to intrinsically harmless materials, or antigens. Most allergens are common environmental antigens. Approximately one in every six Americans is allergic to material such as dust, molds, dust mites, animal dander, or pollen. The effects range from a mere nuisance, such as the rhinitis associated with hay fever allergies or the itching of poison ivy, to the life-threatening anaphylactic shock that may follow a bee sting. Allergies are most often found in children, but they may affect any age group.

Allergy is one of the hypersensitivity reactions generally classified according to the types of effector molecules that mediate their symptoms and according to the time delay that follows exposure to the allergen. There are four types of hypersensitivities. Three of these, types I through III, follow minutes to hours after the exposure to an allergen. Type IV, or delayed-type hypersensitivity (DTH), may occur anywhere from twenty-four to seventy-two hours after exposure. People are most familiar with two of these forms of allergies: Type I, or immediate hypersensitivity, commonly seen as hay fever or asthma; and Type IV, most often following an encounter with poison ivy or poison oak.

TYPE I REACTIONS

Type I hypersensitivities have much in common with any normal immune response. A foreign material, an allergen, comes in contact with the host's immune system, and an antibody response is the result. The response differs according to the type of molecule produced. A special class of antibody, IgE, is secreted by the B lymphocytes. IgE, when complexed with the specific allergen, is capable of binding to any of several types of mediator cells, mainly basophils and mast cells.

Mast cells are found throughout skin and tissue. The mucous membranes of the respiratory and gastrointestinal tract in particular have high concentrations of these cells, as many as ten thousand cells per cubic millimeter. Basophils, the blood cell equivalents of the mast cells, represent 1 percent or less of the total white cell count. Both basophils and mast cells contain large numbers of granules composed of pharmacologically active chemicals. Both also contain surface receptors for IgE molecules. The binding of IgE/allergen complexes to these cells triggers the release of the granules.

Type I allergic reactions begin as soon as the sensitized person is exposed to the allergen. In the case of hay fever, this results when the person inhales the pollen particle. The shell of the particle is enzymatically dissolved, and the specific allergens are released in the vicinity of the mucous membranes in the respiratory system. If the person has had prior sensitization to the materials, IgE molecules secreted by localized lymphocytes bind to the allergens, forming an antibody/antigen complex. Events commonly associated with allergies to pollen—a runny nose and itchy, watery eyes—result from the formation of such complexes.

A sequence of events is set in place when the immune complexes bind to the surface of the mast cell or basophil. The reactions begin with a cross-linking of the IgE receptors on the cell. After an influx of calcium into the cell, two events rapidly follow: The cell begins production of prostaglandins and leukotrienes, two mediators that play key roles in allergic reactions, and preexisting granules begin moving toward the cell surface. When they reach the cell surface, the granules fuse with the cell membrane, releasing their contents into the tissue.

The contents of the granules mediate the clinical manifestations of allergies. These mediators can be classified as either primary or secondary. Thus, clinical responses are divided into immediate and late-phase reactions. Primary mediators are those found in preexisting granules and that are released initially following the activities at the cell surface. They include substances such as histamine and serotonin, associated with increased vascular permeability and smooth muscle contraction. Histamine itself may constitute 10 percent of the weight of the granules in these cells. The result is the runny nose, irritated eyes, and bronchial congestion with which so many are familiar. Secondary mediators, which are released in the late phase, are synthesized following the binding of the immune complexes to the cell surface. These substances include the leukotrienes and prostaglandins. The effects of these chemicals include vasodilation, increased capillary permeability, contraction of smooth muscles in the bronchioles, and, more important, activities that attract white cells in the site to magnify the inflammatory reaction. This is why an allergic reaction is divided into two phases and the late reaction may last for days.

COMMON ALLERGENS

A large number of common antigens can be associated with allergies. These include plant pollens (as are found in rye grass or ragweed), foods such as nuts or eggs, bee or wasp venom, mold, or animal dander. A square mile of ragweed may produce as much as 16 tons of pollen in a single season. In fact, almost any food or environmental substance could serve as an allergen. The most important defining factor as to whether an individual is allergic to any particular substance is the extent and type of IgE production against that substance.

Most individuals are familiar with immediate hypersensitivities as reactions involving a localized area. The most common form of allergy is rhinitis, known as hay fever, which affects approximately 10 percent of the population. When a person inhales an environmental allergen such as ragweed pollen, the result is a release of pharmacologically active mediators from mast cells located in the upper respiratory tract. If the release occurs in the lower respiratory tract, the condition is known as asthma. In both instances, the eyes and nose are subject to inflammation and the release of secretions. In mild cases, the person suffers from watery discharges, coughing, and sneezing. In more severe asthma attacks, the bronchioles may become constricted and obstruct the air passages.

Foods to which one is allergic may trigger similar reactions in the gut. Mast cells in the gastrointestinal tract also contain receptors for IgE, and contact with food allergens results in the release of mediators similar to those in the respiratory passages. The result may be vomiting or diarrhea. The allergen may also pass from the gut into the circulation or other tissues, triggering asthmatic attacks or urticaria (hives).

In severe allergic reactions, the response may be swift and deadly. The venom released during a bee sting may trigger a systemic response from circulating basophils or mast cells, resulting in the contraction of pulmonary muscles and rapid suffocation, a condition known as anaphylactic shock. The leukotrienes, platelet-activating factor, and prostaglandins play key roles in these reactions.

Delayed-type hypersensitivities, also known as contact dermatitis reactions, most commonly occur following exposure to a topical allergen. These may include the catechol-containing oils of poison oak, the constituents of hair dyes or cosmetics, environmental contaminants such as nickel or turpentine, or any of a wide variety of environmental agents. Rather than being mediated by antibodies, as are the other types of hypersensitivities, contact dermatitis is mediated through a special class of T lymphocytes.

Type II and III Reactions

The other classes of hypersensitivity reactions, types II and III, are less commonly associated with what most people consider to be allergies. Yet they do have much in common with Type I, immediate hypersensitivity. Type II reactions are mediated by a type of antibody called IgG. Clinical manifestations result from the antibody-mediated destruction of target cells, rather than through the release of mediators. One of the most common forms of reaction is blood transfusion reactions, either against the A or B blood group antigen or as a result of an Rh incompatibility. For example, if a person with type O blood is accidentally transfused with type A, an immune reaction will occur. The eventual result is destruction of the incompatible blood cells. Rh incompatibilities are most commonly associated with a pregnant woman who is lacking the Rh protein in her blood (that is, Rh negative) carrying a child who is Rh positive (a blood type obtained from the father's genes). The production of IgG directed against the Rh protein in the child's blood can set in motion events that result in the destruction of the baby's red blood cells, a condition known as erythroblastosis fetalis.

Type III reactions are known as immune complex diseases. In this case, sensitivity to antigens results in formation of IgG/antigen complexes, which can lodge in the kidney or other sites in the body. The complexes activate what is known as the complement system, a series of proteins which include vasoactive chemicals and lipolytic compounds. The result can be a significant inflammation that can lead to kidney damage. Type III reactions can include autoimmune diseases such as arthritis or lupus, or drug reactions such as penicillin allergies.

Avoiding Allergens

There exist three methods for dealing with allergies: avoidance of the allergen, palliative treatments, and desensitization. Ideally, one can attempt to avoid the allergen. For example, cow's milk, a common allergen, should not be given to a child at too young an age, and one can stay away from patches of poison ivy or avoid eating strawberries if one is allergic to them.

Yet avoidance is not always possible or desirable, as the problem may be the fur from the family cat. In any event, it is sometimes difficult to identify the specific substance causing the symptoms. This is particularly true when dealing with foods. Various procedures exist to identify the irritating substance, skin testing being the most common. In this procedure, the patient's skin is exposed to small amounts of suspected allergens. A positive test is indicated by formation of hives or reddening within about twenty to thirty minutes. If the person is hypersensitive to a suspected allergen and finds a skin test too risky, then a blood test may be substituted. In addition to running a battery of tests, a patient's allergy history (including family history, since allergies are in part genetic) or environment may give clues as to the identity of the culprit.

The most commonly used method of dealing with allergies is a palliative treatment—that is, treatment of the symptoms. Antihistamines act by binding to histamine receptors on target cells, interfering with the binding of histamine. There exist two types of histamine receptors: H-1 and H-2. Histamine binding to H-1 receptors results in contractions of smooth muscles and increased mucous secretion. Binding to H-2 receptors results in increased vasopermeability and swelling. Antihistamines that act at the level of the H-1 receptor include alkylamines and ethanolamines and are effective in treating symptoms of acute allergies such as hay fever. H-2 blockers such as cimetidine are effective in the symptomatic treatment of duodenal ulcers through the control of gastric secretions.

Many antihistamines can be obtained without a prescription. If they are not used properly, however, the side effects can be serious. Overuse may result in toxicity, particularly in children; overdoses in children can be fatal. Because antihistamines can depress the central nervous system, side effects include drowsiness, nausea, constipation, and drying of the throat or respiratory passage. This is particularly true of H-1 blockers. A new generation of H-1 antihistamines, however, are long-acting and are free of the sedative effect of other antihistamines.

Other symptomatic treatments include the use of cromolyn sodium, which blocks the influx of calcium into the mast cell, and thus is called a mast cell stabilizer. It acts to block steps leading to degranulation and the release of mediators. In more severe cases, the administration of steroids (cortisone) may prove useful in limiting symptoms of allergies.

Anaphylaxis is the most severe form of immediate hypersensitivity, and unless treated promptly, it may be fatal. It is often triggered in susceptible persons by common environmental substances: bee or wasp venom, drugs such as penicillin, foods such as peanuts and seafood, or latex protein in rubber. Symptoms include labored breathing, rapid loss of blood pressure, itching, hives, and/or loss of bladder control. The symptoms are triggered by a sudden and massive release of mast cell or basophil mediators such as histamine, leukotrienes, or prostaglandin derivatives. Treatment consists of an immediate injection of epinephrine and the maintenance of an open air passage into the lungs. If cardiac arrest occurs, cardiopulmonary resuscitation (CPR) must be undertaken. Persons in known danger of encountering such a triggering allergen often carry an emergency kit containing epinephrine and antihistamines.

Rather than resulting from the presence of IgE antibody, the symptoms of contact dermatitis result from a series of chemicals released by sensitized

T lymphocytes in the area of the skin on which the allergen (often poison ivy or poison oak) is found. Treatments generally involve the application of topical corticosteroids and soothing or drying agents. In more severe cases, systemic use of corticosteroids may be necessary.

DESENSITIZATION

In some persons, the relief of allergy symptoms may be achieved through desensitization. This form of immunotherapy involves the repeated subcutaneous injection of increasing doses of the allergen. In a significant number of persons, such therapy leads to an improvement in symptoms. The idea behind such therapy is that repeated injections of the allergen may lead to production of another class of antibody, the more systemic IgG. These molecules can serve as blocking antibodies, competing with IgE in binding to the allergen. Because IgG/allergen complexes can be destroyed by phagocytes and do not bind receptors on mast cells or basophils, they should not trigger the symptoms of allergies. Unfortunately, for reasons that remain unclear, not all persons or all allergies respond to such therapy.

The type I immediate hypersensitivity reactions commonly run in families, which is not surprising since the regulation of IgE production is genetically determined. Thus, if both parents have allergies, there is little chance that their offspring will escape the problem. On the other hand, if one or both parents are allergy-free, the odds are at least even that the children will also be free from such reactions.

—Richard Adler; updated by Shih-Wen Huang, M.D.

See also Asthma; Environmental diseases; Food poisoning; Multiple chemical sensitivity syndrome; Poisoning; Poisonous plants; Secondhand smoke; Sick building syndrome; Smog; Snakebites; Zoonoses.

FOR FURTHER INFORMATION:

Cutler, Ellen W. *Winning the War Against Asthma and Allergies.* Albany, N.Y.: Delmar, 1998. This clearly written book provides practical information on all aspects of allergies—what they are, their causes, testing, diagnosis, and treatment, including nontraditional therapies. Preventive measures are covered, as are scenarios for various allergy elimination therapies.

Kuby, Janis. *Immunology.* 3d ed. New York: W. H. Freeman, 1997. The section on hypersensitivity in this immunology textbook is well written and includes a mixture of detail and overview of the subject. Particularly useful are discussions of the various types of hypersensitivity reactions. Some knowledge of biology is useful.

Roitt, Ivan. *Essential Immunology.* 9th ed. Boston: Blackwell Scientific Publications, 1997. Written by a leading author in the field, the text provides a fine description of immunology. The section on hypersensitivity is clearly presented and profusely illustrated. Most of the material can be understood by individuals who have taken high school-level biology. The first choice as a reference for the subject.

Walsh, William. *The Food Allergy Book.* New York: John Wiley & Sons, 2000. In this excellent guide to one highly prevalent form of allergy, the author presents useful background information on food allergies and a pragmatic guide to identifying and eliminating food allergens from your diet.

Young, Stuart, Bruce Dobozin, and Margaret Miner. *Allergies.* Rev. ed. New York: Plume, 1999. An excellent review from *Consumer Reports.* In addition to discussing the diagnosis and treatment of allergies, the authors evaluate the various remedies on the market at the time of publication. Also useful are lists of organizations to contact for further information and various clinics that specialize in allergy treatment.

✧ ALTERNATIVE MEDICINE

Type of issue: Public health, social trends

Definition: A wide variety of medical practices and therapies which fall outside traditional, Western medical practice. The approaches emphasize the individual as a biopsychosocial whole, or, in some cases, as a biopsychosocial-spiritual whole. They deemphasize focusing treatment on specific diseases or symptoms.

Alternative medicine—known also as holistic medicine, complementary medicine, or natural healing—focuses on the relationship among the mind, body, and spirit. The underlying philosophy is that people can maintain health by preventing disease in the first place by keeping the body in "balance" and by utilizing the body's "natural" healing processes when people succumb to disease. Alternative medicine approaches contrast with Western medicine's traditional focus on treating symptoms and curing disease and its underemphasis of preventive medicine. Thought "way-out" at one time, complementary medicines and therapies are gaining wide appeal as their anecdotal efficacy and reputation grow.

Alternative medicine practitioners treat everything from diseases such as cancer and AIDS to chronic pain and fatigue, stress, insomnia, depression, high blood pressure, circulatory and digestive disorders, allergies, arthritis, diabetes, and drug and alcohol addictions.

The major risks associated with alternative medicine include costly delays in seeking appropriate treatment, misinformation, side effects from self-administered remedies, and psychological distress if patients believe that they are responsible for their own illness or lack of recovery. In addition, many alternative medicine practitioners have little or no formal health training and may discourage traditional medical treatment or oppose proved health measures such as immunization and pasteurization.

THERAPIES BASED ON NONWESTERN TRADITIONS

Acupressure and acupuncture are based on the belief that the body has a vital energy that must be balanced in order to maintain good health. Acupressure uses pressure from the fingertips or knuckles to stimulate specific points on the body, while acupuncture uses needles inserted into the skin to restore the balance of energy. Both acupressure and acupuncture have been shown to stimulate the release of endorphins, the body's natural painkillers. Acupressure is useful for relieving chronic pain and fatigue and increasing blood circulation. Acupuncture is used successfully for relieving chronic pain and treating drug and alcohol withdrawal symptoms. Although hepatitis, transmission of infectious disease, and internal injuries have been reported in connection with acupuncture, such risks are uncommon.

Meditation is used to relax the mind and body, to reduce stress, and to develop a more positive attitude. By focusing on a single thought or repeating a word or phrase, a person can release conscious thoughts and feelings and enter deep relaxation. Meditation can affect the pulse rate and muscle tension and so is effective in treating high blood pressure, migraines, insomnia, and some digestive disorders.

Qi gong (pronounced "chee-kung") translates from the Chinese as "breathing exercise." The Chinese believe that exercise balances and amplifies the vital energy force—Ch'i or qi—within the body. Qi gong is used to increase circulation; to reduce stress; to promote health, fitness, and longevity; and to cure illness. The most common exercises involve relaxation, strengthening, and inward training. Because the exercise involves movement done with gentle circular and stretching movements, people with decreased flexibility or disabilities can participate.

Tai Chi Chuan was originally designed as a form of self-defense, but is now practiced as physical exercises based on rhythmic movement, equilibrium of body weight, and effortless breathing. The exercises involve slow and continuous movement without strain. Tai Chi Chuan is beneficial because it demands no physical strength initially. The exercises increase circulation, stimulate the nervous system and glandular activity, and help joint movement and concentration.

The ancient art of yoga seeks to achieve the balance of mind, body, and spirit. Practitioners believe that good health is created through proper breathing, relaxation, meditation, proper diet and nutrition, and exercise. The deep breathing and stretching exercises bring relaxation, release of tension and stress, improved concentration, and oxygenation of the blood. The exercises can also provide muscle toning and aerobics, which is beneficial to the heart.

MIND/BODY THERAPIES WITHIN THE WESTERN TRADITION

Biofeedback involves learning to control automatic physiological responses such as blood pressure, heart rate, circulation, digestion, and perspiration in order to reduce anxiety, pain, and tension. The patient concentrates on consciously controlling the body's automatic responses while a machine monitors the results and displays them for the patient. Biofeedback can be useful in treating asthma, chronic pain, epilepsy, drug addiction, circulatory problems, and stress.

Chiropractic treatment uses traditional medicine techniques such as X rays, physical examinations, and various tests in order to diagnose a disorder. Muscle spasms or ligament strains are treated by manipulation or adjustment to the spine and joints, thus reducing pressure on the spinal nerves and providing relief from pain. Recent research suggests chiropractic should be considered in treating certain types of lower back pain, as it is often superior to conventional interventions. Practitioners should be state licensed, and caution should be taken with practitioners who often repeat full-spine X rays or who ask patients to sign contracts at any time during treatment. Chiropractic is practiced either "straight," involving only spinal manipulation, or "mixed," involving other biomedical technologies such as electrical stimulation. Chiropractic treatment can be harmful if it is practiced in patients with fractures or undetected tumors or if it is practiced incorrectly.

The use of water for healing or therapeutic purposes is termed hydrotherapy. It is used to treat chronic pain; to relieve stress; to improve circulation,

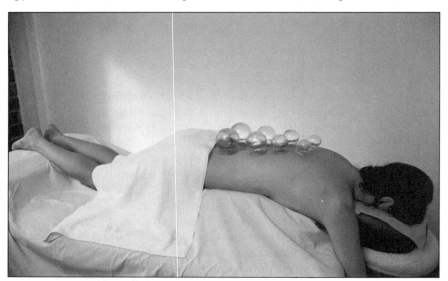

Chinese medicine may employ a technique called cupping, the application to the back of cups that create a vacuum, in order to restore proper circulation. (PhotoDisc)

mobility, strength, and flexibility; to reduce swelling; and to treat injuries to the skin. Because the buoyancy of water offsets gravity, more intense exercise can be done when standing in water, while a lower heart rate is maintained and pain is decreased. The risks associated with hydrotherapy are minimal (such as overdoing exercise) or rare (such as slipping or drowning).

Phototherapy, or light therapy, is used to treat health disorders that are related to problems with the body's inner clock, or circadian rhythms. These rhythms govern the timing of sleep, hormone production, body temperature, and other biological functions. People need the full wavelength spectrum of light found in sunlight in order to maintain health. If the full wavelength is not received, the body may not be able to absorb some nutrients fully, resulting in fatigue, tooth decay, depression, hostility, hair loss, skin conditions, sleep disorders, or suppressed immune functions. Treatment involves spending more time outdoors, exercising, and using light boxes that mimic natural sunlight. It is commonly used to treat seasonal affective disorder, a recognized subtype of depressive illness.

Hyperbaric oxygenation therapy, or oxygen therapy, is used to treat disorders in which the oxygen supply to the body is deficient. This therapy can help with heart disease, circulatory problems, multiple sclerosis, gangrene, and strokes. Oxygen therapy is also used for traumas such as crash injuries, wounds, burns, bedsores, and carbon monoxide poisoning. Treatment consists of exposing the patient to 100 percent pure oxygen under greater-than-normal atmospheric pressure. The body tissues receive more than the usual supply of oxygen and so can compensate for conditions of reduced circulation. The increased oxygen helps keep the tissues alive and promotes healing.

Sound therapy involves the use of certain sounds to reduce stress, lower blood pressure, relieve pain, improve movement and balance, promote endurance and strength, and overcome learning disabilities. The body has its own rhythm, and illness can arise when the rhythm is disturbed. Tests have shown that particular sounds can slow breathing and a racing heart, create a feeling of well-being, alter skin temperature, influence brain-wave frequencies, and reduce blood pressure and muscle tension.

Used extensively in Europe and Japan, aromatherapy involves the use of the essential oils or essence from the flowers, stems, leaves, or roots of plants or trees. These essences can be absorbed through the skin, eaten, or inhaled in vapor form. There is evidence that inhaling some scents may help prevent secondary respiratory infections and reduce stress. Practitioners believe that aromatherapy can benefit people suffering from muscle aches, arthritis, digestive and circulatory problems, and emotional or stress-related problems. Absorption through the skin and inhalation are considered safe, but eating any essence could result in poisoning.

Although not approved in the United States, cell therapy is widely used worldwide. It involves the injection of cells from the organs, fetuses, or embryos of animals and humans. These cells are used for revitalization purposes; that is, they promote the body's own healing process for damaged or weak organs. Cell therapy seems to stimulate the immune system and is used to treat cancer, immunological problems, diseased or underdeveloped organs, arthritis, and circulatory problems.

Bioenergetic medicine, or energy medicine, uses an energy field to detect and treat health problems. A screening process to measure electromagnetic frequencies emitted by the body can detect imbalances that may cause illness or warn of possible chemical imbalances. One of several machines is then used to correct energy-level imbalances. Energy medicine claims to relieve conditions such as skin diseases, headaches, migraines, muscle pain, circulation problems, and chronic fatigue.

Enzyme therapy uses plant and pancreatic enzymes to improve digestion and the absorption of nutrients. Since enzymes provide the stimuli for all chemical reactions in the body, improper eating habits may cause a lack of certain enzymes, resulting in general health problems.

Homeopathy is based on the belief that "like cures like"; homeopathy is thought to provide relief from most illnesses. During therapy, the patient receives small doses of prepared plants and minerals in order to stimulate the body's own healing processes and defense mechanisms. These substances mimic the symptoms of the illness. While studies on this approach remain inconclusive, homeopathic medicine has wide appeal, possibly because most (but not all) homeopathic practitioners are traditionally trained medical physicians.

Kinesiology employs muscle testing and standard diagnosis to evaluate and treat the chemical, structural, and mental aspects of the patient. The principle behind kinesiology is that certain foods can cause biochemical reactions that weaken the muscles. Diet and exercise, as well as muscle and joint manipulation, are part of the treatment. There are risks of injury caused by an unqualified practitioner.

Herbal medicine uses plants and flowers to treat most known symptoms of physical and emotional illnesses. Almost 75 percent of the world's population relies on herbal remedies as their primary source of health care, and much of traditional medicine is derived from plants. Herbal medicine mixtures can be complicated, however, and some, like any medications, are toxic if taken incorrectly.

Colon therapy technique involves the cleaning and detoxification of the colon by flushing with water, using enemas, or ingesting herbs or other substances. A healthy colon will absorb water and nutrients and eliminate wastes and toxins. Most modern diets, however, are low in fiber, a substance which helps clean out the colon. If not completely eliminated, layers of wastes can build up in the colon and toxins can leak into the bloodstream, causing many health problems. Although not a specific cure for any disease, colon therapy removes the source of toxins and allows the body's natural healing processes to function properly. Practitioners claim that symptoms related to colon dysfunction, such as backaches, headaches, bad breath, gas, indigestion and constipation, sinus or lung congestion, skin problems, and fatigue can be relieved when the toxins are removed from the colon.

Detoxification focuses on ridding the body of the chemicals and pollutants present in water, food, air, and soil. The body naturally eliminates or neutralizes toxins through the liver, kidneys, urine, and feces and through the processes of exhalation and perspiration. Detoxification therapy accelerates the body's own natural cleansing process through diet, fasting, colon therapy, and heat therapy. Symptoms of an overtaxed body system include respiratory problems, headaches, joint pain, allergy symptoms, mood changes, insomnia, arthritis, constipation, psoriasis, acne, and ulcers.

Magnetic field therapy, also called biomagnetic therapy, uses specially designed magnets or magnetic fields applied to the body. Electrically charged particles are naturally present in the bloodstream, and when magnets are placed on the body, the charged particles are attracted to the magnets. As a result, currents and patterns are created that dilate the blood vessels, allowing more blood to reach the affected area. Magnetic field therapy is used to speed healing after surgery, to improve circulation, and to strengthen and mend bones. It is also used to improve the quality of healing in sprains, strains, cuts, and burns, as well as to reduce or reverse chronic conditions such as degenerative joint disease, some forms of arthritis, and diabetic ulcers.

Neural therapy is used to treat chronic illness or trauma (injury) caused by changes in the natural electrical conductivity of the nerves and cells. Every cell has its own frequency range of electricity, and tissue remains healthy as long as the energy flow through the body is normal. Neural therapy uses anesthetics injected into the body to deliver energy to cells blocked by disease or injury. Conditions that respond to neural therapy are allergies; arthritis; asthma; kidney, liver, and heart disease; depression; head and back pain; and muscle injuries.

INCREASING INVESTIGATION OF ALTERNATIVE THERAPIES

Many alternative or complementary therapies, while new to Western society and medicine, are ancient and derive from nontechnologically based understandings of how the human body and the world work. What specifically works for whom, when, and for what conditions remains a complex problem. Anecdote and hearsay, and the limits and failures of Western medicine, guide and motivate interest in these approaches.

Renewed interest in alternative therapies occurred in the 1970's and has grown since. By 1998, an estimated one-third of all Americans had used some form of complementary therapy. In 1992, with Americans spending more than 14 billion dollars annually on alternative medicine, the U.S. government established the Office of Alternative Medicine as a part of the National Institutes of Health (NIH). This office evaluates complementary treatments on a scientific basis and provides public information. Health insurers maintain a key interest in alternative medicine, and an increasing number are paying for it. Many traditionally trained physicians are prescribing or recommending some form of alternative medicine as a complement to their own.

—*Virginia L. Salmon; updated by Paul Moglia*

See also Acupuncture; Holistic medicine; Homeopathy; Hypnosis; Light therapy; Meditation; Pain management; Stress; Yoga.

FOR FURTHER INFORMATION:

The CQ Researcher 2, no. 4 (January 31, 1992). This entire issue discusses the topic of alternative medicine. Offers a balanced viewpoint and contains a valuable bibliography for further reading.

Goldberg, Burton, comp. *Alternative Medicine: The Definitive Guide.* Tiburon, Calif.: Future Medicine Publishing, 1999. A well-written reference work which includes long, illustrated entries on various treatments. Provides sources of further information and recommended readings.

Jacobs, Jennifer, ed. *The Encyclopedia of Alternative Medicine: A Complete Family Guide to Complementary Therapies.* Rev. ed. Boston: Journey Edition, 1997. Discusses current alternative medicine approaches.

Kastner, Mark, and Hugh Burroughs. *Alternative Healing: The Complete A-Z Guide to over 160 Different Alternative Therapies.* New York: Henry Holt, 1996. The encyclopedic, one-page to four-page entries are brief but include sources of additional information. Also offers a useful resource section and bibliography.

Mauskop, Alexander, and Brill Marietta Abrams. *The Headache Alternative: A Neurologist's Guide to Drug-Free Relief.* New York: Dell Paperbacks, 1997. A practical review of how to apply complementary and alternative approaches to treating migraine, sinus, and tension headaches. Contains excellent resources and a bibliography section.

✧ ALZHEIMER'S DISEASE

Type of issue: Elder health, mental health, social trends
Definition: A progressive degenerative disorder of the brain characterized by loss of cognitive, visual-spatial, and language skills.

Dementia, a disorder that mainly affects people aged sixty-five and older, may be thought of as a gradual decline of mental function. The most common form of dementia is the Alzheimer's type. Alzheimer's dementia is more fully characterized as a pathological condition in which there is progressive loss of cognitive, visual-spatial, and language skills.

Alzheimer's disease is an acquired condition, the exact causes of which are unknown. Approximately 6 to 8 percent of all people older than sixty-five have Alzheimer's dementia; roughly 1.7 percent of people from sixty-five to seventy years of age have Alzheimer's disease. The prevalence of this disorder doubles every five years after age sixty; thus, about 30 percent of people older than eighty-five have Alzheimer's disease. While Alzheimer's dementia typically begins late in life, a small percentage of sufferers experience its onset in their thirties or forties.

Although some mild decline in memory, primarily demonstrated as slowness of recall, may be considered a normal part of aging, this must be distinguished from the debilitating condition of Alzheimer's disease. Because of the progressive decline that it causes in its victims' ability to function in all aspects of daily life, Alzheimer's dementia eventually results in the need for care and supervision twenty-four hours a day.

It was estimated that four million Americans had Alzheimer's disease in the late 1990's. It was predicted that fourteen million Americans would have Alzheimer's disease by 2050. While the average life expectancy is eight to ten years after diagnosis, some patients may live twenty years or more. In 1999, the average lifetime cost per patient was about $174,000, and this cost was expected to rise. Contrary to public perception, 75 percent of people with Alzheimer's disease receive care at home, often by family members. Nevertheless, nearly half of all nursing home residents have Alzheimer's disease.

The very elderly (those aged eighty and older), as the most rapidly growing segment of the American population, are changing the way in which society copes with this disease. To adjust to the increasing needs and demands for care, assisted-living centers and nursing homes dedicated to the exclusive care of people with Alzheimer's disease are on the rise. Since most of this long-term care is not covered by Medicare or private insurance policies, families are expected to cover the expenses. The cost to families can be devastating, both financially and emotionally.

Signs and Symptoms

Since the rate of cognitive decline in Alzheimer's disease can be slowed with medications, early recognition of the signs and symptoms is imperative. With proper medical guidance and quality care at home or in staffed facilities, one can minimize the dehumanization and suffering that Alzheimer's disease inflicts upon its victims.

Three specific areas of decline found with Alzheimer's disease are in the learning of new information; in complex task completion, organization, and daily planning; and in communication and interactions.

The earliest symptoms of Alzheimer's dementia are noted with difficulty remembering where common items have been placed or recalling basic details of recent conversations. Common examples are forgetfulness concerning appointments with physicians, family gatherings, or meetings that were previously well known and anticipated. For example, a woman who normally goes weekly for salon appointments on a certain day and at a set time might begin to arrive on the wrong day or not at all. Additional early warnings may include inability to recall important recent family events, such as weddings or the birth of new family members.

Unfortunately, it is at this stage that family and friends are prone to dismiss these difficulties as normal aging, part of "getting older." The reluctance to recognize dementia early may arise, in part, from the tendency to dismiss abnormal behaviors as normal, particularly in loved ones. For example, most people can recall a time when, perhaps during a particularly stressful or sad time, they too had been forgetful. Nevertheless, there is a great difference between the minor and time-limited forgetfulness that nearly all people have experienced and the ever-worsening, irreversible forgetfulness of Alzheimer's disease.

Other areas of daily life become increasingly problematic as the dementia progresses. Tasks that require several steps—such as cooking a meal, doing laundry, or balancing a checkbook—may be poorly performed with erosion of the cognitive skills necessary to organize these tasks mentally and physically. Reasoning may decline so that unsound or ill-advised contracts may be signed, perhaps jeopardizing the victim's financial security. There is an inability to devise coping strategies or to develop solutions when problems arise. As such, relatively minor problems such as a burned-out light bulb, a leaky faucet, or a flooded basement can be viewed as insurmountable. Moreover, the skills of knowing one's space and orientation within that space, or visual-spatial awareness, also wane. As a result, navigating through a once-familiar neighborhood or within one's own home becomes increasingly difficult. Even on simple trips, demented individuals are at great risk of getting lost or endangering themselves and possibly others. While this situation is of concern when these individuals are wandering on foot, it is even more problematic when those with dementia are still driving.

Personal grooming and hygiene may also decline with Alzheimer's disease. This may start with subtle cues, such as fingernails not being polished or trimmed. The individual may forget how to shave or shampoo or be unable to remember the last time that bathing occurred. Articles of clothing may be worn in uncharacteristically bizarre or clashing combinations, such as a winter coat with summer sandals, that heretofore would have never been combined by that person. A decline in personal appearance and habits strongly suggests a problem with cognitive skills.

Increasingly, words and sentences become difficult to organize for the person with Alzheimer's disease. Often, the first sign of language decline is the inability to remember words for simple items, such as the palm of the hand or the band of a wristwatch. This inability to find the word to identify an object is called anomia, literally meaning "without name." When speaking, the patient may experience a sense of frustration while halting to recall a word or even the topic of conversation. Substituted phrases or stammering until someone rescues the patient by speaking for him or her become awkward but adaptive ways to communicate with others.

Associated with declining language skills may be an increasing tendency to withdraw from conversations and be uncommonly passive. Alternatively, previously well-mannered people may become socially inappropriate—for example, speaking only in a loud voice. As the ability to modulate behavior deteriorates, social graces are lost. Some people may develop an irritable demeanor; others may become combative or blatantly aggressive with words and actions. These behaviors almost always lead to medical attention if none was previously sought.

Alzheimer's dementia ultimately robs individuals of their personality. At first, this may appear subtly as a loss of interest in once-pleasurable things. Often, there is progression to a more socially withdrawn state, with less expression of mood and feelings evident. Eventually, people who were once full of life, each with unique facial expressions and senses of humor, somehow end up looking very similar—with expressionless, blank faces and eyes that seem to stare deeply into nothing. This flattening of expression and loss of personality usually occur late in Alzheimer's disease.

Diagnosis

Dementia of the Alzheimer's type currently cannot be diagnosed by laboratory tests or imaging techniques such as computed tomography (CT) or magnetic resonance imaging (MRI). As a medical diagnosis, Alzheimer's dementia is a diagnosis of exclusion. As such, the possibility must be evaluated that the presenting symptoms of confusion, memory loss, and poor ability to take care of oneself derive from other causes. First, other forms of dementia, some of which may be reversible, are explored. In addition, medical conditions such as delirium or depression are carefully considered, as both are generally reversible and, with medical treatment and management, of limited duration. The physician will need to know what medical problems, if any, the patient may have, as well as what prescription and over-the-counter medications are being taken. If a fall has occurred that may coincide with the onset of symptoms, it will be important to assess and evaluate the patient for possible head trauma or injury, including intracranial bleeding. Any history of excessive alcohol consumption or illicit drug use is important; such information can clarify certain health issues, such as vitamin deficiencies, that may be contributing to the clinical picture.

Once such factors are identified and resolved or found to be noncontributory, the physician can explore the possibility of Alzheimer's disease more completely. This diagnosis is made primarily from the doctor's suspicion and from clinical findings. Thus, the physician will consider the patient's symptoms as described by family and friends. The physician will observe, engage, and monitor the patient's ability to perform simple tasks, such as social greetings and recalling names of people in the family, important dates, or current events. The evaluation may include the Mini-Mental Status Exam, the Blessed Information-Memory-Concentration Test, a clock drawing test, a functional activities questionnaire, or other diagnostic aids. While helpful tools, these diagnostic assessments alone cannot diagnose Alzheimer's dementia definitively.

The physician will also ask questions regarding certain risk factors for Alzheimer's disease. Known risk factors include a family history of Alzheimer's dementia, increasing age (especially after age eighty), and head trauma in the past that caused a loss of consciousness. An additional risk factor for Alzheimer's disease is found in people who have been diagnosed with Down syndrome (trisomy 21), as almost all people with trisomy 21 who survive to age forty-five will develop early onset of Alzheimer's dementia. Although it remains unclear as to the role of estrogen as it may relate to Alzheimer's disease, the physician may want to know whether female patients are using or have used estrogen replacement therapy after the menopause.

Late in the disease, other signs and symptoms may appear as a consequence of neuron (brain cell) loss and the biochemical dysfunction of surviving neurons. One of these is hallucinations, such as hearing voices or seeing images of people or things that are not present yet believing fully that they are real. This condition is known as psychosis. Another familiar psychotic feature is paranoid delusions. This often presents itself in moderate dementia, typically revolving around unfounded beliefs that family members are stealing items. Sometimes the items "stolen" have no value, such as a hat or glove; more important, such paranoia is a demonstration of the confusion that results from the chaos of not having memory.

A careful history of the patient's decline and the severity of symptoms will help to establish the relative rate of cognitive loss. From these data, a prognosis for the patient in terms of both quality and, to a lesser extent, quantity of life may be made.

TREATMENT AND MANAGEMENT

There is no known cure for or prevention of Alzheimer's dementia. As a consequence, treatment focuses on managing symptoms, slowing the rate of cognitive decline, and improving quality of life.

The most commonly prescribed medications used to abate the progression of Alzheimer's dementia come from a category of pharmaceutical agents known as cholinesterase inhibitors, including tacrine and donazepril. Although the exact role of cholinergic neurons within the central nervous system is not well understood, it has been demonstrated that in Alzheimer's disease, there is both a loss in the number of cholinergic neurons and dysfunction in the cholinergic neurons that remain viable. Thus, Alzheimer's dementia is characterized by a net deficit of cholinergic neurotransmitters.

The enzyme cholinesterase biochemically degrades cholinergic neurotransmitters within the central nervous system. In health, this poses no problem, but in Alzheimer's disease, this process exaggerates symptoms. Even a little reduction of already depleted amounts of cholinergic neurotransmitters worsens the condition. Therefore, an inhibitor that halts the enzyme activity helps to increase the amount of cholinergic neurotransmitter, which, in turn, improves cognition. The optimal benefit from cholinesterase inhibitors is obtained when the medication is started as early in the dementia process as possible. With medications, some people will have improvement of cognition that is evident in their mood, speech, and self-care or in their ability to perform daily tasks. Even in moderate to severe forms of Alzheimer's disease, where cognitive decline is marked, these medications have been helpful in reducing symptoms of agitation, aggression, or restlessness.

About 25 to 30 percent of all people diagnosed with Alzheimer's disease will experience depression. Since loss of brain cells occurs with Alzheimer's disease, it is no surprise that some cells which produce neurochemicals to regulate mood are also lost. Thus, depression should be looked for in all stages of Alzheimer's disease, as it can be identified and treated with antidepressant medications. In the past, tricyclic antidepressants were used for this illness in the elderly, but because tricyclics have multiple side effects, other medications are increasingly receiving favor. Side effects and drug interactions can be particularly problematic in the elder patient who is frequently taking several medications for other medical conditions.

Additional therapies target particular symptoms. For example, paranoia can be managed and often resolved with antipsychotic medications. With the elderly, special efforts are made by physicians to use the lowest dose possible, as well as to select medications that have minimal side effects. Two other common concerns are lack of impulse control or lability of mood and disruption of sleep patterns. Often, the former can be managed with mood stabilizers, such as valproic acid, as well as environmental controls, so that the patient is not overly stimulated by activities or sounds that occur in everyday life. The latter can be managed with "sleep hygiene." This therapy helps to reset the biological clock by establishing fixed hours to go to and awaken from sleep and not allowing napping. Additional aids may include medications, but caution should be exercised because some commonly used agents, such as benzodiazepines, may have paradoxical effects in the elderly. Another caution is to avoid the use of the anticholinergic medications often used to induce sleep, such as diphenhydramine, as this can worsen dementia symptoms.

HOW FAMILIES COPE

Although Alzheimer's disease afflicts individuals, entire families are affected by the cruel and prolonged course of this disease. Enormous emotional costs are paid by family members who care for and attend to a loved one who increasingly grows to depend on others for safekeeping. More often than not, it is adult women, many of whom are working mothers of young children or teenagers, who find themselves in the role of providing care for family members with Alzheimer's disease. In fact, studies indicate that greater than 90 percent of those providing care for patients with Alzheimer's disease in their or a family member's home are women. This role is far more demanding than simply providing meals or getting someone to a doctor's appointment. For example, traveling or even being alone is no longer a safe option for the person with Alzheimer's disease; constant supervision to prevent wandering from the home and getting lost is needed. Cooking or ironing is no longer safe for someone with Alzheimer's disease because of the potential for self-injury or household fires, yet these activities are often attempted when a brief lapse of supervision occurs. Unlike children, who lack good judgment but are small and manageable, adults with Alzheimer's disease may be physically strong and sizable. This fact makes keeping them in safe spaces a real challenge. Families need to "Alzheimer-proof" the home to reduce the risk of injury or tragedy, such as accidental death, for the patient with Alzheimer's disease and other family members. It is helpful to contact local police and fire departments and to advise them that someone with Alzheimer's disease lives at that residence. This allows ease of filing a missing person's report with police or getting a rapid response to home fires, as neither event is uncommon when someone with Alzheimer's disease lives in a family home.

At variable rates, but in a predictable manner, dependence needs grow to include making phone calls to family or friends, finding belongings, grooming and dressing, or using simple appliances such as electric shavers, lamps, or toasters. As the progressive loss of cognition continues, simple housekeeping tasks such as clearing a table or depositing trash into proper receptacles cannot be performed. Assistance with toileting or changing adult diapers also becomes necessary. In the late stage of Alzheimer's disease, assistance with eating, sitting upright, and walking is required as the disease leads a fully debilitating course.

As may be anticipated, caregivers are at risk for emotional burnout and physical fatigue. To alleviate this problem, many areas offer adult day care programs. In these programs, people with Alzheimer's disease are assisted by trained staff in physical, social, and creative activities that help to optimize the overall well-being of participants. In better programs, such activities are tailored specifically to meet the unique needs of Alzheimer's patients. These programs also promote improved mood through socialization and offer a sense of independence from family members. Such programs are beneficial not only to participants but also to their caregivers. Clearly, adult day care offers a reprieve to the caregiver who, for a specified number of hours a day, will be relieved from the burden of having to monitor and care for an ill loved one constantly.

INSTITUTIONAL CARE

Although 75 percent of people with Alzheimer's disease are cared for by family members, 50 percent or more of all nursing home residents have Alzheimer's disease. This shift occurs as debility consumes the very life of the Alzheimer's patient, to the point that safety can no longer be maintained without professional supervision, proper medical care, and careful medication management. When this point is reached, family members become resigned to placing loved ones in facilities where assisted-living and medical services can be provided. With guidance from support groups, doctors, and other professionals, good to excellent facilities can be found that meet the emotional, physical, and medical needs of the family and yet fit within their financial constraints.

In 1999, the average monthly cost of caring for a family member with Alzheimer's disease in either an assisted-living facility or a nursing home was $3,100. When the care was provided in the family home, the average monthly cost was $1,500. These numbers, when multiplied by twelve for the months per year and then by eight for the years of possible life expectancy, give a conservative estimate of $144,000 to $297,000 for lifetime care per person with Alzheimer's disease. Because most families do not have such resources available, great measures are taken to afford care for loved ones, sometimes at great economic risk to these families.

Another consideration is the matter of competency. In Alzheimer's disease, the ability to make important personal decisions such as writing wills or making financial and health care choices is lost. Therefore, early in the course at the disease, families are encouraged to have court-appointed guardianship or executorship established. This allows the appointed person, usually a spouse or child of the patient, to make financial, health care, and medical choices for the demented person. Court actions can assist many families with the economic aspect of Alzheimer's disease as they can manage the patient's financial matters.

As for the emotional toll, support from others who have endured or are enduring the same problem can be found in many communities at Alzheimer's Association chapters. Many turn to lifelong friends and their religious beliefs for further support and guidance.

The cruel reality of Alzheimer's disease is that at the end of the twentieth century, it was the fourth-leading cause of death in adult Americans. Therefore, end-of-life choices need to be addressed, including the "do not resuscitate" (DNR) status and the personal choice of life support. Some families are lucky to have had the patient with Alzheimer's disease designate, while fully competent, his or her wishes through drafting a living will or giving someone trusted durable power of attorney. Such actions give chosen individuals the responsibility for making important decisions for patients in the event that they are unable to do so themselves. DNR status allows a person to die without resuscitation if such measures will simply delay death rather than maintain life in anticipation of recovery. Some members of society consider resuscitation an intrusion of modern medicine into the natural course of dying; others want everything done to sustain life, regardless of the ultimate outcome. Often these emotions are based on deeply held personal beliefs. DNR requests are generally made by the patient (while in good health) or by family members to the patient's physicians without court involvement. Rather, dialogue about prognosis, the pros and cons of DNR status, and family meetings with doctors and other professionals contribute to the family's decision.

Alzheimer's dementia is a progressive, abnormal loss of one's ability to think, learn, communicate, and care for oneself. The illness leads to full debility and a dependence on others in order to sustain life. By the end of the twentieth century, because of the prolonged course of Alzheimer's disease and the need for medical and high-level nursing care, it was the third most costly medical condition, ranked after heart disease and cancer. As people live longer and the "aging of America" continues, the number of people with Alzheimer's disease will increase. As a result, more nurses and physicians will be needed in geriatric medicine.

—*Mary C. Fields*

See also Aging; Dementia; Depression in the elderly; Living wills; Memory loss.

FOR FURTHER INFORMATION:
Larkin, Marilynn. *When Someone You Love Has Alzheimer's.* New York: Dell, 1995. An excellent resource for caregivers. Offers tips on daily management of people with Alzheimer's disease, including diet, toileting, exer-

cise, and medical care. A comprehensive resource list is provided.

Mace, Nancy L., and Peter Rabins. *The Thirty-six-Hour Day: A Family Guide to Caring for Persons with Alzheimer's Disease, Related Dementing Illnesses, and Memory Loss Later in Life.* 3d ed. Baltimore: The Johns Hopkins University Press, 1999. An excellent resource for caregivers who find comfort in fighting this disease with knowledge. The book also offers tips on coping with typical problems encountered in caring for someone with Alzheimer's disease.

Markin, R. E. *Coping with Alzheimer's: The Complete Care Manual for Patients and Their Families.* Secaucus, N.J.: Carol, 1998. A quick read that is helpful in the organization process for caring for someone with Alzheimer's disease. Some of the medication information is outdated, but otherwise this is a good, practical guide.

Nolan, K. A., and R. C. Mohs. "Screening for Dementia in Family Practice." In *Alzheimer's Disease: A Guide to Practical Management, Part II*, edited by Ralph W. Richter and John P. Blass. St. Louis: Mosby-Year Book, 1994. The source from which the clock drawing test was obtained. Although this book is written for physicians, some of the information can be comprehended easily by laypeople who may have a diagnostic interest in Alzheimer's disease.

Powell, Lenore S., and Katie Courtice. *Alzheimer's Disease: A Guide for Families.* Rev. ed. Reading, Mass.: Addison-Wesley, 1993. This excellent book is divided into three sections: "The Burden of Love," "Understanding and Dealing with the Patient's Problem," and "Taking Care of Yourself." Nontechnical chapters about the nature of this disease are helpful. Examples of a living will and a resident's bill of rights (for nursing homes or assisted-living facilities) are given.

✧ AMNIOCENTESIS

Type of issue: Children's health, medical procedures, prevention, women's health

Definition: The removal of amniotic fluid from a pregnant woman for analysis; this fluid provides biochemical and genetic information about the fetus, enabling physicians to identify hereditary problems in the baby well before it is born.

Amniocentesis is used to provide diagnostic information before a fetus is born. It is performed most often on fourteen- to sixteen-week-old fetuses because, at that stage of development, the procedure can be carried out very safely, amniotic fluid samples large enough for detailed genetic and biochemical analysis may be obtained without harming a fetus, and adequate time is available both to obtain data and to use them to solve any problems that are encountered.

The procedure is usually carried out in six consecutive steps. First, the position of the placenta in the uterus is located using ultrasonography. Then, the physician who will carry out the procedure locates the fetus by gentle, careful palpation of the mother's abdomen. Next, the mother is usually, but not always, given a dose of a local anesthetic. This is followed by the careful insertion of a long hypodermic needle through the abdominal wall and into the amniotic sac. As soon as amniotic fluid is seen in an attached sterile hypodermic syringe, a twenty-milliliter sample (about four teaspoons) of fluid is carefully drawn up into the syringe. Finally, the needle and syringe are removed from the mother's abdomen.

Amniocentesis is reported to be almost painless: Even when patients are subjected to the procedure without being given an anesthetic, most report only an initial needle prick and a feeling of pressure during the process. Amniocentesis is also deemed to be very safe for both mother and fetus: Even if repeated several times, it has been reported to produce a risk factor of well under 1 percent.

Amniotic Fluid as a Diagnostic Tool

The amniotic fluid of early pregnancy is very like the blood serum from which it arises. As pregnancy continues, the content in the fluid of substances derived from fetal urine and other fetal secretions increases greatly. Amniotic fluid also contains fetal cells arising from the skin, the stomach and other parts of the gastrointestinal organs, the reproductive organs, and the respiratory organs. Consequently, this fluid is a very valuable diagnostic tool. Immediately after the amniotic fluid is collected, these fetal cells are separated out to be used for genetic analysis. The remaining, cell-free amniotic fluid is examined using a wide variety of biochemical techniques.

Important tests of the amniotic fluid and the cells that it contains include the determination of lecithin and sphingomyelin content, sex determination, and the identification of chromosomal diseases. Lecithins and sphingomyelins are two kinds of fatlike molecules known as lipids. Lecithins are the essential components of the pulmonary surfactant that acts, at lung surfaces, to prevent the collapse and dysfunction of tiny lung air sacs (alveoli) when a person exhales. Subnormal production of the pulmonary surfactant in a fetus may indicate the presence of the potentially fatal respiratory distress syndrome or hyaline membrane disease. Thus an important measurement made after amniocentesis is the ratio of lecithin and sphingomyelin content in the amniotic fluid. Lecithin-sphingomyelin ratio values of about 2.0 are deemed to be healthy, and those of 1.5 or less indicate a likelihood of risk to the fetus. Many other biochemical problems can be identified by similar analysis of other components of the amniotic fluid.

Both the sex of the fetus and the presence of chromosomal diseases can be diagnosed by examining the hereditary material, the deoxyribonucleic acid (DNA), from fetal cells grown in tissue cultures derived from the cells that were obtained by amniocentesis. Sex is determined, and the presence of some diseases caused by abnormal chromosomes is identified, by examination of the number and shape of the chromosomes in the fetal cells, a process known as karyotyping. Human beings usually possess twenty-three pairs of chromosomes, each of which has a characteristic size, shape, and overall appearance. A number of chromosomal diseases are associated with the presence of too many or too few chromosomes. A classical example is Down syndrome, which is always caused by the presence of an extra copy of chromosome number 21 (that is, there are three such chromosomes instead of the usual pair).

Some chromosomal abnormalities are caused by much more subtle DNA changes that do not alter human chromosome numbers. Rather, they are attributable to changed DNA in a chromosome that alters a small part of that chromosome. These diseases are discovered using DNA sequence analysis, which identifies existing abnormalities in the organization of parts of DNA molecules. A gene—a piece of DNA in a chromosome that carries genetic information—can be likened to the bar code used in supermarkets to identify a product at the cash register. Changes in that gene are like the changes in the bar code that indicate another, similar product. The bar code in a gene is a sequence of chemical units, and its alteration may signal the presence of a severe disease.

CHOOSING WHO WILL BE TESTED

The use of amniocentesis can replace or minimize the uncertainty of indirect genetic counseling. The decision to choose or to exclude a particular course of action in family planning had been based entirely on a calculation of the mathematical odds of an inheritable disease being passed on to the children of those who were counseled. For example, when a family history indicated that both of the prospective parents carried a harmful gene—that is, when there was a history of the frequent occurrence of a disease in past generations—some risk was identifiable. On the other hand, if one or both of the parents actually suffered from a genetic disease, the odds of its being passed on increased to a point at which it was assumed that a child would develop that disease.

The use of amniocentesis is most valuable when, because of parental genetics, such a disease is likely but not assured. Genetic and/or biochemical information obtained by testing can either confirm the existence of the problem and suggest a corrective course of action or put the prospective parents' minds at rest. In such testing, it is important to identify the appropriate maternal group to test for each of the many diseases that are detectable by amniocentesis. Testing only the appropriate cases will ensure that the accompanying small but existent risks of amniocentesis to mothers and their fetuses are minimized.

Amniocentesis is usually indicated when an Rh-negative woman and an Rh-positive man conceive a child because of the chance of hemolytic anemia in Rh-positive offspring. In fact, this use of amniocentesis was the basis of the pioneering effort, by Douglas Bevis in the 1950's, that first demonstrated the great predictive value of this procedure.

Additional group selection of subjects appropriate for amniocentesis is possible in many other cases. For example, the use of the procedure to identify Down syndrome is most important in mothers over the age of thirty-five, for whom the risk to a fetus is much higher than that seen in younger women. Likewise, the exploration of the possibility of respiratory distress syndrome is very valuable when there is a family history of previous premature children because premature infants are always at high risk for developing the disease.

A test, via amniocentesis, of the lecithin-sphingomyelin ratio is also quite important in pregnant women who suffer from diabetes mellitus. The babies of such mothers are very likely to have subnormal lecithin levels and thus be at risk for various lung disorders. When amniocentesis identifies an at-risk lecithin-sphingomyelin ratio value, the potentially endangered fetus is injected with hormones that help it to produce mature lungs by raising the lecithin-sphingomyelin ratio value. The success or failure of such efforts is confirmed by the repetition of the amniocentesis. Numerous other biochemical problems that may be present in fetuses can be identified through a similar analysis of other components of the amniotic fluid.

Pregnancy in women who are more than thirty-five years old is currently viewed as the best reason for carrying out amniocentesis. The main fear, in this circumstance, is the presence of severe chromosomal diseases, the incidence of which is far greater for older women than for younger women. For example, the severe mental retardation caused by Down syndrome occurs in 3 percent of all live births of children to mothers over forty-five, an incidence about one thousand times greater than that in the offspring of twenty-year-old women.

Some other chromosomal diseases that can be identified by amniocentesis and DNA analysis are spina bifida, anencephaly, sickle-cell anemia, cystic fibrosis, muscular dystrophy, Huntington's chorea, and Klinefelter's syndrome. A number of these potentially devastating diseases can be corrected while a fetus is in the uterus, if they are diagnosed quickly enough. Where such treatment is not possible, an early diagnosis will usually make it possible either to choose whether to undergo a therapeutic abortion or to have the baby within a time window that ensures the safety of the former option.

ACTING ON THE RESULTS

Where amniocentesis identifies an exceptionally severe chromosomal disease in a fetus, the parents are informed concerning what to expect. In some cases, the decision to terminate the pregnancy may be made, and in others the pregnancy is continued with knowledge regarding the child's likely physical and mental status. A second amniocentesis procedure is often carried out to confirm the existence of the problem before any kind of action is taken by the parents.

It is important to note that, in many cases, amniocentesis will identify a treatable disease that can be handled while the fetus is still in the uterus. One such example is respiratory distress syndrome. When this disease is diagnosed early in the third trimester of a pregnancy, it can be treated successfully with hormones. In such cases, the amniocentesis procedure is then repeated at appropriate intervals after treatment, to assure both the parents and the physician that the problem has been solved.

THE FUTURE OF FETAL TESTING

Numerous consequences of improvements in the methodologies associated with amniocentesis have produced still more effective avenues of exploration of the state of the fetus in the uterus. One example is the use of telescope-like fetoscopes to examine fetuses directly. In a procedure similar to that used to enter the uterus for amniocentesis, a fetoscope is utilized to examine the fetus for physical defects. In some cases, these defects are repaired via surgery, hormone administration, or chemotherapy. Such avenues of fetal monitoring and care are components of the medical specialty called fetology.

Another technique of obtaining fetal cells is chorionic villus sampling. It arose from the demonstration of the clear value of the information derived from fetal cells obtained from amniotic fluid. This useful procedure was devised to shorten the several-week-long time period, after amniocentesis, that is needed to grow enough fetal cells in tissue culture to provide the amount of tissue required for successful karyotyping or DNA sequencing work. Another advantage of the chorionic villus sampling procedure is that it can be carried out with younger fetuses, as young as twelve weeks old, although the risk to such fetuses is somewhat higher than that which is seen after amniocentesis. When an abortion or another type of corrective action is indicated by the results of chorionic villus sampling, moreover, it is often safer to carry out such actions because the testing procedure was performed much earlier in the pregnancy.

In chorionic villus sampling, a catheter is usually inserted into the uterus through the vaginal opening. This catheter is then guided by ultrasonography until its tip reaches the many chorionic villi that edge the placenta at its connection to the uterus. Gentle suction is applied, and a few of the villi are sucked out, first into the catheter and then into a sampling device. The cells that are obtained are tested in the same manner as with cells obtained after amniocentesis.

—Sanford S. Singer

See also Abortion; Birth defects; Disabilities; Down syndrome; Genetic counseling; Genetic diseases; Genetic engineering; Mental retardation; Multiple births; Pregnancy among teenagers; Prenatal care; Preventive medicine; Screening; Spina bifida.

FOR FURTHER INFORMATION:

Filkins, Karen, and Joseph Russo, eds. *Human Prenatal Diagnosis.* 2d ed. New York: Marcel Dekker, 1990. This book attempts to "clarify and rationalize aspects of diagnosis, genetic counseling, and intervention." It is meant as a guide for health professionals and is useful to general readers. The fourteen chapters cover a wide range of useful topics, including DNA analysis.

Holtzman, Neil A. *Proceed with Caution: Predicting Genetic Risks in the Recombinant DNA Era.* Baltimore: The Johns Hopkins University Press, 1989. This quite technical text describes the use of karyotyping and numerous other forms of hereditary material testing for identifying genetic problems. Included among these topics are applications associated with amniocentesis.

Rapp, Rayna. *Testing Women, Testing the Fetus: The Social Impact of Amniocentesis in America.* New York: Routledge, 1999. Rapp, an anthropologist, combines personal experience and professional expertise. She has interviewed women of many different racial, cultural, religious, educational, and financial backgrounds for this study, in which she also explores the role of the genetic counselor.

Sherwood, Lauralee. *Human Physiology: From Cells to Systems.* 4th ed. Pacific Grove, Calif.: Brooks/Cole, 2000. This college textbook contains useful biological information about pregnancy and genetic defects, as well as facts useful to understanding amniocentesis and its advantages and disadvantages. Provides many valuable definitions and diagrams. Clearly written, the book is a mine of information for interested readers.

Verp, Marion S., and Albert B. Gerbie. "Amniocentesis for Prenatal Diagnosis." *Clinical Obstetrics and Gynecology* 24 (1981): 1007-1021. This concise, technical review of amniocentesis covers much material, including genetic counseling, the composition of amniotic fluid, the risks associated with amniocentesis, and Rh sensitization. Seventy-five references are made available to interested readers.

✧ ANOREXIA NERVOSA

Type of issue: Children's health, mental health, social trends, women's health
Definition: Self-induced malnutrition resulting in a body weight 15 percent or more below normal for age and height, and, in women, characterized by the absence of three or more consecutive menstrual periods.

Anorexia nervosa is an obsessive-compulsive disorder characterized by a body weight at or below 85 percent of normal and an intense fear of weight gain. Anorexia nervosa is typically a physical manifestation of underlying emotional conflicts such as guilt, anger, and poor self-image. Eating disorders such as anorexia nervosa are the third most common chronic condition among girls ages fifteen to nineteen. Approximately 95 percent of anorexics are female.

Anorexia nervosa often occurs following a successful dieting experience, and frequent dieting may contribute to the development of the disorder. Dieters may experience positive feedback regarding weight loss and feel compelled to continue losing weight.

Although the term "anorexia" means "loss of appetite," most anorexics continue to experience hunger but ignore the body's normal craving for food. Anorexics frequently identify specific areas of the body that they believe are "fat," despite their emaciated condition. Secrecy and ritual eating habits may be signs of anorexia nervosa. Sufferers often lie to family and friends to avoid eating meals and may eat only a set diet at a specific time of day.

THE PSYCHOLOGICAL ASPECTS OF ANOREXIA

Many anorexics are high achievers, exhibiting perfectionist or "people-pleasing" personalities. In addition, a strong correlation exists between anorexia nervosa and athletic activities that emphasize the physique, such as track, tennis, gymnastics, cheerleading, and dance. Anorexics may demonstrate additional obsessive-compulsive behaviors such as weighing themselves and/or examining themselves in the mirror several times per day, being overly concerned with calorie or fat content, exercising compulsively, maintaining unusually consistent eating patterns, and kleptomania (compulsive stealing).

Anorexia nervosa is frequently a symptom of depression, and the accompanying weight loss can be seen as a cry for help. Eating disorders tend to run in families, particularly those that equate thinness with success and happiness. The condition may also occur as a result of a traumatic situation such as death, divorce, pregnancy, or sexual abuse.

Results of Anorexia

Symptoms and resulting physical conditions include amenorrhea, the abnormal interruption or absence of menstrual discharge, which can occur when body fat drops below 23 percent. Anorexia nervosa may also be characterized by a distended abdomen as a result of a buildup of abdominal fluids and the slowing of the digestive system.

Resulting malnutrition can impair the immune system and cause anemia or decreased white blood cell counts. Brain and central nervous system functions may also be affected, resulting in forgetfulness, attention deficits, and confusion. Anorexics frequently experience fatigue, apathy, irritability, and extreme emotions.

Additional symptoms can include thyroid abnormalities, fainting spells, irregular heartbeat, brittle nails, hair loss, dry skin, cold hands and feet, hypotension (low blood pressure), infertility, broken blood vessels in the face, and the growth of downy body hair called lanugo as the body attempts to insulate itself because of the loss of natural fat.

The occurrence of eating disorders in adolescents is especially dangerous because the condition can retard growth and delay or interrupt puberty. Anorexia nervosa can also result in the erosion of heart muscle, which lowers the heart's capacity and can lead to congestive heart failure. Anorexics may experience musculoskeletal problems such as muscle spasms, atrophy, and osteoporosis as a result of potassium and calcium deficiencies. In extreme cases, patients may also experience kidney failure.

Treating the Disease

It is frequently necessary first to treat the acute physical symptoms associated with anorexia nervosa. Most patients—especially those with severe cases—benefit from treatment in a controlled environment that allows medically supervised "refeeding" to achieve a target rate of weight gain. Less severe cases may be treated on an outpatient basis.

During the initial phase of refeeding, the patient may receive a low-calorie diet to avoid overwhelming low-functioning organs. Patients who do not comply with the recommended diet may receive caloric supplements and, in serious cases, intravenous feeding.

Successful treatment also involves resolution of underlying emotional conflicts through individual and/or family counseling and may also include use of antidepressants such as fluoxetine (Prozac).

Anorexia nervosa is extremely difficult to treat, with a fatality rate of 5 percent to 10 percent within ten years. Nearly half of all sufferers never recover fully from the condition.

The Problem of Body Image

Anorexia is both an emotional and a cultural phenomenon. More than three-quarters of adolescent girls in the United States report being unhappy with their bodies and, on average, 25 percent of women are on a diet at any given time.

Most eating disorders were not recognized as illnesses until the late nineteenth century. Conditions such as anorexia nervosa gained the attention of medical professionals during the 1960's and beyond as a result of the media's obsession with thinness.

The media are prime contributors to this trend. Television and magazines send confusing messages to young consumers, such as depicting painfully thin models promoting high-fat snacks. Most models weigh about 23 percent less than the average American woman, and up to 60 percent of models suffer from eating disorders. In addition, the media frequently portray overweight people as having a lower socioeconomic status than people who are thin. Obese people are generally portrayed as comical, while thin people are often depicted as more intelligent, sophisticated, successful, and happier with their lives.

It appears likely that the incidence of eating disorders will continue to escalate as the media persist in depicting an idealized female body image significantly below normal body weight.

—Cheryl Pawlowski

See also Addiction; Children's health issues; Depression; Depression in children; Eating disorders; Malnutrition among children; Menstruation; Nutrition and women; Obesity; Obesity and children; Stress; Women's health issues.

For Further Information:
Broccolo-Philbin, Anne. "An Obsession with Being Painfully Thin." *Current Health 2* 22, no. 5 (January, 1996): 23.
Costin, Carolyn. *The Eating Disorder Sourcebook.* Los Angeles: Lowell House, 1996.
_____. *Your Dieting Daughter: Is She Dying for Attention?* New York: Brunner/Mazel, 1997.
Goodman, Laura J. *Is Your Child Dying to Be Thin? A Workbook for Parents and Family Members on Eating Disorders.* Pittsburgh: Dorrance, 1992.
Vredevelt, Pam, Deborah Newman, Harry Beverly, and Frank Minirth. *Thin Disguise: Overcoming and Understanding Anorexia and Bulimia.* Nashville: Thomas Nelson, 1992.

✧ Antibiotic resistance

Type of issue: Epidemics, public health, treatment
Definition: The ability of a pathogen, formerly susceptible to a particular
medication, to change in such a way that it is no longer affected by it.

Drug resistance occurs whenever pathogens—microscopic organisms such
as bacteria, viruses, and fungi, or larger organisms such as parasites—that
have been successfully eradicated with a certain agent develop the ability to
resist that agent. The most common and most important form of drug
resistance is the ability of bacteria to develop resistance to antibiotics.

An antibiotic attacks a bacterial cell by binding to the cell wall and
penetrating it to reach the interior of the cell, where it interferes with a vital
biochemical process. Bacteria can develop resistance to an antibiotic in
several ways. The bacterial cell may develop the ability to produce a substance that inactivates the antibiotic. The structure of the cell wall may be
altered so that the antibiotic can no longer bind to or penetrate it. The cell
may increase the activity of the biochemical process being attacked, or it may
develop a new process to replace the old one.

Resistance to a particular antibiotic arises in a bacterial cell by random
genetic mutation. Because this cell survives antibiotic treatment that destroys other bacteria of the same kind, it is able to reproduce, resulting in
numerous offspring that are also resistant. The bacteria that were formerly
susceptible to the antibiotic are now resistant.

Even if an antibiotic is completely successful at eradicating a particular
type of bacteria, problems with drug resistance can arise. The human body
contains billions of bacteria of many different kinds. When one or more of
these kinds of bacteria are eliminated by an antibiotic, those kinds that
happen to be resistant will multiply in greater numbers. Even if these
resistant bacteria are harmless, they often have the ability to transfer antibiotic resistance to harmful bacteria.

Use of multiple antibiotics or antibiotics that attack many kinds of bacteria, known as broad-spectrum antibiotics, can cause other problems. By
eliminating a large number of the bacteria normally present, powerful
antibiotics encourage the growth of fungi such as *Candida albicans*. Fungal
infections are resistant to antibiotics and require special antifungal drugs.

An important factor in the emergence of antibiotic resistance is the
misuse of antibiotics. For example, antibiotics have no effect on viruses but
are often used on viral illnesses. A study published in 1997 revealed that at
least half of all patients in the United States who visited doctors' offices with
colds, upper respiratory tract infections, and bronchitis received antibiotics,
even though 90 percent of these illnesses are caused by viruses. The same
study showed that almost a third of all antibiotic prescriptions written in

doctors' offices were used for these kinds of illnesses. Similar problems are also seen in hospitals. A 1997 study of the misuse of the antibiotic vancomycin in U.S. hospitals revealed that 63 percent of vancomycin orders violated guidelines set up by the Centers for Disease Control.

PUBLIC HEALTH CONCERNS

Several public health concerns have arisen as a result of drug resistance. One of the earliest serious problems to arise was an outbreak of dysentery caused by bacteria resistant to four antibiotics in Japan in 1955. From the 1950's to the 1990's, multiple antibiotic resistance emerged in bacteria that caused pneumonia, gonorrhea, meningitis, and other serious illnesses.

A case documented in Nashville, Tennessee, from 1973 to 1974 demonstrates the severity of the problem. A patient with a history of being treated with broad-spectrum antibiotics was exposed to bacteria known as *Serratia* while in the hospital. The *Serratia*, normally susceptible to many antibiotics, picked up the genetic information encoding for multiple antibiotic resistance from otherwise harmless bacteria in the patient's body. The newly resistant *Serratia* spread to other patients in the hospital and to patients in other nearby hospitals. Meanwhile, the *Serratia* transferred resistance to bacteria known as *Klebsiella*. By the end of 1974, more than four hundred patients in four hospitals were infected with multiply resistant *Serratia* or *Klebsiella*. Seventeen of these patients died.

In the 1980's, drug-resistant tuberculosis emerged as a public health concern. In New York City in 1991, for example, 33 percent of all tuberculosis infections were resistant to at least one drug, and 19 percent were resistant to both of the two most effective drugs used to treat the disease. Because of resistance, many tuberculosis patients require treatment with four drugs for several months. Because of public health concerns and the difficulty of taking so many drugs properly for such an extended period of time, some patients are required to be directly observed by a health care worker every time that they take a dose of medication. The use of multiple drugs and the need for increased numbers of health care workers greatly increase the cost of treating tuberculosis.

A new challenge appeared in 1997, when patients in Japan and the United States developed infections caused by bacteria known as *Staphylococcus aureus* that were partially resistant to the drug vancomycin. These patients required multiple antibiotics for extended periods of time. *Staphylococcus aureus* is an organism normally found on human skin that can cause potentially fatal infections when it enters the blood. Many of these bacteria are resistant to multiple antibiotics, leaving vancomycin as the only effective treatment. Medical researchers fear that if *Staphylococcus aureus* with full resistance to vancomycin appears in the near future, it could cause infections that would be nearly impossible to treat.

ADDRESSING THE PROBLEM

Several different strategies have been suggested for dealing with the problem of antibiotic resistance. In general, these strategies involve educating the public and health care workers, monitoring antibiotic use, and promoting research into methods to deal with resistant bacteria.

The general public should be aware of the proper use of antibiotics. Many patients expect to be given antibiotics for illnesses that do not respond to them, such as viral infections. They may pressure physicians into prescribing antibiotics even when physicians are aware that they are useless. Some patients may use another person's antibiotics or may use old supplies of antibiotics that they have saved from previous illnesses. Even when antibiotics are properly prescribed, patients who begin to feel better may fail to take the entire amount prescribed, leading to an increased risk of drug resistance without completely eliminating the original infection. Public education is even more critical in those nations where many antibiotics can be purchased without a prescription.

All health care workers should be aware of the importance of avoiding the spread of resistant pathogens from one patient to another. In the late 1990's, about two million Americans per year acquired new infections while in hospitals. These infections, known as nosocomial infections, were responsible for about eighty thousand deaths per year. The most important factor in reducing the rate of nosocomial infections is frequent, thorough handwashing with effective disinfectants.

Physicians need to be aware of the proper ways to use antibiotics. Experts have suggested better education in antibiotic use in medical schools, more continuing education in the subject for practicing physicians, and the development of computer programs to aid physicians in selecting antibiotics. Some have suggested that all physicians prescribing antibiotics in hospitals be required to consult with physicians who specialize in infectious diseases. Standardized order forms that include guidelines for proper use of each antibiotic have also been proposed.

Pharmacists need to be aware of appropriate antibiotic use. They must be able to tell patients how to use antibiotics properly and to use them only under the direction of a physician. Some hospitals have given pharmacists the authority to make changes in antibiotic therapy when appropriate.

REDUCING THE USE OF ANTIBIOTICS

Experts agree that monitoring antibiotic use is critical to fighting drug resistance. A study published in 1997 demonstrated the effectiveness of education and monitoring in reducing resistance. Physicians in Finland were educated in the proper use of the antibiotic erythromycin, and use of the drug was monitored. In 1992, 16.5 percent of bacteria known as group A streptococci were resistant to erythromycin. In 1996, only 8.6 percent were resistant. Some experts have proposed using computers to share information about antibiotic use and resistance among as many health care facilities as possible.

Faster development of new antibiotics for use on multiply resistant bacteria has been proposed. Experts stress, however, that these new antibiotics must be used only when necessary in order to avoid promoting resistance to them.

Increased use of vaccines and the development of new vaccines would reduce the need for antibiotics by preventing certain types of bacterial infections. The vaccine that provides protection against pneumonia caused by bacteria known as pneumococci, for example, is recommended for use by all elderly persons in the United States. Despite this suggestion, in 1985 less than 15 percent of older Americans had received the vaccine.

Research into less familiar ways of fighting infections has also been suggested. These methods include developing drugs that strengthen the human immune system. Drugs may also be developed to attack the bacterial genes that encode for drug resistance or to attack the genes that cause certain bacteria to be pathogens. By the late 1990's, these methods remained mostly speculative.

Other methods have been proposed for minimizing antibiotic resistance. Because patients often expect or demand prescriptions when they visit physicians, some experts have suggested that the physician write a "lifestyle" prescription when drug use is not appropriate. Such a prescription would explain why antibiotics should not be used in a particular situation and would give the patient specific instructions on how to treat the illness without them.

—Rose Secrest

See also Childhood infectious diseases; Children's health issues; Epidemics; Hospitalization of the elderly; Iatrogenic disorders; Illnesses among the elderly; Influenza; Medications and the elderly; Meningitis; Necrotizing fasciitis; Overmedication; Tuberculosis.

FOR FURTHER INFORMATION:
Fisher, Jeffrey A. *The Plague Makers: How We Are Creating Catastrophic New Epidemics—and What We Must Do to Avert Them.* New York: Simon & Schuster, 1994. A discussion of antibiotic resistance and steps that can be taken to prevent it. Includes controversial chapters on AIDS and on antibiotic use in animals.
Lappe, Marc. *Germs That Won't Die: Medical Consequences of the Misuse of Antibiotics.* New York: Anchor Press, 1982. A clear and concise description of the mechanisms by which antibiotic resistance arises in bacteria.
Levy, Stuart B. *The Antibiotic Paradox: How Miracle Drugs Are Destroying the Miracle.* New York: Plenum Press, 1992. A wide-ranging, in-depth study of the problem of antibiotic resistance by the founder of the Alliance for

Prudent Use of Antibiotics. Includes clear diagrams explaining the methods by which resistance transfers between bacteria.

Murray, Barbara E. "Can Antibiotic Resistance Be Controlled?" *New England Journal of Medicine* 330, no. 17 (April 28, 1994): 1229-1230. An editorial that outlines the future consequences of increasing drug resistance and offers several suggestions for fighting it.

Smaglik, Paul. "Proliferation of Pills." *Science News* 151, no. 20 (May 17, 1997): 310-311. An account of the frequent misuse of antibiotics, with opinions from several experts.

✧ Arteriosclerosis

Type of issue: Prevention, public health, social trends
Definition: A general term for the progressive thickening and hardening of the arterial walls.

The most common type of arteriosclerosis is atherosclerosis, which is often the cause of heart attacks and strokes. Collectively, arteriosclerosis and other types of heart disease, such as congestive heart failure, are the leading cause of death in the United States for those over the age of sixty-five as well as for all age groups combined.

The Development of Arteriosclerosis

The changes that lead to atherosclerosis involve the arterial wall, which is the inside lining of the arteries. There are three parts to the arterial wall: the intima, the media, and the adventitia. The intima is a single layer of endothelial cells that line the artery. It rests on connective tissue of the media, which is the thickest layer of the wall. The intima and media are both involved in atherosclerotic changes. The third and outer segment of the arterial wall is the adventitia. It contains collagen, blood vessels, nerves, and lymphatic tissue.

Most scientific evidence supports the concept that injury to the epithelial cells of the intima begins the atherosclerotic process. An important function of the epithelial cells is to provide a barrier to keep blood and its components within the artery. Injury to these cells leads to increased permeability, which can allow components that would normally be kept out to pass through the intima and into the media. One of these components is low-density lipoproteins (LDLs).

LDLs are composed of protein, triglyceride, and cholesterol. The quantity of LDLs secreted from the liver is determined by several factors, including genetics and dietary fat. Fat is absorbed in the gastrointestinal tract and secreted into the blood and lymphatics as chylomicrons. The chylomicrons are partially degraded, leaving a chylomicron remnant. This remnant is taken up by the liver and secreted back into the blood as very low-density lipoproteins (VLDLs). The VLDLs are degraded to LDLs. Therefore, the more chylomicrons that are secreted in response to a high-fat diet, the higher the production of LDL.

After the LDLs have been transported into the intima of the arterial wall, they may become oxidized. The consequences of oxidation include recruitment of white blood cells. The white blood cells then initiate synthesis of adhesion molecules on the surface of the endothelial cells. The adhesion molecules attract proteins and fats in the blood to also adhere to the inside of the arterial wall. This produces a narrowing and inflexibility in the artery.

The earliest visible lesions in the arterial wall are fatty streaks, which do not protrude or disturb blood flow. Fatty streaks have been found to begin in early adulthood or even childhood. They do not contain the adhesion molecules or white blood cells.

Fibrous plaques appear to develop from fatty streaks after the LDLs have permeated the intima. They may protrude into the artery, making the diameter of the vessel narrower. They can also make the arterial wall thicker and less flexible, and thus more easily injured. Plaque may partially or totally block the blood's flow. Bleeding into the plaques can also occur, or a blood clot can form on the plaque's surface. In any of these situations, a heart attack or stroke may result. A heart attack occurs when the blood is blocked at the heart, while a stroke occurs when blood is blocked going to the brain. Left undisturbed, fatty streaks develop very slowly, becoming widespread only in old age. However, fatty streaks may be triggered into plaque development during middle age.

RISK FACTORS FOR ATHEROSCLEROSIS

Several factors have been associated with the progression or development of plaques in the artery and subsequent heart disease. Elevated levels of blood cholesterol or LDLs, high blood pressure, cigarette smoking, diabetes mellitus, obesity, and genetic disposition toward heart disease are all risk factors for the development of atherosclerosis. The Framingham Heart Study, begun in 1948, was the first to identify cardiovascular risk factors. The Framingham reports also include advancing age as a risk factor.

The National Institutes of Health (NIH) divides cardiovascular risk factors into those that one can do something about and those factors that cannot be changed. The latter category includes age: being forty-five years old or older for men and fifty-five years old or older for women. (Estrogen plays a protective role for women until they are past the menopause.) Another risk factor that cannot be changed is having a family history of early heart disease: a father or brother who developed heart disease before the age of fifty-five, or a mother or sister who developed heart disease before the age of sixty-five.

Risk factors that can be changed include high blood cholesterol, high LDL levels, low high-density lipoprotein (HDL) levels, high blood pressure (hypertension), diabetes, being physically inactive and overweight, and smoking. All these factors have been shown to be associated statistically with atherosclerosis. However, there is also a physiological basis for their being associated statistically. High blood cholesterol and LDL levels are thought to increase the probability that LDL will adhere to or permeate the epithelial cells of the intima. The HDL transports excess cholesterol in the blood back to the liver. Therefore, a higher level of this lipoprotein is a "risk reducer." Although people cannot be cured of high blood pressure or diabetes, having their blood pressure or blood sugar under control reduces the risks of high blood pressure or elevated blood sugar. Physical inactivity is believed to decrease the levels of HDL in the blood, to decrease uptake of LDL, and to contribute to obesity. Cigarette smoke is thought to directly injure the epithelial cells of the intima in the arterial wall, thus making them more susceptible to LDL adherence to the intima and invasion of the media of the arterial wall.

Because fatty streaks are believed to continue to develop throughout life, health policy has aimed at reducing those behaviors that may contribute to the acceleration of the fatty streaks into dangerous plaque formation. National health campaigns and health policies have suggested the elimination of smoking and the control of high blood pressure as ways to decrease the morbidity and mortality associated with atherosclerosis. Professional organizations have also promoted increasing physical activity, screening and treating those with diabetes, and achieving an optimal weight.

The reduction of dietary fat is also a national health guideline. Dietary fat is more of a risk factor in the development of atherosclerosis than is dietary cholesterol. Dietary cholesterol is also transported in the intestinal chylomicrons, but there is much less of it. Usual intakes of cholesterol fall well within the recommended 300 milligrams per day. In contrast, even a low-fat diet of 30 grams of calories from fat will result in an intake of 66,000 milligrams of fat when consuming a 2,000 calorie diet. It is clear that dietary fat has more of an impact than dietary cholesterol.

Other foods and nutrients continue to be investigated for their role in the prevention and treatment of atherosclerosis. Omega-3 fatty acids may have a role in the prevention or treatment of atherosclerosis, although their contribution remains to be clarified. In general, guidelines suggest that consuming fish once per week as a source of omega-3 fatty acids may be of benefit. Increasing the fiber in the diet can also help in lowering blood cholesterol and LDLs. Soluble fiber reduces blood cholesterol by decreasing absorption of cholesterol or fatty acids. Soluble fiber can be found in some fruits and grains, most notably oats. A variety of other dietary manipulations continue to be investigated. These include soy protein, garlic, isoflavones, and several vitamins.

Medications can also be used to lower elevated blood cholesterol or LDLs. Generally, dietary modification is recommended before medications are used because diet changes have no appreciable side effects. Medications for treating elevated blood lipids include a classification of drugs known as the statins, which work to decrease liver synthesis of cholesterol. Bile acid sequestrants reduce the reabsorption of bile acids and cholesterol. Nicotinic acid is a vasodilator that has been used to decrease blood lipids.

Prevention of atherosclerosis begins during young adulthood and continues into old age. Maintaining the integrity of the arteries is a process that must continue over the life span. When arteries are damaged, treatment and repair is much easier if they have been kept in good shape all along.

—*Karen Chapman-Novakofski*

See also Cholesterol; Heart attacks; Heart disease; Heart disease and women; Hypertension; Malnutrition among the elderly; Nutrition and aging; Nutrition and women; Obesity; Obesity and aging; Strokes.

FOR FURTHER INFORMATION:

American Heart Association. *American Heart Association Guide to Heart Attack: Treatment, Recovery, and Prevention.* New York: Times Books, 1996.

Bennett, J. Claude, ed. *Cecil Textbook of Medicine.* 21st ed. Philadelphia: W. B. Saunders, 2000.

Kris-Etherton, Penny, and Julie Burns, eds. *Cardiovascular Nutrition: Strategies and Tools for Disease Management and Prevention.* Chicago: American Dietetic Association, 1998.

Rutherford, Robert B., ed. *Vascular Surgery.* 5th ed. Philadelphia: W. B. Saunders, 2000.

Tierney, Lawrence M., Jr., et al., eds. *Current Medical Diagnosis and Treatment.* 39th ed. New York: McGraw-Hill, 2000.

✧ ARTHRITIS

Type of issue: Elder health, occupational health
Definition: A number of diseases causing joint difficulties ranging from discomfort and limitation of motion to loss of motion and extreme pain.

Arthritis (from the Greek *arthron,* or "joint," and *itis,* a suffix referring to inflammation) is not one but a number of diseases with the common factor that they affect joints in some way. The term itself is misleading, because joint inflammation is absent in most forms of arthritis. Swelling around the affected joint is not uncommon, and pain is frequent, particularly with extreme muscular effort or range of motion. These symptoms, however, are characteristic of only certain kinds of arthritis. Other kinds can produce growth of nonjoint-type tissue in joints, causing pain and sometimes immobilization of joints; can produce secondary effects such as fatigue or fever; or can operate through interference with the immune system.

Osteoarthritis

Osteoarthritis is the most common form of arthritis. In 1999, it affected an estimated sixteen million Americans, about three-quarters of them women. Osteoarthritis usually occurs in older persons ("older" is a flexible term, as osteoarthritis can appear in one's forties or may appear two decades or more after that) and is often thought of as the result of wear and tear on the material of joints. In most of the joints in the body, the bone ends that come together are padded with cartilage on each side. Cartilage, or gristle, is a protein somewhat similar to that which forms the matrix of bones; this matrix is filled with calcium salts for load-bearing strength. Cartilage has no calcium salts and is porous, spongy, and elastic. With age, joint cartilage can lose its elasticity or develop rough surfaces. This makes for slowed or restricted motion, sometimes with accompanying pain. In addition, the tendons and ligaments that hold the joint together may loosen, allowing slippage in the joint and further wear on the cartilage pads.

With the restricted motion of the worn cartilage padding, the surrounding muscles get less exercise, and a slow decay in strength results. This brings on the problems often ascribed merely to age, such as a slowed gait, limited motion in limbs or neck, and loss of hand strength so that opening jars and bottles becomes difficult. Osteoarthritis can occur in any joint in the body— knees, hips, shoulders, fingers, or toes—but usually is confined to a relatively small number: one hip, or a thumb or a few fingers, for example. Debilitation is rarely complete but can be a thoroughgoing nuisance.

Rheumatoid Arthritis

Rheumatoid arthritis is the second most common type of arthritis. In 1999, there were an estimated two million sufferers in the United States, two-thirds to three-quarters of them women. This is the affliction that many people think of as "arthritis," typified by swollen joints, crooked fingers, and slow and painful movement. Unlike osteoarthritis, rheumatoid arthritis can affect many (or all) joints at once, usually symmetrically—that is, if the left knee and hip are affected, the right ones are almost certain to be affected also. Rheumatoid arthritis is a disease of the synovial membrane, which is the membrane that surrounds the joint (somewhat in the fashion of the rubber boot that seals the joint of the gear lever in a stick-shift car). The synovial membrane holds in the fluid that lubricates the joint, nourishes the joint cartilage, and keeps the joint flexible. The origin of the disease is

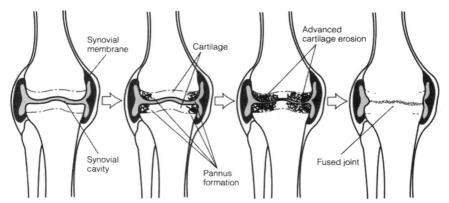

Rheumatoid arthritis begins with the inflammation of the synovial membrance and progresses to pannus formation and erosion of cartilage; eventually, the joint cavity is destroyed and the bones (here, the knee bones) become fused. (Hans & Cassidy, Inc.)

unknown (a virus has been suggested), but the results are clear: the synovial membrane is invaded by inflammatory cells that cause it to thicken and release enzymes that initially irritate the joint cartilage but that can eventually cause it to dissolve. It is often replaced by scar tissue, which can restrict the joint's normal motion and sometimes freeze it altogether. Pain is chronic to acute. Rheumatoid arthritis usually begins in the patient's forties; it can be a one-time (though damaging) bout of a few weeks or months, or a series of recurrences, or an ongoing condition. The synovitis can be treated, and even in chronic cases the disease tends to lessen its effects over time—but the initial damage remains regardless.

JUVENILE RHEUMATOID ARTHRITIS AND GOUT

Despite its name, this form of arthritis is not related to the adult form of rheumatoid arthritis. Three kinds are known: a form that affects only one or a few joints and that usually goes away without recurrence; a form that shows itself as very high fever with little joint involvement (though this can occur in later life); and the form known as rheumatic fever, which is not an arthritis but a streptococcal infection that sometimes invades the joints. All these forms do not usually persist into adulthood.

Gout is a crystalline form of arthritis, in which crystals of uric acid actually deposit in the joint and cause excruciating pain, though usually for only a few days. Sufferers are mainly male. The joints most often affected are those of the foot, usually the big toe, and sometimes the third (metatarsal) joint of the little toe. It was at one time thought that this was a disease of excess—of rich food, much drink, and little exercise. Current thinking suggests that these excesses may be involved but also implicates genetic factors. As animals at the top of the food chain, most humans ingest too many amino acids, from plant and animal sources, that they cannot use in building proteins. The excess nitrogen from these amino acids must be excreted. This is done by passing water-soluble urea in the urine. Some uric acid passes also, but uric acid is only slightly water-soluble; thus, it persists in relatively high concentration in the blood. Some persons are genetically predisposed to precipitate this uric acid, and for some this occurs in the joints, leading to gout. A pseudogout, in which the precipitated crystals are calcium phosphate, is also known. This usually occurs after age seventy, in both men and women; though it may recur, it tends to disappear spontaneously.

ANKYLOSING SPONDYLITIS

Ankylosing spondylitis (AS) is an arthritis mainly of the spine, though it sometimes affects other joints in the central part of the body. The name means an inflammation of the vertebrae (spondylitis) that results in ankylosis (stiffening of a joint, with the bones fusing together in late stages). AS is a genetically connected disease, and the gene site is known and can be detected by standard DNA analysis. AS shows up in early adulthood, predominantly in men. Most cases begin with fusion of the sacroiliac joint, immobilizing the lower back. Many never go beyond this stage, and the majority of persons with AS lead perfectly active lives. A few percent of cases progress to general spinal fusion, but even in these cases, mobility is not seriously impeded. Perhaps one case in a hundred freezes the entire spine, the neck, and even the cartilage of the ribs and breastbone, which restricts breathing but is rarely life-threatening. Most AS victims, in fact, have full lives and die of natural causes, despite the agonizing appearance of spinal rigidity and deformity in extreme cases.

It should be noted that kyphosis, the "dowager's hump" seen in elderly women and in some men, is not a result of this or any other arthritis; rather, it comes from osteoporosis, or loss of bone density, which leads to compression and partial collapse of vertebrae.

SYSTEMIC LUPUS ERYTHEMATOSUS AND OTHER FORMS OF ARTHRITIS

Systemic lupus erythematosus is an autoimmune disease—that is, one in which the system's tissues are attacked by its own antibodies. Arthritis results when the synovium or the joint cartilage is attacked. The symptoms resemble those of rheumatoid arthritis but are much milder and usually do not result in the bone damage of rheumatoid arthritis. On the other hand, the arthritis and its pain persist for the duration of the disease, which can be five to ten years or longer. The overwhelming majority of lupus victims are women.

More than a hundred other kinds of arthritis are known, but they affect relatively fewer people. They include psoriatic arthritis; Reiter's syndrome; fibromyalgia; arthritis associated with gonorrhea, tuberculosis, or Lyme disease; and polymyositis. Descriptions, treatment, and prognosis of these and other forms of arthritis can be found in the books cited at the end of this entry.

MEDICAL TREATMENT FOR ARTHRITIS

Until the mid-1990's, most of the medications used for arthritis were pain-killers. The most notable exceptions were the corticosteroids, which gave dramatic results in relieving inflammation and swelling, though not without undesirable side effects.

The most common pain relievers are the nonsteroidal anti-inflammatory drugs (NSAIDs). They have have no chemical similarity to one another except that they are not steroids. NSAIDS include some of the oldest and cheapest drugs in the pharmacopeia, as well as some newer and correspondingly more expensive drugs. The oldest NSAID is aspirin (acetylsalicylic acid). Other over-the-counter analgesics include acetaminophen, ibuprofen, and naproxen. Although these drugs are available in such brand-name pain relievers as Tylenol and Advil, most of these NSAIDs are available as generic or in-house drugs. They are generally effective pain relievers, but they can cause side effects; for example, all except acetaminophen can cause ulcers and gastric bleeding, sometimes unexpectedly after many months' use. Acetaminophen in protracted high dosage has been shown to cause liver and kidney damage. In addition, NSAIDs can further damage joint cartilage, an effect that has also been demonstrated with the prescription NSAID indocin (indomethacin).

All the standard NSAIDs are cox (short for "cyclooxygenase") inhibitors that interfere with the production of prostaglandins, which control cell chemistry. Only recently was it found that what had been thought to be a single cox that controlled both inflammation and pain as well as ulceration of the stomach and duodenum was in fact two separate compounds: Cox-1, which protected the stomach lining from acid degradation, and Cox-2, which produced joint inflammation. Thus, a compound that inhibited only Cox-2 could relieve arthritis symptoms without irritating the stomach. In 1999, two Cox-2 inhibitors were submitted for Food and Drug Administration (FDA) approval: celecoxib (Celebrex) and rofecoxib (Vioxx).

Two other osteoarthritis drugs are available that work on a totally different principle. These are hyaluronan (Hyalgan) and hylan G-F20 (Synvisc). Both are substitutes for hyaluronic acid, which appears to lubricate and increase the viscosity of joint fluid. As such, they must be injected directly into the joint in question, in a weekly series that typically costs from five hundred to seven hundred dollars. Large joints such as the knee fare best in this treatment; small joints are nearly impossible to inject with the large needle required for the viscous fluid. Relief is reported to last for six months to a year.

The NSAIDs are used extensively in osteoarthritis treatment, although they may be recommended in any case where pain must be controlled. Drugs to treat rheumatoid arthritis have been less effective than the NSAIDs, often merely reducing inflammation and performing a holding action on development of the disease. Historically, the first of these was a cortico-steroid. With its use, inflammation and pain were virtually eliminated, and the disease appeared to be arrested. Side effects soon occurred, however, and in ensuing decades have been well documented: possible ulcers, mental changes, fat accumulation in the body, muscular weakness and wasting, loss of bone calcium, and other symptoms. Steroids are now used sparingly and as a kind of last resort.

A variety of treatments has sprung up to lessen swelling and ease other symptoms of rheumatoid arthritis: methotrexate, injectable gold salts, peni-cillamine, azsulfidine, and hydroxychloroquine, among others. Some of these have serious side effects, and in any case they do not reverse the effects of the disease; moreover, it is generally unclear whether they actually arrest the arthritic damage or merely slow it down. Three newer drugs may actually halt the disease. The first of these, leflunomide (Arava), is an immune suppressor that targets the cells of the joint. General immunosup-pressors like methotrexate have been used, but leflunomide is the first that is tailored to the inflammatory cells that attack the synovium. Standard treatment costs about three thousand dollars per year, however, and re-quires careful monitoring by a physician and laboratory tests to observe effects on the body.

The other two drugs are the anti-TNF (tumor necrosis factor) com-pounds infliximab (Remicade) and etanercept (Enbrel). TNF is a cytokine that seems to cause inflammation and bone damage, so a drug that sup-presses it suppresses its effects. Both drugs are administered by injection—intravenous in the case of infliximab—and both are expensive, about ten thousand dollars per year for etanercept.

One other new treatment for rheumatoid arthritis has been devised, involving blood-serum filtration with a protein called Prosorba, which seems to clear out inflammatory substances. This is a procedure prescribed for those who are getting no help from regular medication; it is very expensive (about twenty thousand dollars per year). None of these drugs or proce-dures had received FDA approval by the end of the 1990's.

Drugs and treatments for other types of arthritis are usually some combi-nation of those given for osteoarthritis and rheumatoid arthritis. No herbal, naturopathic, homeopathic, or other "alternative" treatment has been shown by laboratory testing to give reproducible results other than occasional pain relief.

—Robert M. Hawthorne, Jr.

See also Aging; Canes and walkers; Disabilities; Medications and the elderly; Mobility problems in the elderly; Nursing and convalescent homes; Pain management.

FOR FURTHER INFORMATION:

Dunkin, Mary Ann. "The New Drugs: What to Expect." *Arthritis Today* 12, no. 6 (November/December, 1998): 31-35. Fuller discussion of new drugs mentioned above. *Arthritis Today*, published by the Arthritis Foundation (http://www.arthritis.org), contains well-balanced popular articles on all aspects of the disease.

Fries, James F. *Arthritis: A Take-Care-of-Yourself Guide to Understanding Your Arthritis.* 5th ed. Reading, Mass.: Addison-Wesley, 1999. Thorough discussion of types of arthritis, treatments, and prognoses, followed by an extensive guide to personal management methods and suggestions for problem-solving.

Gordon, Neil F. *Arthritis: Your Complete Exercise Guide.* Champaign, Ill.: Human Kinetics, 1993. The author is eminently qualified to discuss and illustrate the various types of exercise modalities; he suggests a schedule of frequencies and durations for each. The illustrations are easily understood and followed.

Lorig, Kate, and James F. Fries. *The Arthritis Helpbook: A Tested Self-Management Program for Coping with Your Arthritis.* 5th ed. Reading, Mass.: Addison-Wesley, 2000. Gives a brief introduction to the disease along with much valuable advice on exercise, pain management by self-suggestion, sleep, depression, nutrition, medication, working with one's physician, and other topics. Less technical than the preceding text.

Sands, Judith K., and Judith H. Matthews. "Medications: Arthritis Drugs Hit Their Mark." *Harvard Health Letter* 24, no. 4 (February, 1999): 4-5. Evaluates new arthritis drugs.

✧ ASBESTOS

Type of issue: Environmental health, industrial practices, occupational health, public health

Definition: The industrial term for certain silicate minerals that occur in the form of long, thin fibers.

The adverse health effects of breathing high concentrations of asbestos over many years have been known since the early 1970's. The Clean Air Act classified asbestos as a carcinogenic material, and in 1990 the U.S. Environmental Protection Agency (EPA) established a broad ban on the manufacture, processing, importation, and distribution of asbestos products.

Asbestos-form minerals are natural substances that are common in many types of igneous and metamorphic rocks found over large areas of the planet. Erosion continually releases these fibers into the environment; most people typically inhale thousands of fibers each day, or more than 100 million over a lifetime. Asbestos fibers also enter the body through drinking water. Drinking water supplies in the United States typically contain almost 1 million fibers per quart, but water in some areas may have as many as 100 million or more fibers per quart.

Many silicate minerals occur in fibrous form, but only six have been commercially produced as asbestos. In order of decreasing commercial importance, these are chrysotile (white asbestos), crocidolite (blue asbestos), amosite (brown asbestos), anthophyllite, tremolite, and actinolite. All the minerals except chrysotile are members of the amphibole group of minerals, which have a chainlike arrangement of the atoms. In contrast, chrysotile, as a member of the serpentine family, has atoms arranged in a sheetlike fashion.

Uses and Hazards

Although these minerals differ greatly from one another in individual properties, they share several characteristics that make them useful and cost-effective. These include great resistance to heat, flame, and acid attack; high tensile strength and flexibility; low electrical conductivity; resistance to friction; and a fibrous form, which allows them to be used for the manufacture of protective clothing. Therefore, asbestos was widely used until the 1970's in a great variety of building and industrial products. Such common materials as vinyl floor tiles, appliance insulation, patching and joint compounds, automobile brake pads, hair dryers, and ironing board covers all might have contained asbestos. Most such products now contain one or more of several substitutes for asbestos instead of asbestos itself. However, many of the substitutes may not be hazard-free, a fact that is starting to be recognized by legislators. For example, in 1993 the World Health Organization (WHO) stated that all substitute fibers must be tested to determine their carcinogenicity. Germany now classifies glass, rock, and mineral wools as probable carcinogens.

The U.S. Department of Health and Human Services classifies asbestos as a carcinogen. Studies leading to this determination were mostly based on asbestos workers who were exposed to extremely high levels of fibers for many years. These studies concluded that the asbestos workers have increased chances of developing two types of cancer: mesothelioma (a cancer of the thin membrane surrounding the lungs) and cancer of the lung tissue itself. These workers were also at increased risk of developing asbestosis, an accumulation of scarlike tissue in the lungs that can cause great difficulty in breathing and permanent disability. None of these diseases develops immediately; instead, they have long latency periods, typically fifteen to forty years. Despite the common misconception, exposure to asbestos does not cause muscle soreness, headaches, or any other immediate symptoms. The effects typically are not noticed for many years.

DEGREES OF RISK

It is generally agreed that the risk of developing disease depends on the number of fibers in a person's body, how long the fibers have been in the body, and whether one is a smoker, since smoking greatly increases the risk of developing disease. There is no agreement on the risks associated with low-level, nonoccupational exposure. The EPA has concluded that there is no safe level of exposure to asbestos fibers, but the Occupational Safety and Health Administration (OSHA) allows up to one thousand fibers per cubic meter during an eight-hour work day.

Another area of controversy stems from scientific studies showing that all forms of asbestos are not equally dangerous. Evidence has shown that the amphibole forms of asbestos, and particularly crocidolite, are hazardous, but the serpentine mineral chrysotile—accounting for 95 percent of all asbestos used in the past and 99 percent of current production—is not. For example, one case study involved a school that was located next to a 150,000-ton rock dump containing chrysotile. Thousands of children played on the rocks over a one-hundred-year period, but not a single case of asbestos-related disease developed in any of the children. The difference seems to be in how the human body responds to amphibole compared to chrysotile. The immune system can eliminate chrysotile fibers much more readily than amphibole, and there is also evidence that chrysotile in the lungs dissolves and is excreted. This remains a controversial area, and the U.S. government still treats all forms of asbestos the same. This is not true of some European governments.

The risk of developing any type of disease from exposure to normal levels of asbestos fibers in outdoor air or the air in closed buildings is extremely low. Melvin Benarde's 1990 calculations show that the risk of dying from nonoccupational exposure to asbestos is one-third the risk of being killed by lightning. The Health Effects Institute made similar calculations in 1991 and found that the risk of dying from asbestos is less than 1 percent the risk of dying from exposure to secondary tobacco smoke.

—*Gene D. Robinson*

See also Cancer; Environmental diseases; Lung cancer; Occupational health.

FOR FURTHER INFORMATION:
Benarde, Melvin, ed. *Asbestos: The Hazardous Fiber.* Boca Raton, Fla.: CRC Press, 1990.

Harben, Peter W., and Robert L. Bates. *Industrial Minerals: Geology and World Deposits.* London: Industrial Minerals Division, Metal Bulletin, 1990. A good general discussion of asbestos.

McDonald, J. C., et al. "The Health of Chrysotile Asbestos on Mine and Mill Workers of Quebec." *Archives of Environmental Health* 28 (1974). An example of a study conducted to determine the health effects of chrysotile.

Skinner, H. Catherine W., Malcolm Ross, and Clifford Frondel. *Asbestos and Other Fibrous Minerals.* New York: Oxford University Press, 1988. A balanced look at the health effects of asbestos.

✦ Asthma

Type of issue: Children's health, environmental health, public health
Definition: A chronic inflammatory obstructive pulmonary disease that obstructs the airways to the lungs and makes it difficult or, in severe attacks, nearly impossible to breathe.

Asthma is a Greek word meaning "gasping" or "panting." It is a chronic obstructive pulmonary (lung) disease that involves repeated attacks in which the airways in the lungs are suddenly blocked. The disease is not completely understood, but asthma attacks cause the person to experience tightening of the chest, sudden breathlessness, wheezing, and coughing. Death by asphyxiation is rare but possible. Fortunately, the effects can be reversed with proper medication.

The severity of symptoms and attacks varies greatly among individuals, and sufferers can be located on a continuum running from mild to severe. Mild asthmatics have fewer than six minimal attacks per year, with no symptoms between attacks, and they require no hospitalizations and little or no medication between attacks. Severe asthmatics have more than six serious attacks each year, have symptoms between attacks, lose more than ten school days or workdays, and require two or more hospitalizations per year. Attacks are typically spaced with symptom-free intervals but may also occur continuously. Rather than focusing only on the specific attacks, one should view and treat asthma as a chronic disease, a nagging, continuing condition that persists over a long period of time.

The Mechanism of an Asthma Attack

During inhalation, air travels into the nose and mouth and then into the trachea (windpipe); it then divides into the two tubes called bronchi and enters the lungs. Inside each lung, the tubes become smaller and continue to divide. The air finally moves into the smallest tubes, called bronchioles, and then flows into the millions of small, thin-walled sacs called alveoli. Vital gas exchange occurs in the alveoli. This gas exchange involves two gases in particular, oxygen and carbon dioxide. Oxygen must cross the membrane of the alveoli into the blood and then travel to all the cells of the body. Within the cells, it is used in chemical reactions that produce energy. These same reactions produce carbon dioxide as a by-product, which is returned by the blood to the alveoli. This gas is removed from the body through the same pathway that brought oxygen into the lungs.

The parts of this airway that are involved in asthma are the bronchioles. These tubes are wrapped with smooth, involuntary muscles that adjust the amount of air that enters. The lining of the bronchioles also contains many cells that secrete a substance called mucus. Mucus is a thick, clear, slimy fluid produced in many parts of the body. Normal production of mucus in the lungs catches foreign material and lubricates the pathway to allow smooth airflow. People suffering from asthma have very sensitive bronchioles.

Three pathological processes in the bronchioles contribute to an asthma attack. One is an abnormal sensitivity and constriction of the involuntary muscles surrounding the airways, which narrows the diameter of the airway. Another is an inflammation and swelling of the tissues that make up the bronchioles themselves. The third is an increased production of mucus, which then blocks the airways. These three mechanisms may work in combination and are largely caused by the activation of mast cells in the airways. The result can be extreme difficulty in taking air into the lungs until the attack subsides. The characteristic "wheeze" of asthma is caused by efforts to exhale, which is more difficult than inhaling. In the most serious attacks, the airways may close down to the point of suffocating the patient if medical help is not given.

Attacks can vary in severity at different times because of variations in tension within the bronchiole muscles. Although there is still debate about the general function of these muscles, they probably help to distribute the air entering the alveoli evenly. Control of the tension in these smooth muscles is involuntary and follows a circadian (twenty-four-hour) rhythm influenced by neurohormonal control. Accordingly, for most people this cycle causes maximum constriction to occur at about 6:00 A.M. and maximum relaxation to occur at about 6:00 P.M. Hence, asthma attacks tend to be more severe in the late night and early morning.

Following a given asthma attack, patients are sometimes susceptible to additional, more severe attacks. This period of high risk, called a late-phase response, occurs five or six hours after the initial symptoms pass and may last as long as several days. Some researchers believe that the increase in deaths from asthma in the United States may be tied to this danger, which often goes unrecognized.

ASTHMA TRIGGERS

The initial cause and mechanism of an asthma attack can vary from person to person. Accordingly, asthma is usually divided into two types. One type is extrinsic, that is, caused by external triggers that bring about an allergic response. Allergic reactions involve the immune system. Normal functioning of the immune system guards the body against harmful substances. With an allergy, the body incorrectly identifies a harmless substance as harmful and reacts against it. This substance is then called an allergen. If the symptoms of this reaction occur in the lungs, the person has extrinsic or allergic asthma. Pollens, dust, dust mites, animal dander, molds, cockroaches, and feathers are common allergens.

When allergens enter the body, the white blood cells make specific IgE antibodies that can bond with the invaders. Next, the IgE antibodies attach to the surfaces of mast cells; these cells are found all over the body and are numerous in the lungs. The allergens attach to the IgE antibodies located on the mast cells, and the mast cells are stimulated to produce and release chemicals called mediators, such as histamine, prostaglandin D_2, and leukotrienes. These mediators cause sneezing, tighten the muscles in the bronchioles, swell the surrounding tissues, and increase mucus production.

The second type of asthma is intrinsic and does not involve allergies. People who suffer from intrinsic asthma have hyperactive or twitchy airways that overreact to irritating factors. The mechanism for this form is not always understood, but no IgE antibodies for the irritant are placed on the mast cells. Examples of such nonallergic stimuli are cigarette smoke, house dust, artificial coloring, aspirin, ozone, or cold air. Odors from insecticides, cleaning fluids, cooking foods, and perfume can also trigger attacks. Also included in this category are attacks that are caused by viral infections (including colds and flu), stress, and exercise. Asthma can be triggered by many different substances and events in different people. While the symptoms are the same whether the asthma is intrinsic or extrinsic, asthmatics need to identify what substances or events trigger their attacks in order to gain control of the disease.

CAUSES OF ASTHMA

Why people develop asthma is not well understood. Asthma can begin at any age, but it is more likely to arise in childhood. While it is known that heredity predisposes an individual to asthma, the pattern of inheritance is not a simple one. Most geneticists now regard allergies as polygenic, which means that more than one pair of genes is involved. Height, skin color, and intelligence are other examples of polygenic traits. Exposure to particular external conditions may also be important. The children who develop asthma are more likely to be boys, while girls are more likely to show signs of the disease at puberty (about age twelve). Childhood asthma is also most likely to disappear or to be "outgrown" at puberty; about half of the cases of childhood asthma eventually disappear.

Early exposures to some triggers may be a key in the development of asthma. Smoking by mothers can cause children with a genetic disposition to develop asthma. Apparently, the early exposure to secondhand smoke develops an allergy. Early studies in this area were confusing until the data were sorted by level of education. Lung specialist Fernando Martinez of the University of Arizona believes that less-educated women who smoke are more likely to cause this effect because their homes are likely to be smaller and therefore expose the children to more smoke. Another study, this one in Great Britain, indicated that more frequent and thorough housecleaning might keep children from developing asthma. Early exposure by genetically susceptible children to dust and the mites that thrive in dust may also cause some to develop asthma.

CONTROLLING ASTHMA

The key to gaining control of asthma is discovering the particular factors that act as triggers for an attack in a given individual. These factors vary and at times can be surprising; for example, one person found that a mint flavoring in a particular toothpaste was a trigger for his asthma. Nevertheless, most common triggers fall in the following groups: allergies; irritants, including dust, fumes, odors, and vapors; air pollution, temperature, and dryness; colds and flu; and stress. Even types of food may be important. Diets low in vitamin C, fish, or a zinc-to-copper ratio, as well as diets with a high sodium-to-potassium ratio, seem to increase the risk of asthma attacks and bronchitis. There have also been correlations between low niacin levels in the diet and tight airways and wheezing.

Various medications are available to keep the airways open and to lower their sensitivity. In an emergency, drugs may be injected, but medications are usually either inhaled or taken orally as pills. Because inhaling transports the medication directly to the lungs, lower doses can be used. Many asthmatics carry inhalers, which allow them to breathe in the medication during an attack. Because this action requires a person to coordinate inhaling with the release of the spray, young children are sometimes better off with a device that requires them to wear a mask. The choice and dosage of medicine vary with the patient, and physicians need to determine what is safest and most effective for each individual. Self-treatment with nonprescription drugs should be avoided.

Some of the most commonly prescribed drugs are bronchodilators, inflammation reducers, and trigger-sensitivity reducers. The bronchodilators include albuterol, metaproterenol, and terbutaline. They are beta-agonists that mimic the way in which the body's nervous system relaxes or dilates the airways. (Any drug that functions as a beta-blocker should be avoided by asthmatics because of its opposite effects.) Another bronchodilator is adrenaline (or epinephrine), but it is a less specific drug that also affects the heart and pulse rate. Theophylline, a stimulant chemically related to caffeine, relaxes the airways and also helps clear mucus. The use of corticosteroids (or steroids) for asthma has been increasing because they reduce inflammation and relax airways. Initially, corticosteroids were used if other drugs were ineffective, but in 1991 they were strongly recommended for long-term preventive use. As another way of addressing asthma as a long-term problem, cromolyn sodium is sometimes inhaled on a daily basis to prevent attacks by decreasing sensitivity to triggers.

The concern for safety with these medications increases when asthmatics use high doses (more than two hundred inhalations monthly) of beta-agonist inhalers. A higher risk of fatal or near-fatal attacks has been found with a high usage of fenoterol, a beta-agonist that is not used in the United States. Paul Scanlon, a chest physician at the Mayo Clinic, warns that individuals should not exceed their prescribed dosage when using an inhaler. An individual who feels the need to use an inhaler more often to obtain adequate relief should see a doctor. The increased need is a sign of worsening asthma, and a doctor needs to investigate and perhaps change the treatment.

Some doctors have improved their diagnosis of asthma with a tool called the peak flow meter. The meter can also be used by patients at home to predict impending attacks. This inexpensive device measures how fast air can be moved out of the lungs. Therefore, it can be discovered that airways are beginning to tighten before other symptoms occur. The early warning allows time to adjust medications to head off attacks. This tool can help asthmatics take charge of their disease.

Over-the-counter drugs are often used by asthmatics to treat their symptoms. These drugs often use ephedrine, metaraminol, phenylephrine, methoxamine, or similar chemicals. All these drugs are structurally related to amphetamine or adrenaline. Unfortunately, some people may be getting relief without discovering the cause of their asthma. The National Asthma Education Panel (NAEP) maintains that self-treatment without a doctor's guidance is risky.

Asthma is a major health problem in the United States. As many as 20 million Americans may have the disease, and the number has been mysteriously increasing since 1970. While attacks can cause complications, there is no permanent damage to the lungs themselves, as there is in emphysema. Complications include possible lung collapse, infections, chronic dilation, rib fracture, a permanently enlarged chest cavity, and respiratory failure. Furthermore, millions of days of work and school are lost as victims recuperate; asthma is the leading cause of missed school days. Even though attacks can be controlled by medication, occasionally fatalities do occur. The total number of deaths from asthma in the United States reached 4,600 in 1987.

—Paul R. Boehlke; updated by Shih-Wen Huang, M.D.

See also Allergies; Children's health issues; Environmental diseases; Secondhand smoke; Smog; Smoking.

FOR FURTHER INFORMATION:

American Medical Association Essential Guide to Asthma. New York: Pocket Books, 1998. Although sparsely illustrated, this handy book presents the essential details on asthma from diagnosis to treatment and prevention, as well as a chapter covering alternative therapies, a glossary, and a resources list.

Barnes, Peter J., et al., eds. *Asthma.* 2 vols. London: Martin Dunitz, 2000. This text, the core resource in the field, offers a comprehensive overview, incorporating current information related to asthma's pathobiology and clinical aspects. The 148 chapters range from the basic sciences to management of the disease in both adults and children.

Haas, François, and Sheila Sperber Haas. "Living with Asthma." In *The World Book Medical Encyclopedia.* Chicago: World Book, 1988. This special report carefully explains the disease and encourages asthmatics to take control of their lives. A chart details how a house can be asthma-proofed. Side effects and drawbacks of various drugs are charted.

Krementz, Jill. *How It Feels to Fight for Your Life.* Boston: Little, Brown, 1989. A collection of fourteen case studies of children who have serious chronic diseases. In one chapter, Anton Broekman, a ten-year-old, describes what living with asthma is like.

Ostrow, William, and Vivian Ostrow. *All About Asthma.* Morton Grove, Ill.: Albert Whitmany, 1989. A children's book written to inform and encourage. The writers, a boy and his mother, tell about his experience with asthma. He explains causes, symptoms, and ways to lead a normal life. A must for children with asthma.

✧ ATTENTION-DEFICIT DISORDER (ADD)

Type of issue: Children's health, mental health

Definition: A condition characterized by an inability to focus attention or to inhibit impulsive, hyperactive behavior; it is associated with poor academic performance and behavioral problems in children.

Most experts think that 2 to 5 percent of children may have attention-deficit disorder (ADD), which is also known as attention-deficit hyperactivity disorder (ADHD). The cause of ADD is unknown, although the fact that it often occurs in families suggests some degree of genetic inheritance. The condition is more common in boys, but it does occur in girls. ADD is usually diagnosed when a child enters school, but it may be discovered earlier.

Adolescents and even adults who escaped earlier detection may be diagnosed when their symptoms cause particularly severe problems. Some causes of ADD that have been suggested, but never proved, include low blood sugar, food additives, the sweetener aspartame, allergies, and vitamin deficiencies.

THE SYMPTOMS OF ADD

Children who do not have ADD may, at times, have some of the symptoms of this disorder, but children who can be diagnosed with ADD must have most of the symptoms most of the time—in school, at home, or during other activities. The symptoms are usually grouped into three main categories: inattention, hyperactivity, and impulsiveness.

Children who have symptoms of inattention often make careless mistakes at school or do not pay close attention to details in play or work. They may have problems sustaining attention over time and frequently do not seem to listen when spoken to, especially in groups. Children with ADD have difficulty following instructions and often fail to finish chores or schoolwork. They do not organize well and may have messy rooms and desks at school. They also frequently lose things necessary for play or school. Because they have trouble sustaining attention, children with ADD dislike tasks that require this skill and will try to avoid them. One of the key symptoms is distractibility, which means that children with ADD are often paying attention to extraneous sights, sounds, smells, and thoughts rather than focusing on the task that they should be doing. Particularly frustrating to parents is the symptom of forgetfulness in daily activities, in spite of numerous reminders from parents about such common, everyday activities as dressing, hygiene, manners, and other behaviors. Children with ADD have a poor sense of time; they are frequently late or think that they have more time to do a task than they really do.

Not all children with ADD have symptoms of hyperactivity, but many have problems with fidgeting, or squirming. It is common for these children to be constant talkers, often interrupting others. Other symptoms of hyperactivity include leaving their seat in school, church, or similar settings and running around excessively in situations where they should be still. Children with ADD have difficulty playing quietly, although they may watch television or play video games for long periods of time. Some of these children seem to be driven by a motor, or are continuously on the go.

All children with ADD will have some symptoms of impulsiveness, such as blurting out answers before questions are completed or intruding on others by "butting in." They often have difficulty standing in lines or waiting for their turn in games.

Several other neurologic or psychiatric disorders have symptoms that can overlap with ADD, so diagnosis is often difficult. When a child is suspected of having ADD, he or she should have a thorough medical interview with, and physical examination by, a physician familiar with child development, ADD, and related conditions. A psychological evaluation to determine intelligence quotient (IQ) and areas of learning and performance strengths and weaknesses should be obtained. School records need to be reviewed, and teachers may be asked to submit rating forms or similar instruments to document school performance. A thorough family history and a discussion of family problems such as divorce, violence, alcoholism, or drug abuse should be part of the evaluation. Other conditions that might be found to exist along with ADD, or to be the underlying cause of symptoms thought to be ADD, include oppositional defiant disorder, conduct disorder (usually seen in older children), depression, or anxiety disorder. Some physicians, teachers, psychologists, and parents do not believe that ADD is a "real" condition, but this disorder is usually widely accepted in the United States as a credible diagnosis for a child who demonstrates many of the above symptoms at home, at play, and at school.

AN INABILITY TO FOCUS

Children with ADD often make the same mistakes repeatedly because they lack hindsight and forethought. Their primary problem is not that they cannot pay attention but that they pay attention to everything. Consequently, they cannot focus on the most important sensory input, such as a parent's order or a teacher's assignment.

It is important to recognize that children with ADD are not bad children who are hyperactive, impulsive, and inattentive on purpose. Rather, they are usually bright children who would like to behave better and to be more successful in school, in social life with peers, and in family affairs, but they simply cannot. One way to think about ADD is to consider it a disorder of the ability to inhibit impulsive, off-task, or undesirable attention. Consequently, the child with ADD cannot separate important from unimportant stimuli and cannot sort appropriate from inappropriate responses to those stimuli. It is easy to understand how someone whose brain is trying to respond to a multitude of stimuli, rather than sorting stimuli into priorities for response, will have difficulty focusing and maintaining attention to the main task.

It is also important to remember that it is not only the presence of symptoms that categorizes a child as having ADD but also the intensity and prevalence of the symptoms in more than one setting. For example, a child may not seem to pay attention in school and often may be disruptive in class but be a normal child at home, playing Little League baseball, and in church school. This child may have a learning disability without ADD or a specific conflict with the teacher.

Children most likely to be diagnosed correctly with ADD will have many of the following characteristics. They will have a short attention span, particularly for activities that are not fun or entertaining. They will be unable to concentrate because they will be distracted by peripheral stimuli. They will have poor impulse control so that they seem to act on the spur of the moment. They will be hyperactive and usually rather clumsy, resulting in their being labeled "accident-prone." They will certainly have school problems, especially when classwork requires more thinking and planning—often seen about third grade and beyond. They may display attention-demanding behavior and/or show resistant or overpowering social behaviors. Last, children with ADD often act as if they were younger, and "immaturity" is a frequent label. Along with this trait, they have wide mood swings and are seen as very emotional.

ADD as a Developmental Problem

Many experts think that ADD is a developmental problem, caused by the failure of the brain and nervous system to grow and mature normally. Most people would agree that an average, normal two-year-old child is a perfect definition for ADD: short attention span, impulsive, distracted by almost anything new, highly emotional, demanding, often clumsy and reckless, unable to plan well, and sometimes aggressive. All these characteristics are acceptable for the toddler. When those symptoms persist into and beyond kindergarten, however, an unusually slow brain and nervous system development seems likely. This slow development may improve during childhood or may persist into adolescence.

Adolescents who have ADD are usually not hyperactive, although they may have problems with impulsive talking and behavior. They have considerable difficulty complying with rules and following directions. They may be poorly organized, causing problems both with starting projects and with completing them. Their inability to monitor their own behavior leads to problems making and keeping friends and causes them to have conflicts with parents and teachers beyond those normally seen in teenagers. Adolescents with ADD usually have problems in school in spite of average or above-average potential. They may have poor self-esteem and a low frustration tolerance.

The Controversy over Treatment

The medical treatment of ADD is one of the most controversial issues in education and in medicine. Although scientific studies clearly show the value of certain medications, and scores of parents and teachers have noticed remarkable improvement with treatment, some people take issue with using medications to change a child's behavior. Clearly, medications alone are not the answer for ADD. Families and children need guidance and support in the form of counseling, as well as considerable information about the condition. Special accommodations can be arranged with most schools and are mandated by federal law. Once educational adjustments have been made and counseling is in place, however, medications can play an important role.

The most frequently prescribed medications are stimulants; they include dexedrine, methylphenidate (Ritalin), and a combination of dexedrine salts (Adderall). A similar medication, pemoline (Cylert), has been related to side effects, which may limit its usefulness. The stimulant medications may function by influencing chemicals in the brain called neurotransmitters, which help transmit messages among brain and nerve cells. In ADD, it is thought that the medications improve the function of cells that direct the brain to focus attention, resist distraction, control behavior, and perceive time correctly. These medications are generally thought to be safe and effective, although they can have such adverse effects as headache, stomachache, mood changes, heart rate changes, appetite suppression, and interference with going to sleep. All children receiving medication must be monitored at regular intervals by a physician.

Other medications that may be used for ADD include antidepressants and antianxiety medications. Some children are treated with combinations of two medications; in unusual circumstances, there may be even more than two. Some of these medications are Imipramine and Desipramine, antidepressants that act mainly to control impulsiveness and hyperactivity; Bupropion, an antidepressant, and Buspar, an antianxiety medicine, both of which have been used largely in older children and adolescents; and clonidine and guanfacine, which work on brain nerve message transmitters and are sometimes helpful in calming aggressive behavior.

—*Robert W. Block, M.D.*

See also Children's health issues; Health problems and families; Learning disabilities; Stress.

FOR FURTHER INFORMATION:

Barkley, Russell A. *Taking Charge of ADHD*. Rev. ed. New York: Guilford Press, 2000. A comprehensive guide for parents that discusses how to understand ADD, how to be a successful parent, how to cope with the child at home and at school, and how to evaluate medications.

Block, Robert W., and Elaine King Miller. "The Maladroit Adolescent: Learning Disorders and Attentional Deficits." In *Advances in Pediatrics*. Vol. 33. Chicago: Year Book Medical Publishers, 1986. This article was written for parents as well as for medical and educational professionals. It describes ADD and several learning disabilities and recommends appropriate interventions.

Wender, Paul H. *The Hyperactive Child, Adolescent, and Adult*. New York:

Oxford University Press, 1987. This book offers concise information about ADD in children, adolescents, and adults. Clearly defines the characteristics of individuals with symptoms of ADD and discusses the reasons for using medications.

Zeigler Dendy, Chris A. *Teenagers with ADD: A Parents' Guide.* Bethesda, Md.: Woodbine House, 1995. This resource is a workbook for parents and teachers of adolescents who have ADD. Includes useful lists of problem behaviors at home and at school, with practical solutions to these problems.

✧ Autism

Type of issue: Children's health, mental health

Definition: A lifelong mental disability characterized by difficulty with social relationships, difficulty with language and communication, preoccupation with repetitive or stereotyped behaviors and interests, and a general resistance to changes in routine.

Autism is a psychological and behavioral disorder that is characterized by a cluster of symptoms. In the American Psychiatric Association's *Diagnostic and Statistical Manual of Mental Disorders* (4th ed., 1994, DSM-IV), the primary diagnostic handbook used by physicians and psychologists, autism is grouped with Asperger's syndrome and Rett's syndrome under the general classification of pervasive developmental disorder. Children who are diagnosed as having autism can demonstrate a wide range of symptoms; for this reason, physicians and psychologists often refer to "autistic spectrum disorders" to capture the range of symptoms that can be classified as autism. Despite evident differences, all children diagnosed with autism show three basic symptoms: some level of impairment in social functioning, delayed and/or abnormal language development, and a marked participation or interest in restricted and repetitive behaviors or activities.

Austism and Social Interaction

The social interactions of children with autism are strikingly abnormal, ranging from total isolation to inappropriate social behavior. Many autistic children refuse eye contact, show little if any facial expressiveness, and do not engage in social gesturing or body language. While the majority of autistic children develop attachments to their parents and/or other caregivers, there is a marked aloofness and lack of social reciprocity in interactions with autistic children. It is often said that autistic children do not relate to other people as people. They show no empathy for others' emotional expressions; they do not smile in response to others' expressions of happiness, nor do they attempt to comfort others who show distress. Autistic children may treat other people as if they were objects; in so doing, they might produce inappropriate social behaviors such as touching people's bodies, grabbing objects from other people, or bumping into or sitting on people.

The language of autistic children can range from mutism to somewhat deviant speech. Between 25 and 30 percent of children diagnosed with autism never develop spoken language, despite having normal hearing abilities. Those autistic children who do develop language often evidence linguistic disorders such as echolalia, persistent use of neologisms, limited vocabularies, and/or grammatical anomalies. Autistic children who develop fluent speech demonstrate poor conversational skills related to the general lack of social reciprocity seen in autism. Autistic speech is often flat, monotonous, and boring, with autistic speakers tending to focus on their own concerns and showing little regard for the interest or understanding of their conversational partners. Children with autism also evidence deficits in receptive communication. There is reduced attention to human voices in general; poor understanding of nonverbal language, including gesture and vocal intonation; and generalized difficulties with nonliteral language such as metaphors, jokes, and irony.

AUTISTIC BEHAVIORS

Children with autism show a preoccupation with restricted and repetitive behaviors, interests, and activities. This focus on repetition can take a range of forms, from performance of stereotypies to compulsive insistence on daily routines to an intense focus on specific, narrow topics of interest. Common stereotypies seen in autistic children include hand flapping, head banging, and other, more complex whole-body movements. Autistic children sometimes show self-injurious behaviors (such as biting or hair pulling) and/or self-soothing behaviors (such as rocking or stroking). More compulsive, ritualistic behavior patterns might include hand washing, counting, or the arrangement of possessions. This aspect of autism can also include intense preoccupation with highly restricted topics, such as water or pencils. Some children with autism also develop pica, the eating of such nonfood items as paper, paper clips, or dirt.

Another defining characteristic of autism is a lack of imaginative or pretend play. This symptom may be related to the general literalness seen in autistic communication. Autistic children's play tends to be solitary and to involve the repetitive manipulation of objects. The one-sidedness of autistic children's play and their generally impaired social interactions result in a failure to develop peer relationships appropriate to their developmental level. Autistic children are therefore often cut off from their peer groups, which can cause feelings of loneliness and depression, especially as autistic children approach adolescence.

Up to three-quarters of children with autism are also mentally retarded, with an intelligence quotient (IQ) below 70. The mental profiles of autistic children can be unusual, however, with particularly low verbal IQ scores but normal or near-normal scores on measures of mathematical and spatial IQ.

According to the DSM-IV, autism is diagnosed if there is evidence of delay in normal functioning of social interaction, communicative language, or imaginative/symbolic play prior to age three. In some cases, children diagnosed with autism have seemed to develop normally until age two and then apparently lost the beginnings of linguistic and social skills that had been developed up to that point.

The Rise in Autism

In the late 1990's, the incidence of autism was approximately two to three per thousand. Some researchers suggested that the incidence of autism rose over the course of the twentieth century, citing studies from the 1950's and 1960's that listed the incidence of autism at four to five per thousand. It has also been suggested that the apparent rise in the incidence of autism simply reflects a rise in awareness of the disorder and an increase in the accuracy with which the disorder is now diagnosed. Autism is more common in males than in females, with a ratio of 3:1 or 4:1. Autism appears to run in some families, and the concordance of autism or autistic-like symptoms in identical twins is around 50 percent. By the end of the twentieth century, however, autism had not been linked to a single gene.

Asperger's syndrome is thought to represent a subclassification of autism. The psychological and behavioral profiles of children with Asperger's syndrome are very similar to those of children with autism; however, children with Asperger's syndrome evidence normal or above-normal IQ scores and normal language development. Some children with Asperger's syndrome have particular talents, although in restricted domains such as calculation, memorization, or drawing. Children with Asperger's syndrome show the same lack of social awareness and restricted interests that are characteristic of autism.

Forms of Treatment

There is no cure or universal treatment for autism. Because children with autism can show such a wide range of symptoms, the range of available treatments is also wide. In dealing with autism, physicians, psychologists, and other health professionals focus on alleviating the symptoms that are the most disruptive to a particular child. Available treatments include behavior modification, social skills training, speech/language therapy, occupational therapy, music therapy, vitamin therapy, and prescribed medications. Often, a combination of these treatments will be used with a particular autistic child.

One of the most successful treatments for autism has been intensive behavior modification therapy. In his book *The Autistic Child: Language Development Through Behavior Modification* (1977), Dr. O. Ivar Lovaas described a program of intensive, one-on-one behavior modification therapy that was highly effective in alleviating disturbing symptoms and in engendering positive social behaviors in autistic children. Lovaas's technique is controversial because it involves both rewards for such appropriate behaviors as making eye contact or maintaining conversation and punishments for such inappropriate behaviors as self-damaging acts, stereotypies, or pica.

In a well-publicized legal case, the state of Massachusetts banned the use of punishment in a school for autistic children. As a result, the children's levels of self-injurious behavior increased, to the extent that the parents petitioned for punishment to be reinstated in the school's behavior modification program. While the utility of punishment is generally acknowledged, many behavior modification therapists now suggest that the positive reinforcement of rewarding appropriate behavior is effective enough that punishment for inappropriate behavior is not necessary. Despite variations in philosophy and technique, behavior modification aimed at increasing social responsiveness and decreasing inappropriate behaviors is generally an essential component of therapy for autistic children.

Social skills training involves direct teaching of the rules of social interaction. This training encourages autistic children to develop basic interpersonal skills, such as maintaining eye contact, waiting for a turn in conversation, listening to another person's words, and saying "please" and "thank you." Besides working on basic skills, social skills training techniques attempt to educate autistic children about the significance of the behavior, feelings, and thoughts of other people.

Speech therapy has been shown to be effective in improving the communicative and linguistic skills of children with autism. Occupational therapy focuses on teaching skills that allow autistic children to participate in daily life: crossing a street, preparing simple meals, making purchases, or answering the telephone. Music therapy has been used to draw emotional responses from children with autism, with varied levels of success, and vitamin therapy and/or dietary restrictions have also been found in certain cases to alleviate some of the symptoms of autism.

While no drug is specifically prescribed for autism, various medications are sometimes used to treat its symptoms. Stimulants may be used to treat the inattentiveness of autistic children who are particularly isolated and unresponsive. Tranquilizers may be prescribed to manage obsessive-compulsive behaviors that are disruptive to normal functioning. Antidepressants are also sometimes prescribed for autistic children in order to heighten emotional responsiveness and/or to stabilize mood. As many as one-third of children with autism develop seizures, often in adolescence, that are similar to epileptic seizures. These seizures are usually treated with medication.

Children with autism may lead different sorts of lives, depending upon the severity of the symptoms. Autistic children with mild impairments can live at home, learn to participate in family and social life, and go to mainstream schools. Children with more profound autistic symptoms or significant mental retardation may go to special schools or live in residential school settings. Whatever the setting, children with autism respond most positively to a highly structured environment that includes a good deal of one-to-one interaction.

Parents, siblings, and friends of autistic children also benefit from therapy. Life with autistic children can be rewarding, especially when progress is made, but it can also be frustrating and depressing. Often parents, siblings, and friends, as well as medical professionals, feel rejected by autistic children despite continual attempts to make contact. Most professionals suggest that anyone who spends extended periods of time with an autistic child would benefit from some form of training and/or emotional support.

The most recent work on autism has focused on physiological and cognitive aspects of the disorder. Brain studies utilizing magnetic resonance imaging (MRI) and positron emission tomography (PET) scanning have suggested that the cerebellum is abnormal in individuals with autism. A large number of cognitive studies conducted in the 1990's focused on the "theory of mind" hypothesis, which holds that autism results from a congenital inability to understand the minds of others.

—Virginia Slaughter

See also Children's health issues; Learning disabilities.

FOR FURTHER INFORMATION:

Aarons, Maureen, and Tessa Gittens. *The Handbook of Autism: A Guide for Parents and Professionals.* New York: Routledge, 1999. Written by professional speech therapists, this book is a thorough introduction to autism, covering diagnosis, assessments, history, prognosis, and methods of education. It is intended for a British audience.

Cohen, Donald J., and Fred R. Volkmar, eds. *Handbook of Autism and Pervasive Developmental Disorders.* 2d ed. New York: John Wiley & Sons, 1997. This is a scholarly work presenting current information, diverse approaches, and some new areas of investigation that have not been addressed in other sources. There is an extensive review of the literature in all of the chapters and well-documented references based on the research.

Happe, Francesca. *Autism: An Introduction to Psychological Theory.* London: UCL Press, 1994. This readable book gives a historical overview of autism and presents various theories that have been proposed to explain the disorder, including the "theory of mind" hypothesis.

Hart, Charles A. *A Parent's Guide to Autism.* New York: Pocket Books, 1993. A thorough discussion of important issues relevant to parents of autistic children, including chapters on diagnosis, treatment, education, and life choices.

McClannahan, Lynn E., and Patricia J. Krantz. *Activity Schedules for Children with Autism: A Guide for Parents and Professionals.* Bethesda, Md.: Woodbine House, 1999. The authors cover one method of helping autistic children learn: activity schedules. These schedules teach autistic youngsters to follow words, pictures, or other nonverbal prompts to complete all varieties of tasks.

✧ BIOFEEDBACK

Type of issue: Medical procedures, mental health, treatment
Definition: The learned self-regulation of the autonomic nervous system through monitoring of the physiological activity occurring within an individual.

Biofeedback has been utilized in both research and clinical applications. The term itself denotes the provision of information (feedback) about a biological process. It has been found that individuals (laboratory animals included), when given feedback that is reinforcing, are able to change physiological processes in a desired direction; homeostatic processes being what they are, these changes are in a positive direction. In the case of humans, the feedback is provided about a physiological function of which the individual would not otherwise be aware if it were not for the provision—via a biodisplay—of information about that process.

A classic example of biofeedback being used to correct a physiological problem would be the employing of electromyograph (EMG) biofeedback for the correction of a simple tension (or psychophysiologic) headache. The headache is caused by inappropriately high muscle tension in the neck, head, or shoulders. In surface electromyographic biofeedback, the biofeedback practitioner attaches electronic sensors to the muscles of the forehead, neck, or shoulders of the patient. The electronic sensors pick up signals from electrochemical activity at the surface of the skin in the area of the involved muscle groups. The behavior of the muscles being monitored is such that minute changes in the electrochemical activity in the muscles—tension and relaxation—occur naturally.

BIOFEEDBACK INSTRUMENTS

The sensitivity of the biofeedback instrument (the magnification of the signal may be as high as one thousand times) and the display of the signal make the individual aware of these changes via sound or visual signals (biodisplays). When the biofeedback signal indicates that the muscle activity is in the direction of relaxation, the individual makes an association between that muscle behavior and the corresponding change in the strength of the signal. The individual can then increase the duration, strength, and frequency of the relaxation process. Having learned to relax the involved muscles, the individual is able to prevent or abort headache activity.

An electromyograph is an instrument that is capable of monitoring and displaying information about electrochemical activity in a group of muscle fibers. Common applications of surface electromyography (in which sensors are placed on the surface of the skin, as opposed to the insertion of needles into the muscle itself) include stroke rehabilitation. Surface electromyography is also used in the treatment of tension headaches and fibromyalgia.

An electrodermal response (EDR) biofeedback instrument is capable of monitoring and displaying information about the conductivity of the skin. An increase in the conductivity of the skin is a function of moisture accumulating in the space recently occupied by blood. The rate of blood flow depends on the amount of autonomic nervous system arousal present within the organism at the time of measurement. The higher the level of autonomic nervous system arousal, the greater the amount of skin conductivity. Common applications of EDR biofeedback are the reduction of anxiety caused by phobic reactions, the control of asthma (especially in young children), and the treatment of sleep disorders. For example, many insomniacs are unable to drop off to sleep because of higher-than-appropriate autonomic nervous system activity.

An instrument that is capable of monitoring and displaying the surface temperature of the skin, as correlated with an increase in vascular (blood flow) activity in the area of the skin in question, can also be used for biofeedback. Such an instrument is helpful in the treatment for high blood pressure and migraine headaches.

Electroencephalographic (EEG) biofeedback involves the monitoring and displaying of brain wave activity as a correlate of autonomic nervous system activity. Different brain waves are associated with different levels of autonomic nervous system arousal. Common applications of EEG biofeedback are in the treatment of substance abuse disorders, epilepsy, attention-deficit disorders, and insomnia.

COMMON USES OF BIOFEEDBACK

Biofeedback is gaining in popularity because of a number of factors. One of the principal reasons is a growing interest in alternatives to the lifetime use of medications to manage a disorder. The more common usages of biofeedback treatment techniques include migraine headaches, tension headaches, digestive disorders, high blood pressure, low blood pressure, cardiac arrhythmias, Raynaud's disease, epilepsy, and paralysis.

One example worth noting—in terms of the magnitude of the problem—is the treatment of cardiovascular disorders. Myocardial infarctions, commonly known as heart attacks, are one of the major health problems in the industrialized world and an area of special concern to those practitioners with a psychophysiological orientation. In the United States alone, approximately 700,000 persons die of heart attacks each year.

One of the principal causes of heart attacks is hypertension (high blood pressure). Emotions have much to do with the manifestation of high blood pressure (hypertension), which places this condition in the category of a psychophysiological disorder. Researchers have demonstrated that biofeedback is an effective methodology to correct the problem of high blood pressure. The data reveal that many individuals employing biofeedback have been able to decrease (or eliminate entirely) the use of medication to manage their hypertension. Studies also show that these individuals maintain normal blood pressure levels for as long as two years following the completion of biofeedback training.

Because of its noninvasive properties and its broad applicability in the clinical setting, biofeedback is also increasingly becoming one of the more commonly utilized modalities in many fields, such as behavioral medicine. Researchers have provided documented evidence showing that biofeedback is effective in the treatment of so-called stress-related disorders. It is recognized that the four major causes of death and disability in the United States fall into the "stress-related" category. Research has also shown that biofeedback has beneficial applications in the areas of neuromuscular rehabilitation (working with stroke victims to help them develop greater control and use of afflicted muscle groups) and myoneural rehabilitation (working with victims of fibromyalgia and chronic pain to help them obtain relief from debilitating pain).

Research in the 1960's pointed to the applicability of EEG biofeedback for seizure disorders (such as epilepsy). Advanced technology and later research findings, however, have demonstrated EEG biofeedback to be effective in the treatment of attention-deficit disorder, hyperactivity, and alcoholism as well.

Biofeedback appears to have particular applicability for children. Apparently, there is an innate ability on the part of the young to learn self-regulation skills much more quickly than older persons, such as the lowering of autonomic nervous system activity. Since this activity is highly correlated with respiratory distress, biofeedback is often used in the treatment of asthma in prepubescent children. Biofeedback is also being successfully used as an alternative to prescription medications (such as Ritalin) for youngsters with attention-deficit disorder.

BIOFEEDBACK AND SPORTS

The use of biofeedback is also found in the field of athletics and human performance. Sports psychologists and athletic coaches have long recognized that there is an inverted "U" pattern of performance where autonomic nervous system activity and performance are concerned. In the field of sports psychology, this is known as the Yerkes-Dobson law. The tenets of this law state that as the level of autonomic nervous system arousal rises, performance will improve—but only to a point. When autonomic nervous system arousal becomes too high, a corresponding deterioration in performance occurs. At some point prior to an athletic competition, it may be desirable for an athlete to experience an increase (or a decrease) in the level of autonomic nervous system activity (the production of adrenaline, for example). Should adrenaline levels become too high, however, the athlete may "choke" or become tense.

To achieve physiological autoregulation (often referred to in this athletic context as self-regulation), athletes have used biofeedback to assist them with establishing better control of a variety of physiologic processes. Biofeedback applications have ranged from hand-warming techniques for cross-country skiers and mountain climbers to the regulation of heartbeat for sharpshooters (such as biathletes and archers) to the lowering of adrenaline levels for ice-skaters, gymnasts, and divers.

THE ACCEPTANCE OF BIOFEEDBACK

The evolution of biofeedback as a treatment modality has its historical roots in early research in the areas of learning theory, psychophysiology, behavior modification, stress reactivity, electronics technology, and biomedical engineering. The emerging awareness—and acceptance by the general public—that individuals do in fact have the potential to promote their own wellness and to facilitate the healing process gave additional impetus to the development of both the theory and the technology of biofeedback treatment. Several other factors have combined to produce the climate within which biofeedback has gained recognition and acceptance. One of these was widespread recognition that many of the disorders that afflict humankind today have, as a common basis, some disruption of the natural feedback processes. Part of this recognition is attributable to the seminal work of Hans Selye on stress reactivity.

Developments in the fields of electronics, physiology, psychology, endocrinology, and learning theory produced a body of knowledge which spawned the evolution and growth of biofeedback. Further refinement and an explosion of technology have resulted in procedures and techniques that have set the stage for the use of biofeedback as an effective intervention with wide applications in the treatment of numerous disorders.

The practice of biofeedback has extended to a number of disciplines. Included in the membership of the Association of Applied Psychophysiology and Biofeedback (formerly the Biofeedback Society of America) are representatives from the fields of medicine, psychology, physical therapy, social work, occupational therapy, and chiropractic.

—*Ronald B. France*

See also Alternative medicine; Asthma; Attention-deficit disorder (ADD); Cardiac rehabilitation; Exercise; Headaches; Heart attacks; Hypertension; Hypnosis; Meditation; Pain management; Physical rehabilitation; Preventive medicine; Sleep disorders; Stress.

For Further Information:

Basmajian, John V., ed. *Biofeedback: Principles and Practice for Clinicians.* 3d ed. Baltimore: Williams & Wilkins, 1989. A collection of writings dealing with the uses of biofeedback for various disorders. This work contains chapters on instrumentation and theory as well.

Olton, David S., and Aaron R. Noonberg. *Biofeedback: Clinical Applications in Behavioral Medicine.* Englewood Cliffs, N.J.: Prentice Hall, 1980. A practical overview of the applicability of biofeedback in the practice of behavioral medicine. This reference contains a basic overview of the development of biofeedback, as well as fundamental clinical applications in the treatment of various disorders.

Robbins, Jim. *A Symphony in the Brain: The Evolution of the New Brain Wave Biofeedback.* New York: Atlantic Monthly Press, 2000. This work discusses brain-wave biofeedback (or neurofeedback), in which an electroencephalograph measures brain waves, and patients are trained to control them consciously. Robbins interviews many key researchers for this book.

Schwartz, Mark S. *Biofeedback: A Practitioner's Guide.* 2d ed. New York: Guilford Press, 1995. One of the more recent references in the field of biofeedback. The chapters contain updated information concerning the fundamentals of and (as of 1987) state-of-the-art methodologies concerning biofeedback.

Schwartz, Mark S., and Les Fehmi. *Applications Standards and Guidelines for Providers of Biofeedback Services.* Wheatridge, Colo.: Biofeedback Society of America, 1982. A statement of the professional and ethical foundations for the practice of biofeedback. An important reference for anyone considering the employment of biofeedback in a clinical setting.

✧ BIRTH CONTROL AND FAMILY PLANNING

Type of issue: Public health, women's health

Definition: The use of various methods to choose if and when conception will take place, and subsequently the number of children.

Without the ability to determine if they will bear children, women lack self-determination; thus access to safe and reliable birth control and family planning are essential elements in improving their status.

Throughout history, societies have sought to control human fertility. In traditionally agricultural areas, where children represent a source of potential labor and care for aged parents, desired family size has been larger, especially when infant and childhood mortality rates remain high. By contrast, in modern industrialized and urbanized countries where childhood mortality is low and education extends into early adulthood, desired family size is smaller.

METHODS OF BIRTH CONTROL

One way that societies affect the size of families is by encouraging either early or late marriages. Another is by persuading mothers to nurse their infants for extended periods of time; this is not a reliable method of birth control on an individual basis but does lower fertility for groups as a whole. The banning of conjugal relations between spouses during certain times also reduces birthrates. In the United States in the nineteenth century, for example, many couples confined intercourse to a period when they believed women were infertile. This method had limited value, because doctors lacked a clear understanding of the human fertility cycle until 1924. Some couples still use a similar technique, known as the rhythm method, based on careful monitoring of a woman's menstrual cycle and variations in her body temperature. Whatever the success of individual couples, any method that incorporates periods of abstinence lowers the overall birthrate. Finally, many so-

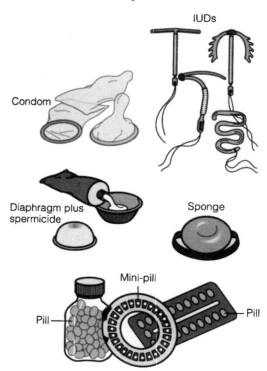

Many different kinds of devices have been designed to prevent pregnancy, from barrier methods such as condoms and diaphragms to hormonal methods such as birth control pills. Each method has its own advantages and disadvantages, and failure rates. (Hans & Cassidy, Inc.)

cieties have resorted to abortion and infanticide when other methods of birth control have failed.

One common form of birth control has been the use of contraception in an attempt to prevent conception in the first place. Perhaps the most widely used method prior to the twentieth century has been male withdrawal before ejaculation, or coitus interruptus. Women, however, often relied on barrier methods such as pessaries, instruments or suppositories placed in the vagina to prevent impregnation. These were more effective when combined with ingredients such as the tips of the acacia shrub. This is a source of lactic acid, an ingredient used in many modern spermicides. Less common until the nineteenth century were douches after intercourse to prevent impregnation.

Although men in primitive tribes sometimes wore sheaths over their penises, scholars believe these served as protection or decoration. By the sixteenth century, however, European men were using the condom, made of silk or from animal bladders or intestines, to prevent the spread of venereal disease. Despite their contraceptive value, these devices were not widely used because they were expensive. By the mid-nineteenth century, the vulcanization of rubber allowed manufacturers to produce condoms at reasonable prices.

Throughout history, individuals have turned to sterilization to prevent conception, a method that is still widely used. Thus, excluding the hormone suppressors developed in the latter part of the twentieth century, the major forms of contraception are centuries old.

THE FIGHT FOR BIRTH CONTROL IN NORTH AMERICA

In North America, the dissemination of birth control information has a controversial history. The U.S. Congress passed a law in 1873 barring the distribution of all matter termed "obscene, lewd, [or] lascivious." Known as the Comstock Law, it had been suggested by Anthony Comstock (1844-1915) and his followers, who feared that urban environments were corrupting youths. They also believed that middle-class women were bearing too few children, and, given the rising tide of immigration from Central and Eastern Europe, the older "Yankee stock" was seen as facing "race suicide." Because of the Comstock Law, any person seeking to mail information about birth control or abortion faced stiff fines and prison sentences. Twenty-two states passed "little Comstock Laws," among them Connecticut. Its 1879 law forbade the use of contraceptive devices and penalized anyone, including physicians, who supplied such devices. In 1892, Canada modified its criminal code by forbidding the dissemination of birth control information, a ban that was not lifted until 1969.

Nevertheless, during the latter decades of the nineteenth century, the Voluntary Motherhood movement came into being, made up of free-love advocates, moral reformers warring against prostitution, and suffragists concerned with raising the status of women. The conviction that wives, as childbearers, had the right to determine when a couple would engage in conjugal relations tied this group together. While Voluntary Motherhood marked the beginning of a true birth control movement in the United States, it opposed contraception. Its adherents believed that separating sexual relations from procreation would expose women to greater exploitation.

Margaret Sanger (1879-1966) initiated the next stage in the drive for freer dissemination of contraceptive information. Sanger, who coined the phrase "birth control," challenged the Comstock Law directly through articles on sexuality in the socialist newspaper, *The Call,* and her own journal, *The Woman Rebel.* Finally, her pamphlet *Family Limitation,* containing explicit information on birth control methods and techniques, led to her arrest in 1914.

After a preliminary hearing, Sanger fled to Europe where she learned the technique of fitting women with diaphragms in Dutch clinics. When she returned to the United States, the groundswell of support for her cause led the government to drop its case against her. New charges were brought after she opened a clinic in Brooklyn. The New York Court of Appeals upheld her conviction in 1918 but affirmed the right of physicians to give contraceptive advice or devices for preventing disease to married persons where not specifically forbidden by law. In the past, doctors had given such information only to men, but now women could also receive it. Many physicians were willing to extend the idea of preventing disease to preventing pregnancy, especially if they were serving middle- and upper-class patients.

When the United States entered World War I, the military, seeking to reduce the incidence of venereal disease, issued condoms for the first time. Afterward, many veterans introduced their wives to contraceptive methods. Nevertheless, by 1930, many poorer women still lacked access to birth control information. During the Great Depression, social workers and health care professionals championed birth control as a way of aiding families on relief. States, beginning with North Carolina, staffed their own clinics, and a 1936 Gallup Poll found that most Americans favored allowing physicians to dispense information on contraception. Similar changes occurred in Canada in this period. In 1942, an organization that Sanger had founded in 1921 to promote greater acceptance of birth control became the Planned Parenthood Federation of America. As the new name suggested, many now saw birth control as a way for couples to space children and achieve their optimum family size. By giving women the power to limit their families, the organization helped lay the foundation for a revived women's movement.

In 1965, the Supreme Court of the United States, in *Griswold v. Connecticut,* overturned the state's "little Comstock Law," passed almost a century earlier. The Court ruled that married couples enjoyed a right to privacy that included access to birth control. Seven years later, in *Eisenstadt v. Baird*, the Court, invoking the same right of privacy, extended similar access to unmarried couples.

The appearance in 1960 of Enovid-10, the first pill that suppressed ovulation, gave women a more effective means of preventing pregnancy while allowing them to separate contraception from sexual intercourse itself. Many women experienced disturbing side effects from the birth control pill, however, including weight gain, rashes, nausea, bloating, and cardiovascular problems. Barbara Seaman, in *The Doctor's Case Against the Pill* (1969), publicized these problems, and a reenergized women's movement pressured the drug companies to manufacture a safer pill. The pharmaceutical companies complied by lowering the dosage of estrogen and progestin, but many women have continued to harbor health concerns about the pill and its long-term usage.

Other birth control methods that initially were promising have since proved problematical. The intrauterine device (IUD), which is inserted into a woman's uterus in order to prevent impregnation, caused serious physical problems for many women, and some types were taken off the market in the United States. Depo-Provera is a synthetic progesterone that prevents pregnancy for several months through injections. Collaboration between a Finnish pharmaceutical company and the nonprofit Population Council resulted in Norplant, a contraceptive implant that releases hormones over time. Although all these methods are highly effective in preventing pregnancy, there are questions about their long-term effects on health.

CONTINUING PROBLEMS AND PROSPECTS

At the beginning of the twenty-first century, many women still relied on the older barrier methods, such as improved diaphragms, cervical caps, spermicides, and even a female condom. These methods are considered to be safer than hormonal treatments but are not as effective. It is not surprising that about half of all unplanned pregnancies occur among women who are using birth control. In that light, the development of RU-486 (first manufactured by the French firm Roussell Uclaf) is germane. It has been used in Europe since 1982 as a way of terminating early pregnancy, and it was finally approved for use in the United States in 2000. RU-486 functions by blocking the body's production of progesterone, the hormone that prepares the uterus to accept the fertilized egg. Other researchers are working on vaccines to cause immune system reactions that would prevent fertilization from occurring in the first place.

Although more governmental and private resources are needed to develop new forms of contraception, technology is only part of the answer. Women usually attain a large measure of control over reproduction only after society has achieved certain necessary preconditions. These include lessening poverty, so individuals gain hope that the future can be different from the past; decreases in infant and childhood mortality; greater educational opportunities for women; and improvements in the status of women so they have chances for achievement beyond the bearing of children.

—Shirley A. Leckie

See also Abortion; Abortion among teenagers; Condoms; Infertility in men; Infertility in women; Morning-after pill; Pregnancy among teenagers; Prenatal care; Sexual dysfunction; Sexually transmitted diseases (STDs).

FOR FURTHER INFORMATION:

Chesler, Ellen. *Woman of Valor: Margaret Sanger and the Birth Control Movement in America.* New York: Simon & Schuster, 1992. This exhaustively researched biography brings this strong-willed birth control pioneer vividly to life, along with the individuals and movements that influenced her work.

Garrow, David J. *Liberty and Sexuality: The Right to Privacy and the Making of "Roe v. Wade."* New York: Macmillan, 1994. More than the title indicates, this prodigiously researched work is invaluable for tracing the fight for reproductive freedom in the United States.

Gordon, Linda. *Woman's Body, Woman's Right: Birth Control in America.* New York: Penguin Books, 1990. Revised and updated edition of Gordon's 1976 work, it places birth control in the context of social history.

Hatcher, Robert A., et al. *Contraceptive Technology.* 17th ed. New York: Irvington, 1998. This frequently revised book offers a thorough and readable discussion of most aspects of contraception.

McLaren, Angus, and Arlene Tigar McLaren. *The Bedroom and the State: The Changing Practices and Politics of Contraception and Abortion in Canada, 1880-1980.* Toronto: McClelland and Stewart, 1986. A valuable overview on the fight for reproductive freedom in Canada.

❖ BIRTH DEFECTS

Type of issue: Children's health, mental health

Definition: Congenital malformations or structural anomalies and their accompanying functional disorders which originate during embryonic development; they are involved in up to 6 percent of human live births.

As the human embryo develops, it undergoes many formative stages from the simple to the complex, most often culminating in a perfectly formed newborn infant. The formation of the embryo is controlled by both genetic factors and interactions between the various embryonic tissues. Because the genes play a vital role as the blueprint for the developing embryo, they must be accurate and the cellular mechanisms that allow the genes to be expressed must also work correctly. In addition, the chemical and physical communications between cells and tissues in the embryo must be clear and uninterrupted. The development of the human embryo into a newborn infant is infinitely more complex than the design and assembly of the most powerful supercomputer or the largest skyscraper. Because of this complexity and the fact that development progresses without supervision by human eye or hand, there are many opportunities for errors that can lead to malformations.

Errors in development can be caused by both genetic and environmental factors. Genetic factors include chromosomal abnormalities and gene mutations. Both can be inherited from the parents or can occur spontaneously during gamete formation, fertilization, and embryonic development. Environmental factors, called teratogens, include such things as drugs, disease organisms, and radiation.

Chromosomal abnormalities account for about 6 percent of human congenital malformations. They fall into two categories, numerical and structural. Numerical chromosomal abnormalities are most often the result of nondisjunction occurring in the germ cells that form sperm and eggs. During the cell division process in sperm and egg production deoxyribonucleic acid (DNA) is duplicated so that each new cell receives a complete set of chromosomes. Occasionally, two chromosomes fail to separate (nondisjunction), such that one of the new cells receives two copies of that chromosome and the other cell none. Both of the resulting gametes (either sperm or eggs) will have an abnormal number of chromosomes. When a gamete with an abnormal number of chromosomes unites with a normal gamete, the result is an individual with an abnormal chromosome number. The missing or extra chromosome will cause confusion in the developmental process and result in certain structural and functional abnormalities. For example, persons with an extra copy of chromosome number 21 suffer from Down syndrome, which often includes mental deficiency, heart defects, facial deformities, and other symptoms. Abnormal chromosome numbers may also result from an egg's being fertilized by two sperm, failure of cell division during gamete formation, and nondisjunction in one or more cells of the early embryo.

Structural chromosomal abnormalities result from chromosome breaks. Breaks occur in chromosomes during normal exchanges in material between chromosomes (crossing over). They also may occur accidentally at weak points on the chromosomes, called fragile sites, and can be induced by chemicals and radiation. Translocations occur when a broken-off piece of chromosome attaches to another chromosome. For example, an individual who has the two usual copies of chromosome 21 and, as the result of a translocation, carries another partial or complete copy of 21 riding piggyback on another chromosome will have the symptoms of Down syndrome. Deletions occur when a chromosome break causes the loss of part of a chromosome. The cri du chat syndrome is caused by the loss of a portion of chromosome number 5. Infants affected by this disorder have a catlike cry, are mentally retarded, and have cardiovascular defects. Other structural chromosomal abnormalities include inversions (in which segments of chromosomes are attached in reverse order), duplications (in which portions of a chromosome are present in multiple copies), and isochromosomes (in which chromosomes separate improperly to produce the wrong configuration).

MUTATIONS

Gene mutations (defective genes) are responsible for about 8 percent of birth defects. Mutations in genes occur spontaneously because of copying errors or can be induced by environmental factors such as chemicals and radiation. The mutant genes are passed from parents to offspring; thus certain defects may be present in specific families and geographical locations. Two examples of mutation-caused defects are polydactyly (the presence of extra fingers or toes) and microcephaly (an unusually small cranium and brain).

Mutations can be either dominant or recessive. If one of the parents possesses a dominant mutation, there will be a 50 percent chance of this mutant gene being transmitted to the offspring. Brachydactyly, or abnormal shortening of the fingers, is a dominantly inherited trait. Normally, the parent with the dominant gene also has the disorder. Recessive mutations can remain hidden or unexpressed in both parents. When both parents possess the recessive gene, there is a 25 percent chance that any given pregnancy will result in a child with a defect. Examples of recessive defects are the metabolic disorders sickle-cell anemia and hemophilia.

ENVIRONMENTAL FACTORS

Environmental factors called teratogens are responsible for about 7 percent of congenital malformations. Human embryos are most sensitive to the effects of teratogens during the period when most organs are forming (organogenetic period), that is, from about fifteen to sixty days after fertilization. Teratogens may interfere with development in a number of ways, usually by killing embryonic cells or interrupting their normal function. Cell movement, communication, recognition, differentiation, division, and adhesion are critical to development and can be easily disturbed by teratogens. Teratogens can also cause mutations and chromosomal abnormalities in embryonic cells. Even if the disturbance is only weak and transitory, it can have serious effects because the critical period for development of certain structures is very short and well defined. For example, the critical period for arm development is from twenty-four to forty-four days after fertilization. A chemical that interferes with limb development such as the drug thalidomide, if taken during this period, may cause missing arm parts, shortened arms, or complete absence of arms. Many drugs and chemicals have been identified as teratogenic, including alcohol, aspirin, and certain antibiotics.

Other environmental factors that can cause congenital malformations include infectious organisms, radiation, and mechanical pressures exerted on the fetus within the uterus. Certain infectious agents or their products can pass from the mother through the placenta into the embryo. Infection of the embryo causes disturbances to development similar to those caused by chemical teratogens. For example, German measles (rubella virus) causes cataracts, deafness, and heart defects if the embryo is infected early in development. Exposure to large doses of radiation can result in death and damage to embryonic cells. Diagnostic X rays are not known to be a cause of birth defects. Some defects such as hip dislocation may be caused by mechanical forces inside the uterus; this could happen if the amnion is damaged or the uterus is malformed, thus restricting the movement of the fetus. About 25 percent of congenital defects are caused by the interaction of genetic and environmental factors (multifactorial), and the causes of more than half (54 percent) of all defects are unknown.

PREVENTING BIRTH DEFECTS

Because many birth defects have well-defined genetic and environmental causes, they often can be prevented. Preventive measures need to be implemented if the risk of producing a child with a birth defect is higher than average. Genetic risk factors for such defects include the presence of a genetic defect in one of the parents, a family history of genetic defects, the existence of one or more children with defects, consanguineous (same-family) matings, and advanced maternal age. Prospective parents with one or more of these risk factors should seek genetic counseling in order to assess their potential for producing a baby with such defects. Also, parents exposed to higher-than-normal levels of drugs, alcohol, chemicals, or radiation are at risk of producing gametes that may cause defects, and pregnant women exposed to the same agents place the developing embryo at risk. Again, medical counseling should be sought by such prospective parents.

Pregnant women should maintain a well-balanced diet that is about 200 calories higher than normal to provide adequate fetal nutrition. Women who become anemic during pregnancy may need an iron supplement, and the U.S. Public Health Service recommends that all women of childbearing age consume 0.4 milligram of folic acid (one of the B vitamins) per day to reduce the risk of spina bifida and other neural tube defects. Women at high risk for producing genetically defective offspring can undergo a screening technique whereby eggs taken from the ovary are screened in the laboratory prior to in vitro fertilization and then returned to the uterus. Some couples may decide to use artificial insemination by donor if the prospective father is known to carry a defective gene.

Detecting Birth Defects

The early detection of birth defects is crucial to the health of both the mother and the baby. Physicians commonly use three methods for monitoring fetal growth and development during pregnancy. The most common method is ultrasound scanning. High-frequency sound waves are directed at the uterus and then monitored for waves that bounce back from the fetus. The return waves allow a picture of the fetus to be formed on a television monitor, which can be used to detect defects and evaluate the growth of the fetus.

In amniocentesis, the doctor withdraws a small amount of amniotic fluid containing fetal cells; both the fluid and the cells can be tested for evidence of congenital defects. Amniocentesis generally cannot be performed until the sixteenth week of pregnancy.

Another method of obtaining embryonic cells is called chorionic villus sampling and can be done as early as the fifth week of pregnancy. A tube is inserted into the uterus in order to retrieve a small sample of placental chorionic villus cells, identical genetically to the embryo. Again, these cells can be tested for evidence of congenital defects. The early discovery of fetal defects and other fetal-maternal irregularities allows the physician time to assess the problem and make recommendations to the parents regarding treatment. Many problems can be solved with therapy, medications, and even prenatal surgery. If severe defects are detected, the physician may recommend termination of the pregnancy.

Treating Birth Defects

Children born with defects often require highly specialized and intense medical treatment. For example, a child born with spina bifida may have lower-body paralysis, clubfoot, hip dislocation, and gastrointestinal and genitourinary problems in addition to the spinal column deformity. Spina bifida occurs when the embryonic neural tube and vertebral column fail to close properly in the lower back, often resulting in a protruding sac containing parts of the spinal meninges and spinal cord. The malformation and displacement of these structures result in nerve damage to the lower body, causing paralysis and the loss of some neural function in the organs of this area.

Diagnostic procedures including X rays, computed tomography (CT) scans, and urinalysis are carried out to determine the extent of the disorder. If the sac is damaged and begins to leak cerebrospinal fluid, it needs to be closed immediately to reduce the risk of meningitis. In any case, surgery is done to close the opening in the lower spine, but it is not possible to correct the damage done to the nerves. Urgent attention must also be given to the urinary system. The paralysis often causes loss of sphincter muscle control in the urinary bladder and rectum. With respect to the urinary system, this lack of control can lead to serious urinary tract infections and the loss of kidney function. Both infections and obstructions must be treated promptly to avoid serious complication. Orthopedic care needs to begin early to treat clubfoot, hip dislocation, scoliosis, muscle weakness, spasms, and other side effects of this disorder.

The medical treatment of birth defects requires a carefully orchestrated team approach involving physicians and specialists from various medical fields. When the abnormality is discovered (before birth, at birth, or after birth), the primary physician will gather as much information as possible from the family history, the medical history of the patient, a physical examination, and other diagnostic tests. This information is interpreted in consultation with other physicians in order to classify the disorder properly and to determine its possible origin and time of occurrence. This approach may lead to the discovery of other malformations, which will be classified as primary and secondary. When the physician arrives at a specific overall diagnosis, he or she will counsel the parents about the possible causes and development of the disorder, the recommended treatment and its possible outcomes, and the risk of recurrence in a subsequent pregnancy. Certain acute conditions may require immediate attention in order to save the life of the newborn.

In addition to treating the infant with the defect, the physician needs to counsel the parents in order to answer their questions. The counseling process will help them to understand and accept their child's condition. In order to promote good parent-infant bonding, the parents are encouraged to maintain close contact with the infant and participate in its care. Children born with severe chronic disabilities and their families require special support. When parents are informed that their child has limiting congenital malformations, they may react negatively and express feelings of shock, grief, and guilt. Medical professionals can help the parents deal with their feelings and encourage them to develop a close and supportive relationship with their child. Physicians can provide a factual and honest appraisal of the infant's condition and discuss treatments, possible outcomes, and the potential for the child to live a happy and fulfilling life. Parents are encouraged to learn more about their child's disorder and to seek the guidance and help of professionals, support groups, family, and friends. With the proper care and home environment, the child can develop into an individual who is able to interact positively with family and community.

—*Rodney C. Mowbray*

See also Amniocentesis; Childbirth complications; Cleft lip and palate; Diabetes mellitus; Disabilities; Down syndrome; Fetal alcohol syndrome; Gene therapy; Genetic counseling; Genetic diseases; Health problems and families; Hydrocephalus; Mental retardation; Phenylketonuria (PKU); Premature birth; Screening; Spina bifida.

FOR FURTHER INFORMATION:

Bloom, Beth-Ann, and Edward Seljeskog. *A Parent's Guide to Spina Bifida.* Minneapolis: University of Minnesota Press, 1988. Designed to assist the parents of children with spina bifida. The book includes chapters on the nature of the disorder and how it is treated, the medical problems associated with spina bifida, and how to help the afflicted child while he or she is growing up. Also includes a useful glossary, a list of organizations and support groups, and an extensive bibliography.

Moore, Keith L., and T. V. N. Persaud. *The Developing Human.* 6th ed. Philadelphia: W. B. Saunders, 1998. An outstanding textbook on human embryonic development. Chapter 8 deals specifically with the causes of congenital malformations, and several other chapters include more detailed information about common defects occurring in each of the body's systems. The book is easy to understand and well illustrated.

Nixon, Harold, and Barry O'Donnel. *The Essentials of Pediatric Surgery.* 4th ed. Boston: Butterworth Heinemann, 1992. Describes in laypersons' terms the surgical treatment of many congenital abnormalities, including birth injuries, imperforate anus, spina bifida, hydrocephalus, pyloric stenosis, birthmarks, cleft lip and palate, hernias, urinary and digestive tract deformities, undescended testis, intersex problems, limb malformations, and congenital heart disease. The book is well illustrated with descriptive line diagrams and includes a thorough discussion of each procedure.

Stray-Gundersen, Karen, ed. *Babies with Down Syndrome.* Kensington, Md.: Woodbine House, 1986. A complete guide for parents with a Down syndrome child, written by doctors, nurses, educators, lawyers, and parents. The book includes a complete medical description of the disorder and extensive coverage of care concerns, child development, education, and legal rights. Contains an extensive glossary, reading list, and resource guide.

Warkany, Josef, Ronald J. Lemire, and Michael Cohen. *Mental Retardation and Congenital Malformations of the Central Nervous System.* Chicago: Year Book Medical Publishers, 1981. A medical reference book that gives complete descriptions of congenital malformations of the nervous system and their effects on the eyes, ears, heart, skeleton, and skin. The authors also include a thorough discussion of congenitally caused mental illness. The book is technical in nature but informative and authoritative. Well illustrated; includes extensive listings of technical articles.

✧ BREAST CANCER

Type of issue: Women's health
Definition: The growth of abnormal cells in the breast, which can spread throughout the body and prevent organs from functioning normally.

It is estimated that one in eight women in the United States will develop breast cancer during her lifetime. Each year, approximately 175,000 new cases of breast cancer are diagnosed, and about 45,000 women die of the disease annually. Although genetic predisposition plays a role in the development of cancer, as many as 80 percent of the women who get the disease have no known risk factor (such as early onset of puberty, having a mother or sister with the disease, or not having given birth before age thirty). Breast cancer is a common cancer in women.

Cancer is caused when normal cells become abnormal and begin to grow out of control. The abnormal cells can spread throughout the body and prevent organs from functioning normally. Breast cancer itself is not fatal; only cancer that has spread outside the breast (to the bones, liver, or brain, for example) can kill.

TYPES AND STAGING

The most common type of breast cancer, about 86 percent of all cases, begins in the drainage ducts of the mammary glands (ductal carcinoma); 12 percent of breast cancers are lobular, meaning they begin in the breast lobules (milk glands). The remainder begin in surrounding tissues. Cancer can also be described as "infiltrating" or "invasive," meaning it has traveled into surrounding tissue from its original site.

Invasive breast cancer is graded from stages 1 to 4 in order to assess treatment possibilities. A number of tests are performed to determine the stage of the disease: chest X rays, blood tests, and a variety of scans (usually of the bones, liver, lungs, and brain). Tumor size, skin swelling, whether the cancer has spread to lymph nodes (lymph node involvement), and results of such tests as hormone receptors and flow cytometry are also considered. Because of more extensive use of mammograms and breast self-examination (BSE), most cancers found are stage 1 or 2, which respond best to treatment.

Stage 1 is a tumor up to two centimeters in size with no lymph node involvement, while stage 2 is a tumor between two and five centimeters with or without lymph node involvement or a tumor larger than five centimeters with no lymph node involvement. Stage 3 cancers have a large (more than five centimeters) tumor with lymph node involvement, and stage 4 describes a tumor that has metastasized, or spread to distant sites in the body (most commonly the liver, lungs, bones, or brain). Breast cancer is detected in several ways: through mammography, needle biopsy (the insertion of a needle to draw out fluid or tissue), and surgical biopsy (the removal of some of the tissue of the breast).

Treatment and Prognoses

Local and systemic treatments are most commonly prescribed for breast cancer. Surgery, including mastectomy and lumpectomy, is generally the first treatment, though research on chemotherapy and/or radiation before surgery continues. Modified radical mastectomy has become the most common treatment for early-stage breast cancer, though an increased number of women opt for lumpectomy, with or without follow-up radiation and chemotherapy. Surgery is used to remove the cancer from the breast; most of the time, underarm lymph nodes are removed and examined to determine whether the disease has spread. Lymph node involvement generally means that radiation and/or chemotherapy are recommended.

Radiation therapy uses high-energy X rays to kill cancer cells; radiation can be given externally by a machine or internally through implants. Chemotherapy, a systemic treatment (able to kill cancer cells outside the breast area) is given by injection, through pills, or both. Hormone therapy can include the use of drugs such as tamoxifen or the removal of hormone-making organs. The aim of adjuvant therapies such as these is to kill any cancer cells that remain after surgery.

Immunotherapy, or biological therapy, was under investigation in clinical trials in the mid-1990's; it uses materials to heighten the body's natural defenses against disease. High-dose chemotherapy followed by bone marrow transplantation (necessary because the chemotherapy destroys the body's bone marrow) has also undergone testing as a new treatment. Complementary treatments can include visualization, diet, exercise, meditation, or alternative therapies and are often used in hopes of strengthening the immune system in its fight against cancer.

Prognoses for breast cancer vary greatly depending on the cancer's stage at detection, the treatment options chosen, and the individual patient. Of stage 1 patients, 85 percent were still alive five years after diagnosis, as opposed to 66 percent of stage 2 patients, 41 percent of stage 3 patients, and 10 percent of stage 4 patients. Mortality rates are difficult to estimate because of constant updating and are highly dependent on a number of variables. Sources tend to disagree given that most survival statistics were compiled before chemotherapy became commonly prescribed as a postsurgery treatment. The most accurate information available suggests very good survival rates for stage 1 and 2 patients, and survival rates for all stages improve over time.

In the United States, for many years the standard treatment was to perform a biopsy, followed immediately by a radical mastectomy if the biopsy results showed cancer. For most of the twentieth century, radical mastectomy, which removes the entire breast, underlying muscles, and lymph nodes, was performed (in more than 90 percent of cases in 1960). This procedure finally began to be questioned, and in Canada and England, surgeons began to perform far less radical procedures. In 1979, the National Cancer Institute (NCI) recommended that the biopsy and follow-up surgery be performed separately, so that women could discuss treatment options and decide on the best course of action to follow. The NCI also declared that radical mastectomy should no longer be the treatment of choice for breast cancer.

The courage of several prominent women who "went public" with their breast cancer played a major role in women's advocacy about the disease and led to widespread questioning of traditional methods of treatment, as well as a dramatic increase in the number of women having mammograms and performing BSE. Many women opt for lumpectomy, usually followed by chemotherapy and/or radiation, in order to preserve their breasts. Numerous studies have shown that survival rates are nearly identical for lumpectomy and mastectomy; in Canada and Europe, statistics show that they have equivalent survival rates for twenty-five years past diagnosis. Increasingly, women are taking a strong role in their treatment: They obtain second and third opinions, assimilate all available information, and make informed decisions.

EMOTIONAL IMPACT

Women's reactions to a diagnosis of breast cancer vary greatly. Some suggest that a woman's first concern is often cosmetic—the possible loss of a breast and the effects of chemotherapy and/or radiation on appearance—whereas others note that a cancer diagnosis is devastating regardless of the area of the body affected. It is certain that rising awareness of breast cancer and support groups for cancer survivors have lessened the stigma of the disease and much of the fear, shame, and isolation felt by breast cancer patients.

Society's stress on perfection of the female body and the Western emphasis on the breasts as an area of eroticism contribute greatly to women's worries about the physical effects of the disease. Losing a breast, or greatly changing its appearance, is one of the biggest fears women face and could be a factor in their apparent reluctance to perform BSE (fewer than 40 percent of women do so). A mastectomy or lumpectomy, by making a woman realize the seriousness of her disease, can also greatly change her self-image. Breast cancer patients often suffer doubts about how this change will affect the rest of their lives, especially regarding intimacy, lifestyle, and personal relationships. Many studies have shown that the attitude of a spouse during a partner's illness has a great impact on the partner's adjustment to the situation.

One of the most common concerns is how a woman's partner will react to her changed body after her surgery. Most sources agree that the specter of a life-threatening illness can have a dramatic impact on a relationship but that, for the most part, the changes are positive, resulting in heightened appreciation of each partner. Another concern springs from the changes in the body wrought by chemotherapy, radiation, and hormonal therapy: nausea, vomiting, hair loss, and mood changes. Hair loss in particular can be a traumatic event, again because of stereotyped ideas of the ideal woman in Western society. Programs such as Look Good, Feel Better, sponsored by the American Cancer Society, can help women deal with their changed appearance.

Many women wear a prosthesis, and increasing numbers have reconstructive surgery to restore their appearance. Although some women are reluctant to put themselves through another surgery, they see reconstruction as an essential step in their recovery, and an increasing number of options are available. Programs such as Reach to Recovery, a peer-visitor organization that provides information and support, and ENCORE, a national discussion and exercise program for breast cancer survivors sponsored by the Young Women's Christian Association (YWCA), are designed to help women cope with the feelings and physical effects of the disease. These programs and I Can Cope, sponsored by the American Cancer Society and the Y-Me National Organization for Breast Cancer Information and Support, emphasize the practical and emotional aspects of dealing with cancer. Breast cancer support groups are common in the United States and are often organized by cancer centers, hospitals, or social service agencies; they are usually led by a nurse or social worker and provide support for cancer survivors and, increasingly, their families. Many women, after facing treatment and recovery, feel the need to help others and join volunteer organizations.

Prevention and Awareness

Breast self-examination is recommended by most physicians to help women detect breast cancer. Many women's groups conduct seminars on this possibly lifesaving skill, given that 85 percent of lumps are found by women themselves. BSE has helped many women detect breast cancer in its early stages. Mammograms (X rays of the breast) are widely used and have been shown to reduce mortality by 30 to 50 percent in women over age fifty.

Research efforts have been aided by the Pink Ribbon Campaign, modeled on the awareness campaign on behalf of acquired immunodeficiency syndrome (AIDS). Wearing a pink ribbon represents awareness of breast cancer and activism for funding research. Sponsored by Avon, *Self* magazine, and other organizations, the Pink Ribbon Campaign has been joined by Race for the Cure, sponsored by the Susan G. Komen Breast Cancer Foundation and the National Alliance of Breast Cancer Organizations, both of which provide information and assistance to breast cancer patients and lobby for heightened public awareness of breast cancer.

—*Michelle L. Jones*

See also Breast surgery; Cancer; Cervical, ovarian, and uterine cancers; Chemotherapy; Hospice; Mammograms; Mastectomy; Pain management; Screening; Women's health issues.

FOR FURTHER INFORMATION:

Berger, Karen, and John Bostwick III. *A Woman's Decision: Breast Care, Treatment and Reconstruction*. 3d rev. ed. St. Louis: Quality Medical Publishing, 1998. Discusses various treatment options with regard to quality of life; combines physicians' perspectives with those of patients. Especially valuable is a section detailing surgical options for breast reconstruction.

Berman, Joel, ed. *Comprehensive Breast Care: Surviving Breast Cancer*. Boston: Branden Books, 2000. A popular work about breast cancer. Includes an index.

Davies, Kevin. *Breakthrough: The Race to Find the Breast Cancer Gene*. New York: John Wiley & Sons, 1996. Chronicles the search for BRCA1, the gene that appears to cause the inheritable form of breast cancer.

Higgins-Lee, Charlotte. *Surviving Breast Cancer*. Pittsburgh: Dorrance, 1997. Written by a psychologist who survived breast cancer. Using a composite client she names Charlie, Higgins-Lee illustrates her therapeutic method as she takes the reader through the emotional stages associated with breast cancer.

Love, Susan, with Karen Lindsey. *Dr. Susan Love's Breast Book*. 3d rev. ed. Reading, Mass.: Perseus Books, 2000. Written by a breast surgeon. A reliable and highly readable analysis of the physical, social, historical, and emotional aspects of breast cancer.

✧ BREAST-FEEDING

Type of issue: Children's health, social trends

Definition: The preferred feeding method for infants, providing optimal nutrition for the infant (including immunologic protection), mother-infant bonding, and enhanced maternal health.

The terms "breast-feeding," "nursing," and "lactation" all refer to the best-known method of infant feeding. Although there are a few rare exceptions, almost every mother can breast-feed and thereby provide low-cost, nutritional support for her infant. Although it is often thought otherwise, the size of the mother's breast has no relationship to successful lactation. In fact, the physiology of successful lactation is determined by the maturation of breast tissue, the initiation and maintenance of milk secretion, and the ejection or delivery of milk to the nipple. This physiology is dependent on hormonal control, and all women have the required anatomy for successful lactation unless they have had surgical alteration of the breast.

Breast and Milk Development

Hormonal influence on breast development begins in adolescence. Increased estrogen causes the breast ducts to elongate and duct cells to grow. (The ducts are narrow tubular vessels that run from the segments of the breast into the tip of the nipple.) More fibrous and fatty tissue develops, and the nipple area matures. As adolescence progresses, regular menstrual cycle hormones cause further development of the alveoli, which are the milk-producing cells.

The elevated levels of estrogen present during pregnancy promote the growth and branching of milk ducts, while the increase in progesterone promotes the development of alveoli. Throughout pregnancy and especially during the first three months, many more milk ducts are formed. Clusters of milk-producing cells also begin to enlarge, while at the same time placental hormones promote breast development.

Shortly before labor and delivery, the hormone prolactin is produced by the pituitary gland. Prolactin, which is necessary for starting lactation and sustaining milk production, reaches its peak at delivery. Another hormone, oxytocin, which is also produced by the pituitary, stimulates the breast to eject milk. This reaction is called the "let-down reflex," which causes the milk-producing alveoli to contract and force milk to the front of the breast. Oxytocin serves an important function after delivery by causing the uterus to contract. Initially, the let-down reflex occurs only when the infant suckles, but later on it may be initiated simply by the baby's cry. An efficient let-down reflex is critical to successful breast-feeding. Emotional upset, fatigue, pain, nervousness, or embarrassment about lactation can interrupt this reflex; these psychological factors, rather than breast size or physiology, are predictive of successful lactation.

The Nutritional Value of Breast Milk

Not only is breast-feeding a natural response to childbirth, but the nutrient content is tailor-made for the human infant as well. More than one hundred constituents of breast milk, both nutritive and nonnutritive, are known. Although the basic nutrient content is a solution of protein, sugar, and salts in which fat is suspended, those concentrations vary depending on the period of lactation and even within a given feeding.

Colostrum, often called "first milk," is produced in the first few days after birth. It is lower in fat and Calories (kilocalories) and higher in protein and certain minerals than is mature breast milk. Colostrum is opaque and yellow because it contains a high concentration of the vitamin A-like substances called carotenes. It also has a high concentration of antibodies and white blood cells, which pass on immunologic protection to the infant.

Within a few days after birth, the transition is made from colostrum to mature milk. There are two types of mature milk. Foremilk is released first as the infant begins to suckle. It has a watery, bluish appearance and is low in fat and rich in other nutrients. This milk accounts for about one-third of the baby's intake. As the nursing session progresses, the draught reflex helps move the hindmilk, with its higher fat content, to the front of the breast. It is important that the nutrient content of breast milk be determined from a sample of both types of milk in order to make an adequate assessment of all nutrients present.

Breast milk best meets the infant's needs and is the standard from which infant formulas are judged. Several nutrient characteristics make it the ideal infant food. Lactose, the carbohydrate content of breast milk, is the same simple sugar found in any milk, but the protein content of breast milk is uniquely tailored to meet infant needs. An infant's immature kidneys are better able to maintain water balance because breast milk is lower in protein than cow's milk. Most breast milk protein is alpha-lactalbumin, whereas cow's milk protein is casein. Alpha-lactalbumin is easier to digest and provides two sulphur-containing amino acids that are the building blocks of protein required for infant growth.

The fat (lipid) content of breast milk differs among women, and even from the same woman, from day to day. The types of fatty acids that make up most of the fat component of the milk may vary in response to maternal diet. Mothers fed a diet containing corn and cottonseed oil produce a milk with more polyunsaturated fatty acids, which are the predominant fatty acids in those oils. Breast milk is higher in the essential fatty acid called linoleic acid than is cow's milk, and it also contains omega-3 fatty acids. About 55 percent of human milk Calories come from fat, compared with about 49 percent of Calories found in infant formulas. In addition, enzymes in breast milk help digest fat in the infant's stomach. This digested fat is more efficiently absorbed than the products that result from digesting cow's milk.

Breast milk contains more cholesterol than cow's milk, which seems to stimulate development of the enzymes necessary for degrading cholesterol, perhaps offering protection against atherosclerosis in later life. Cholesterol is also needed for proper development of the central nervous system.

Vitamin and Mineral Content

The vitamin and mineral content of breast milk from healthy mothers supplies all that is needed for growth and health except for vitamin D and fluoride, and these are easily supplemented. Breast milk and the infant's intestinal bacteria also supply all the necessary vitamin K, but since no bacteria are present at birth, an injection of vitamin K should be given to prevent deficiencies.

Breast milk mineral content is balanced to promote growth while protecting the infant's immature kidneys. Breast milk has a low sodium content, which helps the immature kidneys to maintain water balance. No type of milk is a good source of iron. Although breast milk contains relatively small amounts of iron, about 50 percent of this iron can be absorbed by the body, compared with only 4 percent from cow's milk. This phenomenon is called bioavailability. Because of the high bioavailability of breast milk iron, the introduction of solids, which are given to replace depleted iron stores, can be delayed until six months of age in most infants; this delay may help to reduce the incidence of allergies in susceptible infants. There is also evidence that zinc is better absorbed from breast milk.

The vitamin content of milk can vary and is influenced by maternal vitamin status. The water-soluble vitamin content of breast milk (the B vitamins and vitamin C) will change more because of maternal diet than the fat-soluble vitamin content (vitamins A, E, and K). If women have diets that are deficient in vitamins, their levels in breast milk will be lower. Yet even malnourished mothers can breast-feed, although the quantity of milk is decreased. As the maternal diet improves, the level of water-soluble vitamins in the milk increases. There is a level, however, above which additional diet supplements will not increase the vitamin content of breast milk.

Nonnutritive Advantages of Breast-Feeding

There are many nonnutritive advantages to breast-feeding. A major advantage is the immunologic protection and resistance factors that it provides to the infant. Bifidus factors, found in both colostrum and mature milk, favor the growth of helpful bacteria in the infant's digestive tract. These bacteria in turn offer protection against harmful organisms. Lactoferrin, another resistance factor, binds iron so that harmful bacteria cannot use it. Lysozyme, lipases, and lactoperoxidases also offer protection against harmful bacteria.

Immunoglobulins are present in large amounts in colostrum and in significant amounts in breast milk. These protein compounds act as antibodies against foreign substances in the body called antigens. Generally, the resistance passed to the infant is from environmental antigens to which the mother had been exposed. The concentration of antibodies in colostrum is highest in the first hour after birth. Secretory IgA is the major immunoglobulin that provides protection against gastrointestinal organisms. Breast milk also contains interferon, an antiviral substance which is produced by special white blood cells in milk. Protection against allergy is another advantage of breast-feeding. It is not known, however, whether less exposure to the antigens found in formula or some substance in the breast milk itself provides this protection. Normally, a mucous barrier in the intestine prevents the absorption of whole proteins, the root of an allergic reaction. In the newborn, this barrier is not fully developed to allow whole immunologic proteins to be absorbed. The possibility that whole food proteins will be absorbed as well is greater if cow's milk or early solids are given, and this absorption increases the potential for allergic reactions.

Milk from mothers delivering preterm infants is higher in protein and nonprotein nitrogen, calcium, IgA, sodium, potassium, chloride, phosphorus, and magnesium. It also has a different fat composition and is lower in lactose than mature milk of mothers delivering after a normal term. These concentrations support more rapid growth of a preterm infant.

ADVANTAGES FOR THE MOTHER

Breast-feeding is not only good for the baby but also good for the mother. There is an association between reduced breast cancer rates and breast-feeding, although the reason is not known. In addition, the hormonal influences caused by suckling the infant help to contract the uterus, returning it to prepregnancy size and controlling blood loss. Breast-feeding also helps to reduce the mother's weight. Calories required to make milk are drawn from the fat stores that were deposited during pregnancy. Nevertheless, breast-feeding should be viewed not as a quick weight loss program but as a healthful, natural weight loss process.

If a woman breast-feeds completely, which means that no supplements or solid foods are given until the baby is six months of age, often she will not menstruate. Many women find this lack of menstrual periods psychologically pleasant while not realizing the physiological benefit of restoring the iron stores that were depleted during pregnancy and delivery. An important advantage to breast-feeding in developing countries is that it can help to space pregnancies naturally. Most infant malnutrition occurs when the second child is born, because breast-feeding is stopped for the first child. The first child is weaned to foods that do not supply enough nutrients. By spacing pregnancies out, the first child has a chance to nurse longer.

COMPLICATIONS AND DISORDERS

Some special problems or circumstances can make breast-feeding difficult. The breasts may become engorged—so full of milk that they are hard and sore—making it difficult for the baby to latch onto the nipple. Gentle massaging of the breasts, especially with warm water or a heating pad, will allow release of the milk and reduce pain in the breast. This situation is common during the first few weeks of nursing but will occasionally recur if a feeding is missed or a schedule changes.

Sometimes a duct will become plugged and form a hard lump. Massaging the lump and continuing to nurse will remedy the situation. If influenza-like symptoms accompany a plugged duct, the cause is probably a breast infection. Since the infection is in the tissue around the milk-producing glands, the milk itself is safe. The mother must apply heat, get plenty of rest, and keep emptying the breast by frequent feedings. Stopping nursing would plug the duct further, making the infection worse.

Of concern to many mothers are reports of contaminants in breast milk. Drugs, environmental pollutants, viruses, caffeine, alcohol, and food allergens can be passed to the infant through breast milk. Drug transmission depends on the administration method, which influences the speed with which it reaches the blood supply to the breast. Whether that drug can remain functional after it is subjected to the acid in the baby's digestive tract varies. Large amounts of caffeine in breast milk can produce a wakeful, hyperactive infant, but this situation is corrected when the mother stops her caffeine consumption. Large amounts of alcohol produce an altered facial appearance which is reversible; however, some psychomotor delay in the infant may remain even after the mother's drinking has stopped. Nicotine also enters milk, but the impact of secondhand smoke may pose more of a health threat than the nicotine content of breast milk. Since the human immunodeficiency virus (HIV), the virus that causes acquired immunodeficiency syndrome (AIDS), can also pass through breast milk, HIV-positive mothers should not breast-feed their infants.

Of greater concern is the presence of contaminants that cannot be avoided, such as pesticide residues, industrial waste, or other environmental contaminants. Polychlorinated biphenyls (PCBs) and the pesticide DDT have received the most attention. Long-term exposure to contaminants promotes their accumulation in the mother's body fat, and the production of breast milk is one way to rid the body of these contaminants. Concentrations present in the breast milk vary. Ordinarily, these substances are in such small quantities that they pose no health risk. Women who have consumed large amounts of fish from PCB-contaminated waters or have had occupational exposure to this chemical, however, need to have their breast milk tested. It is also possible for these substances to enter the infant's food supply from other sources.

There are very few instances in which a woman should not breast-feed her infant. Babies with a rare genetic disorder called galactosemia cannot nurse since they lack the enzyme to metabolize milk sugar. Phenylketonuria (PKU), another genetic disorder, requires close monitoring of the infant's blood phenylalanine level, but the infant can be totally or at least partially breast-fed. Breast-feeding is contraindicated for women suffering from AIDS, alcoholism, drug addiction, malaria, active tuberculosis, or a chronic disease that results in maternal malnutrition. The presence of other conditions, from diabetes to the common cold, are not reasons to avoid breast-feeding.

—Wendy L. Stuhldreher, R.D.

See also Children's health issues; Malnutrition among children; Nutrition and children; Nutrition and women; Phenylketonuria (PKU); Women's health issues.

FOR FURTHER INFORMATION:

Huggins, Kathleen. *The Nursing Mother's Companion.* 4th ed. Boston: Harvard Common Press, 1999. This personable book provides comprehensive information about breast-feeding. Topics include preparation, special situations, returning to work, and nursing the older infant.

Mason, Diane, and Diane Ingersoll. *Breastfeeding and the Working Mother.* Rev. ed. New York: St. Martin's Griffin, 1997. This book, written by women who have personal experience in the area, provides a host of practical tips for the working mother who wishes to breast-feed her baby. How-to basics as well as suggestions for practically every job situation are addressed.

Rolfes, Sharon Rady, and Linda Kelly DeBruyne. *Life Span Nutrition: Conception Through Life.* 2d ed. Edited by Eleanor Noss Whitney. St. Paul, Minn.: West, 1998. Chapter 5 of this textbook contains a comprehensive section on breast-feeding. Covers societal support, special medical conditions, physiology, the nutritional characteristics of breast milk, and the nutrient requirements for nursing mothers. An easy-to-read text with illustrations of the physiology of breast-feeding.

Stanway, Penny, and Andrew Stanway. *Breast Is Best.* Rev. ed. London: Pan Books, 1996. Written by two doctors who are also parents, this book provides practical, yet medically sound information about many aspects of breast-feeding. Chapters on etiquette, working, special situations, and readers' questions and answers cover issues not discussed in other books.

The Womanly Art of Breastfeeding. 5th rev. ed. Franklin Park, Ill.: La Leche League International, 1997. This bible of breast-feeding covers preparation, the advantages of breast-feeding, and how to overcome problems. This illustrated manual provides the most up-to-date, comprehensive information, supported by an advisory board of medical experts. A must-read for all nursing mothers.

✧ BREAST SURGERY

Type of issue: Medical procedures, social trends, women's health
Definition: Procedures performed for aesthetic enhancement of the breasts,

which may be undertaken on an elective basis, following surgery to correct defects resulting from a pathological process such as cancer, or to correct genetic deformities.

Breast augmentation, reduction, and reconstruction are procedures that are undertaken for different but related reasons. These procedures are almost always performed using general anesthesia. Augmentation procedures increase the size of breasts and are performed electively to correct hypomastia (abnormally small breasts). Reduction procedures decrease the size and shape of breasts. This is called reductive mammoplasty. Most commonly, reductions are performed on an elective basis for aesthetic reasons, but they can be indicated to relieve back, shoulder, and neck pain. Such abnormally large breast size is called mammary hyperplasia. Reconstruction involves the use of tissues from other parts of the body or prosthetic devices to restore a normal shape and contour.

Surgical Techniques

There are alternative sites for incisions to augment breasts. The site selected depends on the size and shape of the implant to be used. The safest surgical approach is from the underside of the breast (inframammary), with the incision being made in the skin fold formed by the bottom margin of the breast. A small scar will result. A second incision site is around the outer edge of the areola of the nipple (circumareolar). Scarring is minimal and hardly noticeable. A third approach is through an incision under the armpit (axillary). This leaves no scar on the breast but is technically more difficult.

The underlying pectoralis major muscle is separated from the fascia beneath it, creating a pocket for the implant. The implant is inserted and attached to adjacent tissue. The pocket is closed with sutures that will dissolve and do not have to be removed; the skin is carefully closed. The patient is seen approximately a week after surgery for a check-up and removal of any skin sutures.

Surgical reduction involves the removal of tissue. The amount and location of tissue to be removed depends on the initial size of the breast. Commonly, tissue is removed from the most dependent (lowest) portion of the breast. It is important to preserve the nipple and immediately underlying structures: the nerves and lactic ducts.

Vertical incisions are made in the underside of the breast. The excess tissue is removed, preserving the nipple, areola, nerves, and connecting ducts. A wedge-shaped portion of skin is also removed. After all bleeding is stopped, the remaining breast tissue is sutured together and the skin carefully closed. Care in closure and immediate postoperative activity will minimize scarring. The breast should be adequately supported, and stretching should be avoided for the first few weeks after surgery. The patient returns in a week so that the surgeon can monitor healing and remove skin sutures.

Reconstruction of breast tissue for reasons other than those described above is similar. In cases of trauma, damaged tissue is debrided, underlying tissues are replaced and sutured together, and the skin is carefully closed. The nipple, areola, and nerves are protected and preserved to the greatest extent possible. Skin closure may require assistance from a plastic surgeon to minimize scarring.

USES AND COMPLICATIONS

Breast surgery is useful to correct breast ptosis (sagging). Sagging occurs with normal aging and the influence of gravity. The extent and severity of this condition are functions of the size of the breast, the adequacy of undergarment support, and position of the nipple. With minimal ptosis, a prosthesis can be inserted to provide internal support. With severe ptosis, a combination of tissue removal and relocation of the nipple and areola are performed simultaneously. These procedures can usually be done using local anesthesia on an outpatient basis.

Two potential complications of all breast surgery are infection and scarring. Infections are infrequent but must be treated aggressively when they occur. If a prosthesis is involved, it is usually removed and reinserted three to six months later. Scarring is of concern because breast surgery is most often undertaken for cosmetic or aesthetic reasons. The placement of incisions along skin folds and careful skin closure help to minimize scarring. Restricting immediate postoperative activities, especially those that require stretching, also reduces untoward scarring.

Two potential problems exist with the use of prostheses: contracture and leakage. Contracture occurs when the tissue immediately surrounding the prosthesis shrinks and pulls the prosthesis out of position, detracting from the normal appearance of the breast. This condition formerly occurred in approximately 25 percent of cases but has been largely eliminated through the use of a textured outer envelope. Microscopic surface variations provide anchoring points for tissue and deter contracture formation. When both inner and outer envelopes rupture, the implant material can reach adjacent tissues. Silicone is irritating and can lead to the formation of nodules. Saline is now the material of choice for filling breast prostheses. Such leaks have received widespread attention in the media, but they are uncommon. In recent years, the legal climate has led to the virtual withdrawal of all silicone-based products from use in North America. Saline implants have been widely and safely used.

SOCIAL CONTEXTS OF BREAST SURGERY

With the exception of repairing the effects of unexpected trauma, most breast surgery is undertaken for cosmetic or aesthetic reasons. Individuals are influenced by those around them and by messages received from the media concerning what breast size and shape are desirable. Although these values change over time, it is more difficult to alter breast tissue. Aging plays a role. Supportive elements within tissues break down with age, resulting in unwanted but inevitable sagging of tissues.

Breast size, shape, and integrity are intimately related to feelings of self-worth and confidence. Reduction is indicated for massively oversized breasts. Augmentation is indicated in instances of pathology that require removal of a portion of breast tissue. Enlarging genetically small breasts is not a medical reason for augmentation.

—*L. Fleming Fallon, Jr., M.D., M.P.H.*

See also Aging; Breast cancer; Cancer; Cosmetic surgery and aging; Cosmetic surgery and women; Mammograms; Mastectomy; Women's health issues.

FOR FURTHER INFORMATION:

Ball, Adrian Shervington, and Peter M. Arnstein. *Handbook of Breast Surgery.* London: Edward Arnold, 1999. Provides a concise description of the full range of surgical procedures that constitute the practice of a specialist breast surgeon.

Bostwick, John. *Aesthetic and Reconstructive Breast Surgery.* St. Louis: Matthew Medical Books, 1990. This textbook presents an excellent discussion of cosmetic and reconstructive breast surgery.

Georgiade, Nicholas G., ed. *Aesthetic Breast Surgery.* 7th ed. Philadelphia: W. B. Saunders, 1990. This book describes procedures for cosmetic breast surgery. It is written by internationally recognized authorities and well illustrated.

Guthrie, Randolph, and Doug Podolsky. *The Truth About Breast Implants.* New York: John Wiley & Sons, 1994. This book helps to clear away the confusion and anxiety surrounding the silicone implant controversy. The author is a plastic surgeon who details the safest techniques now available to women, tells how to find the right doctor, and explains what women should expect at every step for both breast reconstruction and enlargement.

Stewart, Mary White. *Silicone Spills: Breast Implants on Trial.* Westport, Conn.: Praeger, 1998. Stewart details the experiences of women who suffered devastating, sometimes fatal consequences of silicone breast implants at the hands of doctors and manufacturers seeking monetary gain. Uses sources ranging from medical and court records to face-to-face interviews with survivors.

✧ BROKEN BONES IN THE ELDERLY

Type of issue: Elder health
Definition: A break in the continuity of a bone.

A fracture is a break in the continuity of a bone. Fractures can occur at any age, but there are certain causes and types of fractures that are more common in older people. Internal and external factors influence the development of a fracture. The internal factors include the strength of the bone and whether it is affected by disease. For example, osteoporosis, which is common in the elderly, makes the bone thin and fragile and more likely to break with minimal trauma. External factors include the type of trauma that occurs. In the elderly, falls are the major cause of trauma leading to fractures.

Fractures may be complete or incomplete. Complete fractures involve a break across the entire section of the bone. In incomplete fractures, the break occurs in only a part of the bone. Open, or compound, fractures involve a break in the bone as well as a break in the skin, with an increased risk of acquiring an infection in the wound. In closed, or simple, fractures, the bone is broken but does not pierce the skin. Fractures that occur with minimal but repeated stress on a bone, such as in running, are called stress fractures. Fractures that occur in diseased bones are referred to as "pathologic." Fractures are also named according to the bone affected, such as the femur (thigh bone), humerus (upper arm bone), or vertebra (back bone).

Broken bones begin to heal as soon as they are injured. Bleeding from the blood vessels inside the bone occurs first. Then a clot forms, which later develops into a callus. The callus serves as a bridge or framework in which new bone cells begin to develop. The length of time for complete healing varies with the age of the person and the type of bone injured. In general, older people take longer to heal.

FRACTURES IN OLDER ADULTS

Older people are at special risk for certain types of fractures, including those of the wrist, upper arm, and ankle. Hip fractures frequently occur as a result of injury caused by falls; complications may lead to additional problems and even death. The number of hip fractures that occur each year is expected to increase as the baby-boom population ages. Crush or compression fractures in the backbone may occur with minimal trauma and are related to weakening of the bone because of osteoporosis. The presence of osteoporosis increases the risk of fractures in women after the menopause, as well as in elderly men.

Many factors increase the risk of accidental injury in the elderly. Older adults with mental impairment or other health problems affecting their balance are more likely to fall. The chance of falls increases with the use of tranquilizers and medications to lower blood pressure, and also increases in people who are poorly nourished or do not exercise regularly. Decreases in both mobility and independence that accompany fractures lessen the individual's quality of life. The medical costs related to fractures measure in the billions of dollars each year.

Treatment of Fractures

Prompt recognition and treatment of a fracture increases the likelihood of a better outcome for healing. One of the most common signs of a broken bone is pain in the affected part. The ability to use the injured part may or may not be affected. If a bone in the arm or leg is broken, swelling will become noticeable in the painful area. The extremity may appear abnormal in shape or position because of the break in the normal alignment of the bone. Some fractures do not displace the bones, so the extremity may not appear abnormal except for swelling.

The immediate treatment of fractures involves measures to protect the injured part and person from further injury. If a fracture is suspected after a fall, the most important concern is to watch for signs of shock, including pale, cool, and moist skin. The person may become light-headed or may seem less alert. If these signs are present, it will be necessary to call for emergency assistance; the injured person should remain quiet and should not be moved.

A fractured body part should not be moved. Attempts to put the part back into normal position may cause further injury and pain. If a broken bone is suspected, the injured part should not be used. Ice may be applied to reduce swelling and discomfort. If the suspected fracture is in an arm or a leg, the extremity should be elevated to reduce swelling. People with suspected fractures should be examined by a health professional who can confirm the diagnosis with specialized testing, such as X rays or bone scans.

Fractures must be treated to restore correct position and function of the affected part. A physician who specializes in broken bones is called an orthopedic surgeon or an orthopedist. The physician can diagnose the fracture and determine the best method for treatment. The fractured bone must be properly aligned for proper healing. The physician will return the bone to its normal position if necessary. The bone must be immobilized to prevent movement while healing occurs. Methods of immobilizing the bone include casts, which may be made of plaster or fiberglass. Some fractures may require surgery to insert different types of metal devices into the bone to stabilize the fracture. The healing time varies according to the type of fracture and the age of the individual. Older people generally require a longer time to heal. Rehabilitation after a fracture may involve physical or occupational therapy to help the individual regain maximum function of the affected part.

Prevention of Fractures

Prevention of fractures is extremely important for older people. The development of osteoporosis is one of the major factors related to fractures in the elderly. Measures that may be taken to reduce the effect of this disease include regular weightbearing exercise such as walking, dancing, or stair climbing; sufficient calcium intake; and avoiding smoking. Screening tests are available that measure the density of the bone. Medications and hormones may be ordered by the health care provider for those who are particularly at risk for osteoporosis.

Measures to reduce the chance of falls include safety precautions in the home. The chance of tripping may be reduced by applying nonskid backing to throw rugs and keeping electrical cords or other small objects out of walking areas. The more medications a person takes, the greater the chance that he or she may experience side effects that may affect balance or judgment. Individuals should be aware of these side effects and exercise caution when moving about. The physician should be informed about these side effects to see if changes in the medication could be made.

—*Bobbie Siler*

See also Aging; Exercise and the elderly; Falls among the elderly; First aid; Foot disorders; Injuries among the elderly; Mobility problems in the elderly; Osteoporosis; Safety issues for the elderly; Smoking.

For Further Information:

American Academy of Orthopedic Surgeons, Public Information, Patient Education Brochures. http://www.aaos.org/wordhtml/home2.htm

Horan, Michael Arthur, and Rod A. Little, eds. *Injury in the Aging.* New York: Cambridge University Press, 1998.

Preventing Falls and Fractures. Bethesda, Md.: U.S. Department of Health and Human Services, Public Health Service, National Institutes of Health, National Institute on Aging, 1998.

Siegel, Irwin M. *All About Bone: An Owner's Manual.* New York: Demos Medical Publishing, 1998.

✧ Burns and scalds

Type of issue: Children's health, occupational health, public health
Definition: Damage to tissue caused by exposure to heat, chemicals, electricity, or radiation.

Burns and scalds are caused by exposure to heat, chemicals, electricity, or radiation. Scalds refer specifically to burns caused by hot liquid. Burns are often the result of accidents or carelessness. It is estimated, however, that perhaps as many as 20 percent of all pediatric burns are the result of deliberate abuse. About 97 percent of all pediatric burns are thermal, or caused by heat; of these, between 65 and 85 percent are scalds. Burns and scalds are one of the leading causes of death among children. Neal D. Uitvlugt and Daniel J. Ledbetter report in *Pediatric Trauma: Initial Care of the Injured Child* (1995) that in 1985, for example, burns killed 1,461 children under age nineteen in the United States. Further, about 500,000 children need medical attention each year for burns and scalds, with between 23,000 and 60,000 requiring hospitalization. The average age of children treated for burns is thirty-two months.

Sources of Burns

Common causes of burns in children include defective wiring, cigarettes and matches, defective heating equipment, spilled containers of hot liquids or food, and flammable clothing. Electrical burns in children may be caused by chewing on an exposed electrical cord or sucking on the outlet end of an extension cord. Burns deliberately inflicted on a child are most common in toddlers, and these injuries tend to be more severe than those received accidentally. Uitvlugt and Ledbetter report a five times greater mortality rate for inflicted burns than for pediatric burns in general.

The severity of a burn can be determined by classifying it according to degree and size. A first-degree burn is red and painful, affecting the epidermis. It is a superficial, partial thickness burn. The surface area is unbroken and dry. A second-degree burn affects both the epidermis and the dermis. It can be a superficial or a deep partial thickness burn. The skin is pink or mottled red and blistered, and it is often moist and weeping. Second-degree burns are very painful. Third-degree burns may affect tissue to the bone, damaging or destroying the full thickness of the skin. A third-degree burn may appear charred, white, waxy, or very deep red. The surface area is dry and leathery, with charred vessels apparent. Because such burns do so much nerve damage, it is likely that the victim will not feel pain. Third-degree burns are caused by prolonged exposure to heat or chemicals or short exposure to electricity.

Burn Treatment

Most pediatricians agree that first-degree burns can be treated at home by removing the source of the burning and then dousing the burned area with cold water for about ten minutes. Any jewelry or belts should be removed. A first-degree burn should heal on its own in two to three days. In the past, caregivers often coated the burn area with butter or grease; doctors, however, strongly advise against this practice.

Most doctors also agree that minor second-degree burns smaller than a quarter can be treated at home in the same manner. Nearly all sources agree, however, that any burn affecting the face, hands, feet, or genitals should be treated at a hospital. Likewise, burns caused by smoke inhalation or electricity should be treated at a hospital. Electrical burns are notoriously difficult to assess; the body can conduct the electricity to internal organs, and a wound that has a minor surface appearance can mask a very serious internal injury. Doctors also agree that a victim whose burns total 10 to 15 percent of his or her total body surface area should be hospitalized.

In cases of third-degree burns or where the burn or scald appears to have been inflicted, the victim must be hospitalized. Hospital treatment varies according to the severity of the injury. Generally, emergency personnel remove any remaining clothing or jewelry, debride the wound, and monitor the lungs and the heart. Often, oxygen is administered. If at least 15 percent of the body surface is affected, medical personnel put an intravenous line in place for the replacement of lost body fluids. Doctors also check blood gases in the case of smoke inhalation. In addition, doctors administer a topical therapy designed to reduce the chance of bacterial or fungal infection. Depending on the severity of the injury, a patient might have to undergo several skin grafts, in which sections of the patient's undamaged skin is transplanted over the injured site.

Appropriate and effective treatment of burns has long been of concern to doctors. In 1944, the Lund and Browder chart was developed to regularize the assessment of burn size to the size of the victim's body. An accurate assessment of the burn size helped doctors better determine appropriate treatment. Also, in the early twentieth century, doctors recognized that burn patients have large fluid requirements. Some sources claim that this recognition contributed more to the survival of burn patients than any previous discovery.

Doctors continue to research burn treatment, often focusing their attention on the development of an appropriate covering for burn wounds until the patient is ready for a skin graft. They have tested both frozen cadaver skin and temporary skin substitutes grown in laboratories from human cells.

—*Diane Andrews Henningfeld*

See also Child abuse; Children's health issues; Electrical shock; First aid; Safety issues for children; Sunburns.

For Further Information:

Clayman, Charles B., ed. *American Medical Association Encyclopedia of Medicine*. New York: Random House, 1989. A concise presentation of numerous medical terms and illnesses. A good general reference.

Glanze, Walter D., Kenneth N. Anderson, and Lois E. Anderson, eds. *The Signet Mosby Medical Encyclopedia*. New York: Signet, 1996. Excellent general reference for the layperson. Offers a concise but clear presentation of numerous medical topics.

Hendin, David. *Save Your Child's Life!* New rev. ed. New York: Pharos Books, 1986.

Miller, Benjamin, and Claire B. Keane. *Encyclopedia and Dictionary of Medicine, Nursing, and Allied Health.* 6th ed. Philadelphia: W. B. Saunders, 1997. A good, concise presentation of the topic of burns.

Uitvlugt, Neal D., and Daniel J. Ledbetter. "Treatment of Pediatric Burns." In *Pediatric Trauma: Initial Care of the Injured Child,* edited by Robert M. Arensman et al. New York: Raven Press, 1995.

✧ CANCER

Type of issue: Environmental health, occupational health, public health

Definition: Inappropriate and uncontrollable cell growth within one of the specialized tissues of the body, threatening normal cell and organ function and in serious cases traveling via the bloodstream to other areas of the body.

Cancer is a disease of abnormal growth. All growing cells pass through a strictly regulated series of events called the cell cycle. Most structures of the cell are duplicated during this sequence. At the end of the cycle, one cell is separated into two "daughter cells," each of which receives one copy of the duplicated cellular structures. The most important structures that must be exactly duplicated are the genes, the master blueprints that govern all cellular activities.

Human life starts with a single microscopic cell—a fertilized egg. This cell divides again and again; the adult human body is composed of more than a trillion cells, each with a very specific job to perform. After adulthood is reached, most cells of the body stop duplicating themselves. Some cell types, however, do need to continue dividing to replace worn-out cells; these include cells of the blood, skin, intestine, and some other tissues. Such growth is very accurately controlled so that excess cells are not produced. It is in these cell types, those that normally grow in the adult body, that cancer most often occurs. A small defect arises in one gene so that the cells are able to progress through the cell cycle even though more cells are not needed. This is the start of cancer. Such cancer cells do not need to grow faster than do their normal neighbors; their key feature is simply that they continue growing when no more cells should be produced. At first, these cells very closely resemble their neighbors. For example, newly altered blood cells still look very much like normal blood cells, and in most respects they are.

CANCEROUS DEFECTS

The first defect that gets cancer started is called initiation. It is typically the result of a mutation in one of the genes whose job it is to control some feature of the cell cycle. There are probably several hundred such genes, each of which regulates a different aspect of the cell cycle. These genes have perfectly normal jobs in the life of the cell until they become damaged. When there is a mutation in a controlling gene, the gene functions improperly: It does not govern the cell cycle quite right, and the cell cycle therefore proceeds when it should instead be halted. Such cancer-causing genes are called oncogenes.

After the initiation of cancer, additional mutations and other defects begin to pile up, and the defective cells become increasingly abnormal. Tumor suppressor genes, which normally function to keep cell division from becoming disorganized, are the site of these second-stage mutations. Those cells whose cell division and growth genes have mutated (oncogenes) and whose cell division and growth inhibitor genes (tumor suppressor genes) have also been mutated will become cancer cells. Typically, a second change, called promotion, must take place before cancer cells begin really growing freely. The promotion step typically allows the initiated cell to escape some policing activity of the body. For example, various hormones provide cells with instructions about how to behave; a promotion-type change may allow a cell to ignore such instructions. Both initiation and promotion occur randomly. Many cells that are initiated, however, fail to grow into tumors. It is only those relatively few cells that happen to acquire both defects that become a problem. Fortunately, very few cells will have both their oncogenes turned "on" and their tumor suppressor genes turned "off."

BENIGN AND MALIGNANT TUMORS

At this point, the new cancer cell is dividing and collecting in large numbers. These excess cells make up a mass called a tumor (except in the blood and lymph cancers, in which the cancer cells circulate individually). Nevertheless, all these cells are fairly "normal." Indeed, at this early stage, cancer is relatively easy to control using methods such as surgery. The excess cells may not cause much harm—warts, for example, are excess numbers of growing cells. Such relatively harmless tumors are called benign. If the cancer is detected at this early stage, while it is still relatively harmless, effective treatment and even a cure are still quite possible, which is why early diagnosis is so important in cancer medicine.

Unfortunately, more and more defects accumulate in these cells as they grow, and some of these defects (again by chance) will be particularly harmful. The most harmful changes make the growing cells capable of causing damage to other parts of the body. For example, cancer cells may acquire the ability to digest their way through nearby tissues, a process called invasion. Eventually, the functions of organs containing such cells become impaired. Such an invasion of body parts can be extremely painful as well. Other cancer cells may come loose from the tumor and travel to other parts of the body in the circulatory or lymphatic system: This process is called metastasis. In advanced stages of cancer, a patient may actually have dozens or hundreds of tumors, all of which have developed from a single parent tumor. Cells that can invade or metastasize are called malignant. It becomes increasingly difficult to eradicate cancer cells as they become more malignant. Pathologists are highly skilled at distinguishing benign from malignant cancer cells based on their appearance in a microscope and can provide accurate diagnosis of how far a case of cancer has progressed. Such information is crucial for deciding how best to treat the cancer.

Tendencies Toward Cancer

Most kinds of cancer typically occur during old age. Because each of the events that leads to tumor development is rather uncommon, it takes years for the several required mistakes to accumulate in a single cell, which then grows into a tumor. A few kinds of cancer occur most commonly in children. Such children usually have inherited one or more of the genetic defects that lead to cancer (already mutated oncogenes or tumor suppressor genes) from their parents. It then takes less time before the additional required defects are likely to occur. Thus, a tendency toward certain kinds of cancer can be inherited in families, as with other genetic traits (such as hair and eye color, height, and nose shape).

Cancer occurs when anything causes oncogenes and tumor suppressor genes to function abnormally, allowing cells to continue growing when they should not. The delicate genes in an individual's cells can be modified chemically by a number of different highly active and dangerous chemicals known collectively as carcinogens. Several kinds of radiation also pose a threat to genes. The best-known example is ultraviolet radiation from the sun, which can damage genes of the skin and lead to skin cancer. Finally, certain kinds of viruses can cause oncogenes to function improperly.

Surgery and Chemotherapy

The cancer treatments used most commonly are of three kinds: surgery, chemotherapy, and radiation therapy. First, and most straightforward, is the surgical removal of tumors. If done at an early stage, before cancer has spread, this method can be highly successful. Even so, surgery is much easier and less dangerous for some cancers (for example, skin cancer) than for others (such as brain tumors, which can be difficult to reach and remove safely). Naturally, surgery is much less successful with widely spread cancers such as leukemia (a cancer of blood cells) and in more advanced stages of cancer.

The second type of cancer treatment is chemotherapy. Patients are treated with chemicals that prevent cells from duplicating themselves, or at least limit or slow that process. Such drugs, which are usually injected, reach all parts of the body and so are much more effective than surgery when cancer has reached a later stage of spreading. Different kinds of chemicals work in very different ways to achieve this result. These chemicals can be roughly divided into four categories. First are chemicals that react directly with the substances required for cells to survive and function. Many such agents directly attack a cell's genes, preventing them from passing along information required for a cancer cell to stay alive. Second are antimetabolites, which prevent the chemical reactions that allow cells to produce energy (energy must also be available for cells to stay alive). The third category consists of steroid hormones. Cancer cells in some organs of the body respond to these hormones, which can therefore be used to regulate their growth. Thus estrogens, the female sex steroid hormones, are often used for treatment of breast cancer, whereas the male sex steroids, or androgens, may influence prostate cancer. Fourth are miscellaneous drugs, a few other chemicals that affect cancer cells in some different way. For example, drugs called vinca alkaloids stop the mechanical process of one cell dividing into two, in this way preventing growth. A derivative of the insecticide DDT (dichloro-diphenyl-trichloroethane) prevents unwanted steroid-hormone production and has been useful for treating tumors of the adrenal gland.

ADDRESSING THE SIDE EFFECTS OF CHEMOTHERAPY

The most common and difficult problem with the chemotherapeutic approach to cancer management is that normal cells that happen to be growing are also affected by the same drugs that halt the growth of cancer cells. This reaction causes many difficulties for patients, some serious and some less so. Probably the most serious problems are in the immune system. The growth of blood cells that make antibodies, called lymphocytes, is necessary before antibodies can be produced in response to an infectious disease. Because these cells cannot grow, patients in chemotherapy are much more vulnerable to illnesses caused by bacteria and viruses. Other blood cells, including those that carry oxygen, are also affected, causing additional problems. Skin cells and cells lining the digestive tract stop dividing, causing additional difficulties for the patients. A less serious problem for such patients is hair loss, as hair cells also are prevented from growing.

Designing drug treatments that kill cancer cells while minimizing these problems is a demanding and precise task for oncologists (physicians who specialize in cancer research and treatment). Some drugs affect different cell types in somewhat different ways, allowing normal cells to continue their functions while killing tumor cells. Doses and timing of treatments can be adjusted to maximize the effect of the drugs. It is typical for several drugs that act in different ways to be given in the same treatment, to assure that all cancer cells are halted; this approach is called combination chemotherapy. It is of critical importance that all cancer cells be stopped because a single unaffected cancer cell at any place in the body can begin growing after chemotherapy and develop into a cancer, a process known as relapse.

Another useful approach for improving chemotherapy is drug targeting. The chemical structure of tumor cells is subtly different from that of normal cells, and it is sometimes possible to make use of this difference. For example, a drug can be attached to an antibody molecule that reacts with a tumor protein (antigen) that is not found on normal cells. In this way, most of the drug will be directed to the tumor cells, while normal cells will receive a much lower dose. Hormones and other molecules also attach to specific molecules on cells, and this fact can sometimes be exploited to target drugs if the tumor cells have a particularly high number of such molecules.

Another problem with drug delivery is that the most effective drugs are rapidly degraded by the body's defense systems and secreted from the body. The actual period of exposure to an active drug in the body can be quite brief (a few minutes) for this reason. Methods have been developed for hiding or disguising drugs so they are not removed so rapidly. For example, some drugs can be placed inside fat droplets, and in this way they can escape detection by the immune system and breakdown in the liver.

RADIATION THERAPY

The third type of cancer treatment is radiation therapy. The radiation of choice is X rays, which can penetrate the body to reach a tumor and which can be produced at very high dosages using modern equipment. X rays can be focused on a specific small area or can be given over the whole body in the case of metastasized cancer. Therapeutic radiation damages genes to such an extent that they become physically fragmented and nonfunctional, ending the life of the target cell.

Radiation therapy has some of the same drawbacks as chemotherapy. Again, the most serious problem is that normal cells in the pathway of the radiation will also be killed. Bone marrow, the source of blood cells, is destroyed by whole-body cancer treatments. This problem can be overcome after radiation therapy by transplanting new bone marrow to the patient from close relatives, so that a treated patient can begin to remanufacture blood cells. Ironically, radiation designed to kill cancer cells can also turn normal cells into new cancer cells. Some normal cells may receive a reduced exposure of X rays. The dosage may be just sufficient to damage oncogenes of normal cells, causing them to become cancerous. Thus radiation therapy must be carried out with great care and precision.

—Howard L. Hosick; updated by Connie Rizzo, M.D.

See also Breast cancer; Cervical, ovarian, and uterine cancers; Chemotherapy; Colon cancer; Environmental diseases; Hospice; Hysterectomy; Living wills; Lung cancer; Mammograms; Mastectomy; Prostate cancer; Radiation; Screening; Secondhand smoke; Skin cancer; Smoking; Terminal illnesses.

FOR FURTHER INFORMATION:

Levenson, Frederick B. *The Causes and Prevention of Cancer.* New York: Stein & Day, 1985. A very personal attempt to give an overview of cancer and how it fits into health maintenance in general. Presented as a storylike narrative with the emphasis ultimately on the author's unproved ideas about cancer prevention and its relationship to human life.

Murphy, G., L. Morris, and D. Lange. *Informed Decisions: The Complete Book of Cancer Diagnosis, Treatment, and Recovery.* New York: Viking Press, 1997. This text from the American Cancer Society is intended for the layperson. It is exemplary in its discussion of cancer.

Prescott, D. M., and Abraham S. Flexer. *Cancer: The Misguided Cell.* Sunderland, Mass.: Sinauer Associates, 1986. The authors focus primarily on how cells change during cancer. This book describes more basic biology than most of the other publications listed.

Siegel, Mary-Ellen. *The Cancer Patient's Handbook: Everything You Need to Know About Today's Care and Treatment.* New York: Walker, 1986. Siegel is a physician who explains concepts in simple terms. A very practical discussion of medical procedures related to cancer, including diagnosis and therapy. Provides descriptions of the various kinds of cancer and a useful glossary.

Tierney, Lawrence M., Jr., et al., eds. *Current Medical Diagnosis and Treatment: 2001.* New York: McGraw-Hill, 2000. This text, updated yearly, is the point of reference for physicians and other health care practitioners. It incorporates each year's biomedical research discoveries that have immediate, relevant, and applicable use for the patient.

✧ CANES AND WALKERS

Type of issue: Elder health, treatment
Definition: Devices for temporary or long-term assistance in walking.

Many types of canes and walkers are available for purchase in drugstores and variety stores. Many older individuals using these assistive devices purchased them in such stores or borrowed one from a friend or family member. Often, these devices are prescribed by a physician or therapist for either temporary or long-term use. Regardless of how the device was obtained, proper choice and fit are important for many reasons. A poor choice or fit can result in

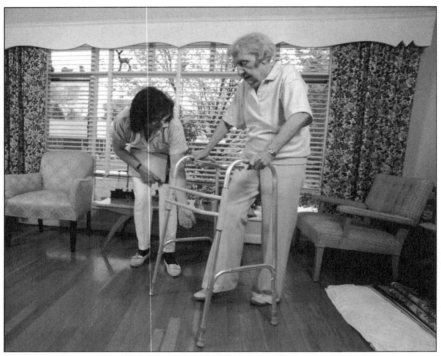

A home care professional instructs a patient in the proper use of a walker. (Digital Stock)

decreased stability, increased energy expenditure needed to walk, and unsafe walking.

A cane or walker properly fit for an individual results in the handgrip of the device being level with the user's wrist crease when the user is standing with arms at the sides. The fit can also be checked by ensuring that the elbow is bent approximately twenty to thirty degrees when the user stands and holds the device. (For individuals with decreased leg strength, walkers may be fit a bit lower to allow greater use of the arms.) A combination of these methods should be used to check for proper fit, since individuals sometimes have proportionally long or short arms. In addition, the device should be measured with the user in the footwear normally worn, since shoe height will affect the fit.

Types of Canes and Walkers

The choice of device should be made considering the user's needs and abilities. Canes are more functional on stairs and in confined areas, and they are easier to transport than are walkers. Canes do not provide as much support, however, and are not recommended for use with any weight-bearing restrictions, such as after total knee or hip replacement surgery.

Walkers offer maximal support and stability, but mobility is somewhat restricted because of their size. Walkers are often prescribed for mobility with weight-bearing restrictions, with the goal of advancing to a cane or another assistive device as healing progresses.

Several styles of canes and walkers are available, and the choice should depend on the user's needs and abilities. Standard *J* canes are inexpensive; most are wooden and can be cut to the proper height. They are not the most stable choice, however, since the user's hand is not directly over the foot of the cane. Offset canes have a bend in the shaft that places the user's hand over the cane's foot, thereby increasing stability. Often, these canes are also adjustable in length and, therefore, can be used with varying footwear or by different individuals. Quad canes have four feet and offer the most stability. They are more difficult to use, however, and can be very unstable if all four feet do not come in contact with the ground with each step.

Standard walkers are the most inexpensive type, but they are relatively awkward and difficult to transport since they do not fold. This problem is solved with folding walkers, but these devices can collapse if they are not set up properly. Wheeled varieties are available for individuals without the arm strength to pick up and advance a walker with each step. They also allow increased speed and provide good stability if used with brakes that activate when the user pushes down with each step.

—Mary Ann Holbein-Jenny

See also Aging; Broken bones in the elderly; Falls among the elderly; Foot disorders; Injuries among the elderly; Mobility problems in the elderly; Osteoporosis; Safety issues for the elderly; Wheelchair use among the elderly.

FOR FURTHER INFORMATION:

Means, K. M., D. E. Rodell, and P. S. O'Sullivan. "Obstacle Course Performance and Risk of Falling in Community-Dwelling Elderly Persons." *Archives of Physical Medicine and Rehabilitation* 79, no. 12 (1998): 1570-1576.

Murray, Ruth Beckmann, and Judith Proctor Zentner. *Health Assessment and Promotion Strategies Through the Life Span.* 7th ed. Englewood Cliffs, N.J.: Prentice Hall, 2000.

Ryan, J. W., and A. M. Spellbring. "Implementing Strategies to Decrease Risk of Falls in Older Women." *Journal of Gerontological Nursing* 22, no. 12 (1996): 25-31.

Walker, Bonnie L. "Preventing Falls." *RN* 61 (May, 1998).

✦ CARDIAC REHABILITATION

Type of issue: Medical procedures, prevention, treatment
Definition: The activities that ensure the physical, mental, and social conditions necessary for returning cardiac patients to good health.

Cardiovascular disease (CVD), or heart disease, is the leading cause of death and disability in most of the industrialized nations of the world. For those persons who survive a cardiac event, discharge from a hospital or medical setting without further assistance may lead to financial, physical, and mental incapacity.

Just as interventional procedures and medical care are important for the initial treatment of acute cardiac events, such as a myocardial infarction (heart attack) or angina (chest pain), cardiac rehabilitation influences long-term morbidity and mortality. Such preventive cardiology assists persons with CVD in three main areas: education, behavior modification, and patient and family support. The two primary goals of the rehabilitation program are to help increase the patient's functional capacity (the ability to perform activities of daily living) and to counteract or arrest the patient's disease process using a multidisciplined educational approach.

MODIFYING RISK FACTORS

In order to provide direction in prevention and rehabilitation, research studies have clearly defined several modifiable risk factors for heart disease, which are presented to patients. Among the most significant are smoking, high serum cholesterol, hypertension, and physical inactivity. Assistance with education about and modification of these risk factors, through risk factor counseling and participation in physical activity, is provided in modern cardiac rehabilitation programs.

Methods for providing education on risk factor modification can vary greatly from program to program, but include such means as didactic lecturing, slide presentations, printed material for patients to read, demonstrations (such as cooking and stress reduction techniques), providing loaner books, and one-on-one counseling.

The exercise portion of the cardiac rehabilitation is most often the time-consuming element of the program. It involves controlling and monitoring four major variables: mode (type of activity, such as bicycling, walking, or stair-stepping), duration (length of time the patient exercises), frequency (number of times per week that exercise is performed), and intensity (exertion level of the patient, usually assessed by the heart rate response).

To become involved in the cardiac rehabilitation program, a patient is initially screened by a physician, nurse, or other clinical specialist and directed to the appropriate level (or phase) of intervention.

There are three to four clinical phases involved with cardiac rehabilitation, as various groups categorize them differently. The Exercise and Cardiac Rehabilitation Committee of the American Heart Association outlines three phases; the American Association of Cardiovascular and Pulmonary Rehabilitation (AACVPR) outlines four phases.

COMBATING BED REST

Phase 1 occurs while the patient is still in the hospital. It begins when the patient's condition is stabilized, sometimes as soon as forty-eight hours after the coronary event or procedure. This phase can begin in the coronary care unit (CCU) or the intensive care unit (ICU). Phase 1 incorporates several disciplines, including physical therapy, nursing, psychiatry, dietetics, occupational therapy, and exercise science. It is designed to prevent the deleterious physiological effects of bed rest.

The physical components of this phase include maintaining a range of motion and gradually returning to activities of daily living. Patients gradually advance through stages until they are able to walk up to 200 or 400 feet. Before discharge, patients are encouraged to walk up and down one flight of stairs while accompanied by a physical therapist or other clinician who monitors heart rate and blood pressure. The level of exertion during the early portion of this phase is normally 1 to 2 METs. Thus, in phase 1, the mode of exercise focuses on motion (sitting, standing, and finally walking), the frequency is seven days per week, the duration of exercise is usually five to ten minutes at a time, and the intensity of activity should not cause the heart rate to exceed twenty beats above the resting rate while standing.

For coronary artery bypass graft (CABG) patients who have not experienced a myocardial infarction, progress during this phase is usually faster than for heart attack patients. Percutaneous transluminal coronary angioplasty (PTCA) patients may receive only a few days of rehabilitation, as they are usually discharged from the hospital sooner than heart attack or CABG patients.

The mental components of phase 1 include risk factor modification education and an introduction to rehabilitation concepts.

EXPOSURE TO EXERCISE

Phase 2 customarily begins within three weeks of discharge from the hospital and lasts for four to twelve weeks. During phase 2, patients are exposed to a level of exertion commensurate with several criteria: the patient's clinical status (stable or unstable, depending on whether the patient is experiencing problems related to the disease); the patient's functional capacity, or fitness level; orthopedic limitations, such as muscle or joint problems; the goals for functional capacity (what tasks the patient wants to be able to perform); and any other special circumstances or situations.

In a given phase 2 program, there are a variety of patients, all with varying levels of physical fitness. Through variations in the mode, duration, frequency, or intensity of exercise, these differing levels of fitness can be accommodated. A variety of exercise modes are presented in the phase 2 program, including walking, stationary cycling, stationary rowing, simulated stair-climbing, water aerobics, swimming, and upper-body ergometry. The exercise for this phase frequency is three to six days per week, the duration consists of twenty to forty-five minutes of continuous aerobic activity, and the intensity should produce a heart rate that is 60 to 85 percent of the symptom-limited maximal heart rate. Exercises are monitored by an exercise specialist and a cardiovascular fitness nurse. Exercise intensity is determined in most cases by heart rate and may be monitored by electrocardiogram (EKG or ECG) telemetry on a number of patients simultaneously.

Outpatient Supervision and Maintenance

Patients move into phase 3 of cardiac rehabilitation, a community-based outpatient program, when cardiovascular and physiological responses to exercise have been stabilized and the patient has achieved the goals initially set. Phase 3 is generally considered to be an extended, supervised program which usually lasts from four to six months but which can continue indefinitely.

Participants in phase 3 programs become more involved in and in charge of their own exercises. Typically, these programs do not include EKG monitoring. Individuals are given more responsibility with respect to maintaining their own heart rates in their training heart rate range. Usually, an exercise specialist, nurse, or physician is available to oversee the exercises. The mode, frequency, duration, and intensity of exercise in this phase is similar to that of phase 2.

Phase 4 is a maintenance program. Although many rehabilitation settings label this a phase 3 program, the phase 4 program is considered to be the longest-term, ongoing phase and is of indefinite length. Many phase 2 cardiac rehabilitation program graduates remain in phase 3 or phase 4 programs for years. The mode, frequency, duration, and intensity of the exercise program for phase 4 is also similar to that of phase 2.

Expanding Participation

Increasing numbers of cardiac rehabilitation programs are accepting unconventional patient populations. These patients now include heart transplant recipients, congestive heart failure patients, individuals suffering from ischemic heart disease, and those with arrhythmias and/or pacemakers.

Although most of the prescribed exercise regimens for these patients parallel those for the conventional cardiac patient, there are subtle differences. In the heart transplant population, for example, heart rate response differs from nontransplant patients. The adjustment of heart rate to various workloads lags in acute heart transplant recipients; that is, the heart rate does not increase as rapidly as it does for normal patients. To accommodate this difference, researchers have suggested that, in place of heart rate response, clinicians use a "rating of perceived exertion" scale to monitor the patients' responses to exercise.

Even patients who have orthopedic limitations, such as arthritis or chronic injuries, may be accommodated in the exercise portion of the cardiac rehabilitation program. Exercises can be adjusted to allow participants to derive cardiovascular benefits without causing them unnecessary discomfort.

Although cardiac rehabilitation is safe in general, several factors may emerge during graded exercise testing (a screening for entry into a cardiac rehabilitation program) that can identify those patients who may be at increased risk. These factors include a significant depression or elevation of the S-T wave segment from a resting EKG, angina, extensive left ventricular dysfunction and severe myocardial infarction, ventricular dysrhythmias, inappropriate blood pressure response to exercise, achieving a peak heart rate of less than 120 beats per minute (if not taking a negative chronotropic medication, which slows down the heart rate), and a functional exercise capacity of less than 4 to 5 METs. Inclusion in one of these categories does not preclude participation in a cardiac rehabilitation program, but it may warrant specific exercise guidelines and close monitoring.

Among the criteria for exclusion from a cardiac rehabilitation program are unstable angina, acute systemic illness, uncontrolled arrhythmias, tachycardia, diabetes, symptomatic congestive heart failure, a resting systolic blood pressure over 200 millimeters of mercury (mm Hg) or a resting diastolic blood pressure over 110 mm Hg, third-degree heart block without a pacemaker, and moderate to severe aortic stenosis.

ASSESSMENT AND RISK STRATIFICATION

For those who meet the criteria for inclusion in a cardiac rehabilitation program, risk stratification (low, moderate, or high) may be employed. This allows an appropriate amount of supervision to be in place based on each patient's goals and condition. Clinical observations and tests allow each patient to be assessed individually. Within each phase, levels of risk may be established. Various proposals have been made for risk stratification prior to entry into a cardiac rehabilitation program, including stratification based on several factors: the degree of left ventricular dysfunction, presence or absence of myocardial ischemia, extent of myocardial injury, and presence of ventricular arrhythmias.

Some of the most widely examined noninvasive assessment tools include the extent of QRS wave abnormalities on a resting EKG and the results of exercise stress testing, twenty-four-hour ambulatory EKG monitoring, radionuclide ventriculography, and echocardiography. A combination of these test results may be used to determine the course of action provided to an individual.

As with any effective therapy, exercise as a form of cardiac rehabilitation is neither without hazard nor always beneficial. If appropriate clinical guidelines are utilized, however, the benefit-risk ratio can be very favorable. In a 1986 study of 51,303 patients from 142 outpatient cardiac rehabilitation programs in the United States (representing 2,351,916 patient-hours of exercise), the incidence rate for fatal and nonfatal cardiac events was 1 in 111,996. This low incidence of cardiac-related events during participation in programs is probably attributable to improved risk stratification, the use of appropriate medical and surgical therapies, and improved exercise guidelines. On the rare occasions when cardiac events occur, reports have indicated that up to 90 percent of all patients with exercise-related cardiac arrest are successfully resuscitated when the patient experiences the event in a properly equipped and supervised program.

—Frank J. Fedel

See also Exercise; Exercise and the elderly; Heart attacks; Heart disease; Heart disease and women; Physical rehabilitation; Preventive medicine; Stress.

For Further Information:

American Association of Cardiovascular and Pulmonary Rehabilitation. *Guidelines for Cardiac Rehabilitation Programs.* 2d ed. Champaign, Ill.: Human Kinetics Books, 1995. This short text is laid out well, with many citations of research studies and books on cardiac rehabilitation. A broad-based book that provides information for existing rehabilitation programs and proposes new programs.

Blocker, William P., and David Cardus, eds. *Rehabilitation in Ischemic Heart Disease.* New York: SP Medical & Scientific Books, 1983. Thoroughly researched, this text is almost a bible for any cardiac rehabilitation program. Provides a broad base of background information, in addition to the history and philosophy of the rehabilitation process.

Gordon, Neil F., and Larry W. Gibbons. *The Cooper Clinic Cardiac Rehabilitation Program.* New York: Simon & Schuster, 1990. Provides a wide array of anecdotes for the layperson, as well as a good foundation for the clinician. Includes personal stories from former cardiac patients regarding the intimate process of cardiac rehabilitation, lending credibility to the book. Written by clinicians who care about their patients, one of the intangible attributes of cardiac rehabilitation.

McGoon, M. *The Mayo Clinic's Heart Book*. New York: William Morrow, 1993. The most respected text for laypeople on heart disease. Covers all aspects of anatomy, physiology, diagnosis, treatment, and prevention.

Pryor, J. A., and B. A. Webber, eds. *Physiotherapy for Respiratory and Cardiac Problems*. 2d ed. Edinburgh, Scotland: Churchill Livingstone, 1998. Provides therapists with a great deal of useful information regarding the treatment of individuals with respiratory or cardiac conditions. The appendix offers normal values for vital signs, arterial and venous blood gases, blood chemistry, and pressures in the circulatory and respiratory systems, as well as common medical abbreviations.

✧ CARPAL TUNNEL SYNDROME

Type of issue: Occupational health

Definition: A common disorder that causes discomfort and decreased hand dexterity via excessive pressure on the median nerve at the wrist, often caused by repetitive wrist and hand movements.

Carpal tunnel syndrome, also known as median nerve palsy, is caused by the transverse carpal ligament compressing the median nerve. This nerve passes through the carpal tunnel alongside nine tendons attached to the muscles that enable the hand to close and the wrist to flex. The tendons have a lubricating lining called the synovium, which normally allows the tendons to smoothly glide back and forth through the tunnel during wrist and hand movements. The median nerve is the softest component within the tunnel and becomes compressed when the tendons are stressed and become swollen. Median nerve compression most often results when the synovium becomes thick and sticky as a result of the wear and tear of aging or repeatedly performing stressful motions with the hands while holding them in the same position for extended periods.

The roots of carpal tunnel syndrome can be traced back to the 1860's, when meatpackers complained of pain and loss of hand function, which physicians initially attributed to reduced circulation. Modern occupations that require repetitive motions for extended periods—such as typing on a computer keyboard, construction and assembly-line work, and jackhammer operation—have caused a dramatic rise in cumulative trauma disorders such as carpal tunnel syndrome, while other workplace injuries have leveled off.

Entrapment of the median nerve is less commonly caused by rheumatoid arthritis, diabetes mellitus, poor thyroid gland function, excessive fluid retention such as during pregnancy or by medications, vitamin B_6 or B_{12} deficiency, or bone protruding in the tunnel from previous dislocations or fractures of the wrist.

Symptoms and Diagnosis

Initial symptoms of carpal tunnel syndrome include tingling and numbness in the hands, often beginning in the thumb and index and middle fingers, that causes the hand to feel as though it were asleep and shooting pain from the thenar region radiating as far up as the neck. Later symptoms include burning pain from the wrist to the fingers, changes in touch or temperature sensation, clumsiness in the hands, and muscle weakness creating an inability to grasp, pinch, and perform other thumb functions. Swelling of the hands and forearms and changes in sweat gland functioning in the hands may also be noted. Symptoms can be intermittent or constant and often progress to the point of regularly awakening the patient at night. Temporary relief is sometimes available by elevating, massaging, and shaking the hand. Although very treatable if diagnosed early, carpal tunnel syndrome can escalate into persistent pain, which can become so crippling that workplace duties and such simple tasks as holding a cup, writing, and buttoning a shirt are compromised.

A clinical examination for confirmation of median nerve impingement includes wrist examination, an X ray for previous injury and arthritis, assessment of swelling and sensitivity to touch or pinpricks, and the reproduction of symptoms by tapping of the median nerve (Tinel's test) and holding the wrist in a flexed position for several minutes (Phalen's test). Nerve conduction tests, which measure nerve transmission speed by electrodes placed on the skin, and electromyogram evaluation, which notes muscle function abnormalities, may also assist in a diagnosis.

Treatment and Therapy

Early diagnosis and the taking of appropriate preventive measures, such as ergonomic modifications in the way that upper extremity movements are performed, often reduce the risk of developing advanced carpal tunnel syndrome. The need to compensate for weak muscles with an inappropriate wrist position can be reduced by maintaining a neutral (straight) wrist position instead of a flexed, extended, or twisted wrist position; utilizing the entire hand and all the fingers to grasp and lift objects, instead of gripping solely with the thumb and index finger; minimizing repetitive movements; allowing the upper extremities regular rest periods; using power tools, instead of hand tools; alternating work activities; switching hands; reducing movement speed; and stretching and using strengthening exercises for the hand, wrist, and arm. Keeping the hands warm to maintain good blood circulation and avoiding smoke-filled environments, which reduce peripheral blood flow, are also recommended.

Treatment generally begins with splinting of the wrist and medication, but surgery may be required if symptoms do not subside within three months. Both nocturnal splints and job-specific occupational splints can effectively keep the wrist in a neutral position, thus avoiding the extreme wrist flexion or extension that narrows the carpal tunnel. Wrist supports lying on the desk in front of a computer keyboard are often helpful, but the benefit of strapping on wrist splints while typing is controversial because disuse atrophy may result, potentially creating a muscle imbalance. Aspirin and other oral nonsteroidal anti-inflammatory drugs (NSAIDs) may reduce swelling and inflammation, relieving some nerve pressure. Corticosteroids and cortisone-like medications injected directly into the carpal tunnel can help confirm diagnosis if the symptoms are relieved. Diuretics and vitamin supplementation may also be beneficial.

If initial symptoms do not subside, pain increases, or the risk of permanent nerve and muscle damage exists, then surgery may be necessary, with subsequent rehabilitation and ergonomic counseling with a physical or occupational therapist. An outpatient surgical procedure called carpal tunnel release involves dividing the transverse ligament to open the carpal tunnel to relieve pressure and removing thickened synovial tissue, with recovery expected in six to ten weeks.

An endoscopic procedure utilizing a much smaller incision and a fiber-optic camera holds considerable promise for alleviating the median nerve pressure that causes carpal tunnel syndrome.

—Daniel G. Graetzer

See also Disabilities; Occupational health; Pain management.

FOR FURTHER INFORMATION:

Johansson, Philip. *Carpal Tunnel Syndrome and Other Repetitive Strain Injuries.* Berkeley Heights, N.J.: Enslow, 1999.

Katz, R. T. "Carpal Tunnel Syndrome: A Practical Review." *American Family Physician* 51, no. 1 (1995): 48-57.

Kulick, R. G. "Carpal Tunnel Syndrome." *Orthopaedic Clinics of North America* 27, no. 2 (1996): 345-354.

Rosenbaum, Richard B., and Jose L. Ochoa. *Carpal Tunnel Syndrome and Other Disorders of the Median Nerve.* Boston: Butterworth-Heinemann, 1993.

✦ CERVICAL, OVARIAN, AND UTERINE CANCERS

Type of issue: Public health, women's health
Definition: The primary cancers of the female reproductive system.

Tumors of the reproductive tract occur in relatively high rates in women. Cervical cancer accounts for 6 percent, ovarian cancer 5 percent, and cancer of the lining of the uterus (endometrial cancer) 7 percent of all cancers in women. A variety of treatments are available for patients with cancers of the reproductive tract: surgical removal of the organ, hormonal therapy, chemotherapy, or radiation therapy.

Cervical Cancer

Cervical cancer is most frequently found in women who are between forty and forty-nine years of age, but the incidence has been steadily increasing in younger women. Several factors appear to be involved in initiating this cancer: young age at first intercourse, number of sexual partners (as well as the number of the partner's partners), infection with sexually transmitted diseases such as herpes simplex type 2 and human papilloma virus, and cigarette smoking. Since most patients do not experience symptoms, regular checkups are necessary. The Pap (Papanicolaou) smear performed in a physician's office will detect the presence of cervical cancer. In this procedure, the physician obtains a sample of the cervix by swabbing the area and placing the cells on a microscope slide for examination.

The treatment of cervical cancer depends on the size and location of the tumor and whether the cells are benign or malignant. If the patient is no longer capable of or interested in childbearing, then she may choose to have her uterus, including the cervix, removed in the procedure known as hysterectomy. The physician may also use a laser, cryotherapy (use of a cold instrument), or electrocautery (use of a hot instrument) to destroy the tumor without removing the uterus. Malignant tumors may require a total hysterectomy as well as the removal of associated lymph nodes, which can trap metastatic cells. This surgery may be followed by radiation or chemotherapy if there is a possibility that all cancer cells have not been removed.

Cervical cancer diagnosed in a pregnant patient can complicate the treatment. Fortunately, only about 1 percent of cervical cancers are found in pregnant women. If the cancer is restricted to the cervix (that is, it has not metastasized), treatment is usually delayed until after childbirth. It is interesting to note that a normal vaginal delivery may occur without harming the mother or the infant. Malignant cervical cancer must be treated in a similar way as in nonpregnant women. If the cancer is found in the first trimester, a hysterectomy or radiation therapy or both is used to help eradicate the malignancy. Obviously, these approaches terminate the pregnancy. During the second trimester, the uterus must be emptied of the fetus and placenta, followed by radiation therapy or removal of the affected reproductive organs. In the third trimester, the physician will typically try to delay treatment until he or she believes that the fetus has developed sufficiently to stay alive when delivered by cesarean section. A vaginal delivery is not recommended, as it has been shown to lower the cure rate of malignant cervical cancer. Treatment after delivery consists of surgery, radiation therapy, and chemotherapy.

The prognosis in patients who have elected surgical removal of the tumor is a five-year survival rate of up to 90 percent. Cure rates for patients undergoing radiation therapy are between 75 and 90 percent. Chemotherapeutic agents have not had as much effect, as they significantly reduce only 25 percent of tumors. It is important to note that the best outcomes are achieved with early diagnosis.

OVARIAN CANCER

Ovarian cancer accounts for more deaths than any other cancer of the female reproductive system. While the cause of ovarian cancer is unknown, the risk is greatest for women who have not had children. Ovarian cancer does not appear to run in families, and its incidence is slightly decreased in women who use oral contraceptives for many years. Ovarian tumors generally affect women over fifty years of age.

There are two major types of ovarian cancer: epithelial and germ cell neoplasms. About 90 percent of ovarian cancers are epithelial and develop on the surface of the ovary. These tumors often are bulky and involve both ovaries. Germ cell tumors are derived from the eggs within the ovary and, if malignant, tend to be highly aggressive. Malignant germ cell neoplasms tend to occur in women under the age of thirty.

Ovarian cancer is generally considered a silent disease, as the signs and symptoms are vague and often ignored. Abdominal pain is the most obvious symptom, followed by abdominal swelling. Some patients also report gastrointestinal disorders such as changes in bowel habits. Abnormal vaginal bleeding may occur but like the other symptoms is not specific for the disease. Diagnosis is made using imaging techniques such as ultrasound, computed tomography (CT) scanning, and magnetic resonance imaging (MRI).

Ovarian cancers are treated with a similar approach. Surgery may involve the removal of the ovaries, uterine tubes, and uterus, as well as associated lymph nodes depending upon the extent of malignancy. Radiation and chemotherapy are usually employed but oftentimes are not effective. The drug taxol is a relatively new agent which shows some promise in treating ovarian cancers. This drug was isolated from the bark of the yew tree and shows some specificity for ovarian tumors. Taxol prevents cell division in ovarian tumors, slowing the progression of the disease.

The outcome for ovarian cancer is usually not as good as for cervical and endometrial cancers, since the disease is usually in an advanced stage by the time that it is diagnosed. The overall survival rate without evidence of recurrence in patients with epithelial ovarian cancers is between 15 and 45 percent. The more uncommon germ cell ovarian cancers have a much more variable prognosis. With early diagnosis, aggressive surgery, and the use of newer chemotherapeutic agents, the long-term survival rate for all ovarian cancer patients approaches 70 percent.

Uterine Cancer

Uterine cancer, also known as endometrial cancer, most frequently affects women between the ages of fifty and sixty-five. Like most cancers, the cause of endometrial cancer is not clear. Nevertheless, relatively high levels of estrogens have been identified as a risk factor. For example, obese women, women who have an early onset of their first period (menarche), and women who never became pregnant tend to have high estrogen levels for longer durations than those without these conditions. Medical scientists believe not only that it is estrogens that are important but also that the other ovarian hormone, progesterone, must be lower than normal for the cancer to develop. Therefore, progesterone appears to have a protective effect in endometrial cancer. Detection of endometrial cancer is accomplished by having a physician take a small tissue sample (biopsy) from the lining of the uterus. The sample can be examined under the microscope to determine if the cells are cancerous.

Surgery is often the treatment of choice for endometrial cancer. As with cervical cancer, however, treatment depends upon the extent of the disease and the patient's wishes relative to reproductive capabilities and family planning. A hysterectomy—removal of the uterine tubes, ovaries, and surrounding lymph nodes—is usually indicated. Chemotherapy and radiation therapy are occasionally utilized as adjunctive therapy, as is progesterone. Progesterone (medroxyprogesterone or hydroxyprogesterone) may benefit patients with advanced disease, as it seems to cause a decrease in tumor size and regression of metastases. In fact, progesterone therapy in patients with advanced or recurrent endometrial cancer leads to regression in about 40 percent of cases. Progesterone therapy also has produced regression in tumors that have metastasized to the lungs, vagina, and chest cavity.

The outcome of endometrial cancer is influenced by the aggressiveness of the tumor, the age of the woman (older women tend to have a poorer prognosis), and the stage at which the cancer was detected. Almost two-thirds of all patients live without evidence of disease for five or more years after treatment. Unfortunately, 28 percent die within five years. For cancer identified and treated early, almost 90 percent of patients are alive five years after treatment.

Increasing Preventive Measures

Scheduling regular checkups with a health care provider may increase the likelihood of detecting cervical, ovarian, and uterine cancers early, even if no symptoms are present. Pelvic examinations should be performed every three years for women under the age of forty and yearly thereafter. Pap smear tests for cervical cancer should be undertaken yearly from the time that a woman becomes sexually active. Some physicians will take an endometrial tissue biopsy from women at high risk and at the time of the menopause.

Some data suggest that modifying lifestyle may help reduce the incidence of cervical cancer. The cervix is exposed to a variety of factors during intercourse, including infections and physical trauma. Multiple sexual partners increases the risk of sexually transmitted diseases which may predispose the cervix to cancer. This factor is compounded by the fact that infectious agents and other carcinogens can be transmitted from one individual to another. Therefore, theoretically the cervix can be exposed to carcinogens from a partner's sexual partners. Regular intercourse begun in the early teens also predisposes one to cervical cancer, as the tissue of the cervix may be more vulnerable at puberty. Barrier methods of contraception, mainly the condom, reduce the risk of developing cervical cancer by reducing the exposure of the cervix to potential carcinogens. Smoking also increases the risk of cervical cancer, perhaps because carcinogens in tobacco enter the blood which in turn has access to the cervix.

Women who are twenty or more pounds over ideal body weight are twice as likely to develop endometrial cancer, and the risk increases with increased body fat. Some estrogens are produced in fat tissue, and this additional estrogen may play a role in the development of endometrial cancer. Therefore, reduction of excess body fat through diet and exercise would be important for a woman who wished to reduce her chances of developing uterine cancer.

—Matthew Berria

See also Cancer; Chemotherapy; Hysterectomy; Pap smears; Radiation; Screening; Women's health issues.

FOR FURTHER INFORMATION:

Epps, R., and the American Medical Women's Association, eds. *The Women's Complete Handbook.* New York: Dell Books, 1995. This book, by the oldest organization of female physicians in the United States, is an invaluable guide for the layperson on female-specific diseases.

Fox, Stuart I. *Perspectives on Human Biology.* Dubuque, Iowa: Wm. C. Brown, 1991. Chapter 14 provides the nonscientist with a basic understanding of cancer biology. Fox explains how oncogenes are thought to act in the formation of neoplasms and how antioxidant vitamins may protect against certain forms of cancer.

Hales, Dianne. *An Invitation to Health.* 9th ed. Belmont, Calif.: Wadsworth Thomson Learning, 2000. This text should be read by anyone who wishes an overview of health topics. Particularly important reading for those interested in the prevention of cancer.

Mader, Sylvia S. *Human Biology*. 5th ed. Dubuque, Iowa: Wm. C. Brown, 1997. Chapter 20 is devoted to a discussion of cancer and provides an excellent overview of cancer biology. This text was written for the nonscientist yet details contemporary theories on cancer formation and treatment.

Murphy, G., L. Morris, and D. Lange. *Informed Decisions: The Complete Book of Cancer Diagnosis, Treatment, and Recovery*. New York: Viking Press, 1997. This text from the American Cancer Society is intended for the lay reader. It is exemplary in its discussion of cancer.

✧ CHEMOTHERAPY

Type of issue: Medical procedures, treatment
Definition: The treatment of a disease, especially cancer, by the use of drugs.

The term "chemotherapy" is used to refer to the use of chemical agents in the treatment of any disease. It is employed most often, however, in reference to the treatment of cancer. Some drugs are capable either of stopping the undesirable spreading of cancer cells or of preventing cancer from occurring at all. These drugs, called chemotherapeutic agents, destroy cells by interfering with their life-sustaining functions. For example, one type of drug prevents cells from forming the proteins and enzymes that keep them alive. Another type kills by disrupting a step in the process of cell division, while a third type upsets the balance of hormones in a patient's body, creating conditions unsuitable for cancer survival. Unfortunately, all drugs that kill cancer cells also kill normal cells. On the other hand, they selectively kill more cancer cells than normal cells.

Chemotherapy is used when cancerous cells have spread through the body, so that their location cannot be precisely determined. Neither surgery nor radiation therapy can destroy widespread cancer, but drugs can circulate throughout the entire body and kill the cells that surgery and radiotherapy miss. Typically, a cancer cell develops resistance or spreads so extensively that an effective drug dose would kill the patient. Even when a cure is not achieved, however, chemotherapeutic agents can be useful in extending the life of patients, in sensitizing a tumor to radiation treatment, and as an adjuvant or precautionary method when doctors cannot determine whether a cancer has spread.

Immediately after a malignancy is diagnosed, it must be appropriately classified before therapy can be delivered. Out of classification comes an appropriate treatment prescription. The crucial decision in pretreatment planning is whether a cure is feasible. If a cure is possible, aggressive therapy is indicated and certain risks are worth taking. If a cure is not possible, then the therapeutic goal is the prolongation of life, the relief of symptoms, and the maintenance of as near-normal function as possible.

THE COURSE OF TREATMENT

The route of administration is an important variable in the delivery of the required dose of chemotherapy. Administration can be oral, intravenous, by continuous infusion, or by intracavity instillation. The optimum drug dosage is also a critical variable. The objective is to provide the patient with the maximum therapeutic benefit and the minimum side effects. For the large majority of anticancer drugs, administered singly or in combination, bone marrow suppression represents the most important dose-limiting factor, and close monitoring of the patient is critical.

The choice of drugs to be used is dependent on the primary site of origin of the malignancy. Over the years, a database has been established that links specific primary tumor types with drugs that have demonstrated reproducible clinical activity. If combination therapy is chosen, the choice of drugs follows the following empirical guidelines: Each drug should be active when used alone against the disease in question; the drugs should have different postulated or known mechanisms of action; and the drugs should not have overlapping toxicity patterns.

TYPES OF CHEMOTHERAPY

Alkylating agents are reactive organic compounds that transfer alkyl groups in chemical reactions. Their effectiveness as anticancer drugs is attributable to the transfer of these alkyl groups to biologically important cell constituents whose function is then impaired. Examples of alkylating agents are cyclophosphamide, used in the treatment of lymphomas, different types of leukemia, and lung cancer; chlorambucil and melphalan, used in the treatment of multiple myeloma and ovarian cancer; and the nitrosoureas, such as carmustine and lomustine, which are useful in the treatment of brain neoplasms, gastrointestinal carcinomas, and malignant melanomas.

Antimetabolites are structurally similar to the naturally occurring compounds required for synthesis of purines, pyrimidines, and nucleic acids. They interfere with DNA synthesis by inhibiting key enzymes in the purine or pyrimidine synthetic pathways or by misincorporation in the DNA, leading to strand breaks or premature chain termination and slow cell division. An example of antimetabolites is 5-fluorouracil, which inhibits the formation of a thymine-containing nucleotide necessary for DNA synthesis; it is used in the treatment of breast cancer. Methotrexate is another antimetabolite; it binds to the enzyme responsible for the reduction of folic acid in the first step of the synthesis of nucleic acids, and is commonly used to treat leukemia. Other antimetabolites used for the treatment of leukemia are 6-thioguanine and 6-mercaptopurine.

Antitumor antibiotics are natural products of microbial metabolism. The singular purpose of these compounds is to afford these microbial organisms a selective advantage in hostile environments by interfering with the growth or proliferation of competing life-forms—therefore their usefulness in destroying cancer cells. Some of these antibiotics have been synthesized, but the naturally occurring ones have proven to be more effective. Antitumor antibiotics are effective against leukemia, lymphomas, sarcomas, carcinomas of most organs, and germ cell tumors. They are normally used as part of a multiagent chemotherapy regimen and also as part of adjuvant protocols. These compounds show a wide array of structures because of the variety of fungal organisms that are their source. They also exhibit a great diversity in mechanisms of action. For example, doxorubicin has been reported to have at least seven different mechanisms of action, and it is very difficult to determine which is the most effective. Daunorubicin acts by inhibition of DNA and ribonucleic acid (RNA) enzymes, idarubicin acts by the generation of oxygen-free radicals, and mitoxantrone's mechanisms of action include single-strand and double-strand DNA breaks, the peroxidation of cell membranes, and cell surface action.

Vinka alkaloids represent natural or semisynthetic drugs derived from the periwinkle plant, and the epipodophyllotoxins are semisynthetic products derived from the roots of the mayapple or mandrake plant. Of the vinka alkaloids, the most important are vincristine and vinblastine. Their general mechanism of action is the binding to dimers of tubulin, a protein subunit of microtubules. Microtubules perform many critical functions in the cell, such as the maintenance of cell shape, mitosis, meiosis, secretion, and intracellular transport. The binding of vinka alkaloids to tubulin causes the microtubule structures to disappear and the cell to die. They are useful in the treatment of Hodgkin's lymphomas and leukemia. Etoposide and teniposide, two of the epipodophyllotoxins, show good clinical activity, although their mechanism of action is not fully understood. Apparently involved in the mechanism are the breakage of single-strand and double-strand DNA and DNA protein cross-links. These compounds are useful in treating pediatric malignancies.

Hormonal therapy is an important and effective means to treat hormonally sensitive tumors, such as breast, endometrium, prostate, ovarian, and renal tumors. Although it is very hard to explain the mechanism of action, it is assumed that the initial step is the binding to a specific cell surface receptor. This can result in the inhibition of the production of factors necessary for tumor growth, the induction of growth inhibitory proteins, or the inhibition of oncogene expression. Examples of compounds employed in this type of therapy are the adrenocorticoids, used to treat leukemia; estrogens, used in breast cancer therapy; progestins, used for breast and endometrial cancer treatment; and androgens, used against breast cancer.

Immune modulation, or biological response modification against malignant disease, has been a long-sought goal. Developments in molecular biology and immunology and refinements in recombinant methodologies have set the stage for this approach to cancer treatment. It involves the modification of the relationship between the tumor and the host, primarily by modifying the host's response to tumor cells, with resultant therapeutic benefit. Among the substances studied is interferon, a simple glycoprotein with profound immunomodulatory, antiviral, and antiproliferative characteristics. There are three types of interferons, which attach themselves to receptors in the cell surface. This receptor-interferon complex initiates a variety of processes that affect DNA synthesis; it may also render a cell as foreign, facilitating the immune system's job of getting rid of it. In adoptive immunotherapy, immune-activated cells (or tumor killer cells) are administered to a host with advanced cancer in an attempt to mediate tumor regression. Tumor necrosis factor also exhibits antitumor activity and has also shown a synergistic effect with interferon.

Platinum analogues such as cisplatin produce high response rates in patients with small cell carcinoma of the lung, bladder cancer, and ovarian cancer. Most of the data are consistent with the hypothesis that the major target of the drug is DNA, although the type of lesions produced in the DNA structure is not clearly established.

SIDE EFFECTS

In addition to being highly toxic, most of the useful chemotherapy agents are themselves carcinogenic. Often, very high doses are necessary for effective treatment. As a result, combination therapy has increased in use because of the success of additive or even synergistic effects when two or more drugs are used, allowing the use of lower doses and reducing side effects.

Side effects of chemotherapy include nausea, vomiting, and diarrhea resulting from damage to the stomach and intestines; dryness and soreness of the mouth from damage to the mucous membranes; and partial loss of hair from damage to the hair follicles. When damage to the bone marrow occurs, the marrow ceases to supply the blood with a normal amount of white blood cells, platelets, and red blood cells, so that the body cannot properly control infection, bruising, or fatigue. Patients may also experience muscular weakness, loss of appetite, rashes, discoloration of the skin, irregular menstrual periods, and sterility. Most of these effects disappear when chemotherapy ends.

Unfortunately, cancer chemotherapy fails to cure most cancer patients because of the growth of resistant cells. Tumor cells are either intrinsically resistant or become resistant to individual drugs. A given chemotherapy regimen is followed until indication of the overgrowth of resistant cells, at which point treatment is ineffective. The development of effective drugs for treating cancer has been a landmark achievement of medical research. The hope for the eventual cure and prevention of malignancy rests with the development of safer agents with enhanced antitumor spectrums, as well as in the study of the synergistic effect of chemotherapy and biological response modifiers.

—Maria Pacheco

See also Breast cancer; Cancer; Cervical, ovarian, and uterine cancers; Colon cancer; Lung cancer; Mastectomy; Pain management; Radiation; Skin cancer.

FOR FURTHER INFORMATION:
Carter, Stephen K., Mary T. Bakowski, and Kurt Hellmann. *Chemotherapy of Cancer.* 3d ed. New York: John Wiley & Sons, 1987. A good reference book with sections on general cancer treatment, clinical trials, drug development, anticancer drugs, treatment of specific types of cancer. Very complete.
Chabner, Bruce A., and Jerry M. Collins, eds. *Cancer Chemotherapy: Principles and Practice.* 2d ed. Philadelphia: J. B. Lippincott, 1996. A compilation of works by more than thirty expert authors in the field of cancer chemotherapy. The book provides both an in-depth reference and a rapid source of critical information. An excellent reference work.
Joesten, Melvin D., David O. Johnston, John Netterville, and James L. Wood. *The World of Chemistry.* 2d ed. Philadelphia: W. B. Saunders College, 1999. A basic chemistry book with a good section on cancer and its treatments. Good for a quick reference.
Murphy, G., L. Morris, and D. Lange. *Informed Decisions: The Complete Book of Cancer Diagnosis, Treatment, and Recovery.* New York: Viking Press, 1997. This text from the American Cancer Society is intended for the layperson. It is exemplary in its discussion of cancer.
Perry, Michael C., ed. *The Chemotherapy Source Book.* 2d ed. Baltimore: Williams & Wilkins, 1996. A compilation of essays by experts in this field. Deals with the practical principles of chemotherapy, commercially available drugs by class (emphasizing their mechanisms of action), chemotherapy drug toxicity, combination therapy programs, and the therapy methods for specific tumors. A complete, thorough reference.

✧ CHILD ABUSE

Type of issue: Children's health, ethics, mental health
Definition: A series of problems that may include child neglect, physical

abuse, sexual abuse, emotional abuse, failure to thrive, and Münchausen syndrome by proxy.

Physical abuse may involve children of any age, but those at greatest risk for death are children under the age of three, especially infants under the age of one. Fatal abuse most often follows head trauma, often with the injuries inflicted during a violent shaking and/or a blunt impact to the head.

SHAKEN INFANT SYNDROME

Injuries related to shaking assume a classic pattern that allows physicians and other health care workers to recognize the abusive situation. Generally, the shaking episode is precipitated by an event such as inconsolable crying that angers and frustrates the caretaker. Often, the caretaker is a male companion of the mother or an inexperienced young babysitter. The infant is usually shaken with rapid successive movements, with the perpetrator's hands encircling the infant's chest. Sometimes, the infant sustains rib fractures. Intracranial injuries follow the rapid centrifugal movement of the infant's head back and forth through an arc. There is both axonal injury to the brain and subsequent bleeding, as small bridging blood vessels are disrupted. The bleeding is usually subdural or subarachnoid in location. In addition, there are hemorrhages into the infant's retinas. The mechanism of formation of these hemorrhages is unclear, although they may form directly as a result of the force being exerted on the retinal blood vessels. Cerebral edema and infarction (brain death) are additional sequelae of the shaking.

Several different clinical patterns may develop as a result of the shaking. The infant may experience apnea, seizures, or signs of increased intracranial pressure such as vomiting. Frequently, there has been a brief interval (sometimes about an hour) between the shaking and when the infant is reevaluated by the caretaker, who then fails to connect the earlier episode with the subsequent symptoms. Paramedics may be summoned, and the caretaker expresses puzzlement that the infant who was sleeping peacefully suddenly experienced medical problems.

At the hospital, an evaluation should include imaging studies such as computed tomography (CT) scanning and magnetic resonance imaging (MRI) of the head, which may reveal the presence of intracranial hemorrhages. A careful fundoscopic examination of the retina of the eye usually also shows hemorrhages. A skeletal survey may reveal the presence of fractures. Classically, rib fractures may be present, especially in younger infants. The absence of either retinal hemorrhages or rib fractures does not preclude the diagnosis of shaken infant syndrome. Other appropriate studies usually include coagulation panels to ensure that there are no underlying blood-clotting problems. Spinal taps, undertaken to exclude meningitis, may reveal the presence of yellow (xanthochromatic) fluid or shrunken (crenated) red blood cells. Skull fractures, when present, usually denote an impact injury, such as would occur if an infant were slammed against a solid surface during or after the shaking episode.

INJURIES DUE TO BLOWS

The second leading cause of death among abused children is abdominal trauma, usually following a direct blow to the abdomen. There may be laceration of the liver or spleen, with subsequent intra-abdominal hemorrhage and shock. Other injuries include rupture of the intestine or laceration of the mesentery (a layer of the peritoneum). In these cases, peritonitis may develop, with death occurring from this complication if medical intervention does not take place. Hematomas of the duodenum are another specific abdominal injury. In this case, the child may experience uncontrollable vomiting such as is seen with pyloric stenosis. An X ray of the abdomen would reveal a "double bubble" pattern as is seen in duodenal atresia (absence of an opening in the duodenum). Occasionally, trauma to the pancreas also occurs. In the absence of overt trauma or the use of medications that are harmful to the pancreas, inflicted injury is the leading cause of pancreatitis in children. The clinical picture in each of these cases may be confusing because of the absence of an overt history or any visual findings on the abdominal wall. The latter is a classic finding because of the force of the blow and the absorption of the impact internally. A high index of suspicion about inflicted abdominal trauma is essential to ensure the appropriate intervention.

External bruising is another manifestation of child abuse. Injuries may take various forms and need to be differentiated from accidental injuries. Normal bruises are noted over bony prominences, including the shins and forehead. Concern should be present when multiple bruises of different ages are present over soft tissue areas. The dating of bruises is somewhat controversial. In general, bruises follow a predictable pattern as they resolve, going from purple-blue (a classic black-and-blue mark) to green, then yellow and brown. The time course for the resolution of bruises is usually about two weeks, and some bruises do not make an appearance until one to two days after the injury. The size and depth of the bruise will affect the rate of resolution, and deeper, larger bruises may take longer to resolve.

Certain bruise patterns are clues to what induced the injury. Slap marks, grip marks, belt marks, paddling, cords, and bind and gag marks are some examples of these patterned injuries. Sometimes, unusual patterns are noted that may represent specific objects such as hairbrushes or wall molding. A search of the home may uncover such objects.

BURNS, BITES, AND BROKEN BONES

Burn injuries are also seen in abused children. Some of these injuries have characteristic patterns that occur because of immersion injuries. These injuries may involve the hands, feet, buttocks, or genitals. Injuries to the latter two areas usually occur in children between the ages of eighteen months and three years, when they are being toilet trained. Accidents during this period may be met with anger by a caretaker who cleans children in a punitive manner by immersing them in a tub filled with hot water. Other burn injuries may occur when a heated object is held in direct contact with the child's skin. The pattern of the object, such as a heating grid, is imposed on the skin. Cigarette burns also produce characteristic injuries. Sometimes, impetigo or resolving chickenpox may be mistaken for an inflicted burn, especially if there is superinfection with *Staphylococcus aureus.* Culturing the skin lesion is helpful in detecting such an infection.

Bites may also be an inflicted injury. Human bites, particularly if the skin is broken, carry the risk of serious infection. Differentiating child from adult bite marks can be facilitated by measuring the distance between the lateral incisors. The space between the lateral incisors in adults is at least 3 centimeters, while in children it is less than 3 centimeters. Additionally, forensic dentists can identify a perpetrator by the bite marks on the victim's skin.

Fractures may involve any bone, particularly long bones. While spiral or oblique fractures are highly suggestive of an inflicted injury (especially in the absence of a credible history), transverse fractures may also be inflicted. Other fractures include injuries to the metaphysis, leading to bucket handle or metaphyseal chip fractures. These injuries usually result from a twisting motion. Accidental fractures that are common during childhood include clavicular fractures, transverse long bone fractures, and supracondylar fractures which are incurred when a child falls from a height. The presence of multiple fractures of different ages is highly suspicious of inflicted injury.

CHILD NEGLECT

Sometimes, a child is injured as a result of neglect. Neglect includes withholding from the child basic needs such as food, clothing, housing, medical care, and education. The issue of medical care is somewhat complex. Some parents do not obtain medical care because of an alternative belief system. Other times, the family has not been compliant in following medical recommendations. For example, some children with asthma or diabetes require hospitalization in an intensive care unit because they do not take their medicines as prescribed. Neglect can also have fatal consequences. An infant left in a bathtub unattended even for a moment can drown. Children left unattended in a home may die as a result of a house fire that sometimes they are responsible for starting. An infant left in a car may overheat and die from hyperthermia. Sometimes, the parent's actions are even more blatant.

A mother may place her unwanted infant in a trash dumpster, where the infant dies as a result of exposure and lack of nutrition.

SEXUAL AND PSYCHOLOGICAL ABUSE

Sexual abuse differs from physical abuse in that the injuries are often not readily apparent. Sexual abuse can occur in many different ways, and for certain situations it would not be expected that the abuse would result in any findings. In general, concern about sexual abuse is raised because of a disclosure by a child or the presence of medical or behavioral problems.

In the past, often a long time interval existed between when the abuse occurred and when the child revealed the details of the events. This was in part related to the fact that children were frequently not believed, and no intervention occurred. With greater investigation and understanding of the nature of the sexual use of children, most adults now accept these disclosures as true, or at least believe that they warrant further evaluation.

Disclosures may be made to different individuals. In school-age children, the disclosure may be made to a teacher. Sometimes, children disclose the abuse to a close friend. Interviewing a child about the possibility of prior sexual abuse requires a skilled interviewer. Such interviews should be kept to a minimum, involve the most expert professionals, and allow for observation by legal agencies such as law enforcement and the district attorney's office. Children may recant their disclosures because of fear or embarrassment. The emotional turmoil associated with disclosure has been described in the writings of Dr. Roland Summit.

Some sexually abused children are brought to medical attention because of behavioral symptoms that they are experiencing. The specific symptoms are age-dependent but include sleep difficulties, bed-wetting (enuresis), soiling (encopresis), acting out behavior, masturbation, and sexually inappropriate behavior. In adolescents, school problems, running away, promiscuity, suicide gestures, and eating disorders (particularly bulimia) have also been reported. None of these problems is specific for prior sexual abuse and may be associated with other stressors, such as parental divorce or familial dysfunction.

Medical conditions may also bring sexually abused children to medical attention. In a child who has been recently abused, genital injuries may be present, and the child will have pain or bleeding in either the genital or anal areas. Sexually transmitted diseases (STDs) may develop in children who have been sexually abused. They may include gonorrhea, chlamydia, herpes, genital warts, and human immunodeficiency virus (HIV). Suspicion about an STD is usually aroused by the presence of lesions in the anogenital area or the appearance of a vaginal discharge. Not all discharges are caused by sexually transmitted conditions, however, and careful laboratory assessment is needed to ensure a correct diagnosis.

The medical assessment of the sexually abused child calls for a careful interview and a full medical evaluation. The examination of the anogenital area is frequently done with the use of magnifying equipment, most commonly a colposcope. Colposcopes usually include recording devices such as a video or still camera. The value of magnification is that it permits the examiner to differentiate normal variation from changes attributable to scarring and prior injuries. Most children with a history of prior sexual abuse have normal anogenital examinations because many abusive acts, such as fondling or oral-genital contact, do not produce physical injuries and because injuries to the anogenital area may heal without leaving residual findings. In girls, a hymen that has been injured may show evidence of disruptions, be reduced in amount, or have scars.

There are also medical conditions that affect the anogenital area which are not related to abuse. Accidental injuries, including straddle injuries, may cause bleeding in the genital area. Skin conditions can cause changes that may be mistaken for trauma. Other medical conditions that have been mistakenly diagnosed as sexual abuse include urethral prolapse (in which the urethra extrudes through the urethral orifice) and inflammatory bowel disease.

TREATING CHILD ABUSE

In all cases where an injured child is suspected of having been abused, an assessment must be made about the possibility of accidental trauma or some medical condition contributing to the findings. Such a determination is made after obtaining a full history, performing a comprehensive physical examination, and reviewing the appropriate diagnostic studies.

In cases of head trauma, a history of a minor fall or an unwitnessed event is often elicited. Simple falls do not result in significant intracranial hemorrhage. Occasionally, an epidural hemorrhage will occur following a minor fall, especially if there is an associated parietal skull fracture with disruption of the middle meningeal artery. The classic symptoms in this situation include a period of clearheadedness following the fall, after which the child becomes increasingly lethargic. Surgical intervention is essential and lifesaving. Similar surgical intervention with evacuation of a blood clot is sometimes needed with hemorrhages related to shaking. Management of cerebral edema is complicated and requires placement in an intensive care unit.

In children with multiple bruises, a medical condition that could account for easy bruising needs to be eliminated. In general, coagulation studies should include a complete blood count, including a platelet count and blood smear, a prothrombin time (PT), an activated partial thromboplastin time (aPTT), and a bleeding time. These studies will detect most, but not all, bleeding disorders, in addition to leukemia and thrombocytopenic conditions. Other medical conditions, such as Henoch-Schönlein purpura, may be misdiagnosed as inflicted trauma by the inexperienced clinician.

Children with bruises related to conditions other than abuse need to be managed accordingly.

In cases of abuse involving children under the age of two, there is consensus that skeletal surveys should be obtained to detect occult fractures. Such fractures are clinically apparent in older children, although some experts recommend trauma series in cases of abuse involving children up to the age of five. Children with fractures resulting from abuse need to have their fractures evaluated by orthopedists and then managed like fractures that result from accidental injuries, usually with casting, traction, and/or open reduction.

Children who have been sexually abused sometimes have medical problems that need to be addressed. Such problems may include the presence of STDs that warrant the use of antibiotics. Acute genital injuries may require surgical repair in the operating room.

In all cases of inflicted injuries, documentation of the findings is critical. The examiner should record carefully all physical findings, as well as diagnostic studies, in the medical records. In addition, photographs should be obtained. If law enforcement is available, a police photographer should photograph the child using a color index recorded on the photograph. Alternatively, a hospital photographer or the examiner should obtain photos of the injuries.

Long-term management of a child who has been abused needs to address the psychological trauma that has been experienced. As a rule, such children should be given counseling, which may include group sessions with other abused children, individual counseling, and family sessions.

Another component of the child abuse process involves the interaction with the legal system. The child, family, and physician may be called upon to testify in court about the events surrounding the alleged abuse. Testifying in court may be a stressful event for the child, but preparation, including speaking to the attorney ahead of time, may make the experience less traumatic.

THE PREVALENCE OF CHILD ABUSE

Child abuse was initially reported by American pediatrician John Caffey in 1946, when he described a series of children with chronic subdural hematomas and multiple fractures in long bones. The battered child syndrome was first reported by Henry Kempe and colleagues in 1962 in a classic article in which they described the multiple types of injuries that could be inflicted on a child.

The pervasiveness of abuse is evidenced by the fact that in the United States in 1996, there were approximately 1 million cases of abuse and an additional 1 million cases of neglect that were identified through the National Incidence Survey. It is unclear how many additional cases are not recognized through this surveillance mechanism.

Although many would choose to believe that child maltreatment is restricted to poor and inner-city populations, this is not the case. Children from all socioeconomic classes may be the victims of abuse. Some of the most publicized cases involve families not affected by the stresses of poverty and unemployment.

The understanding and knowledge of the nature of child abuse has grown since the 1960's, but areas remain that need further research and assessment. The mechanism of injury in shaken infant syndrome is still being evaluated. The resiliency of some children to abuse and neglect is being assessed in a longitudinal follow-up study. There are many unanswered questions related to child sexual abuse. What are the long-term medical effects of sexual abuse? Studies have suggested that women with functional bowel disease, chronic pelvic pain, and obesity have a higher incidence of having been abused as children. What happens to boys who are sexually abused? Do they experience medical problems or sexual dysfunction as adults?

The area of child abuse prevention is a challenging one to address. While the ability to recognize abuse and intervene has improved, no evidence exists that society has made any progress in the arena of child abuse prevention. This issue is very much linked to violence and how pervasive it has become in society. While poverty, substance abuse, and unemployment all have a role in predisposing people to child abuse, the ability of individuals to care for and parent children is also a contributing factor. The challenge for society is to interrupt the cycle of abuse and empower parents with the skills to nurture their children in a safe and caring environment.

—*Carol D. Berkowitz, M.D.*

See also Burns and scalds; Children's health issues; Domestic violence; Ethics; Falls among children; Malnutrition among children; Münchausen syndrome by proxy.

FOR FURTHER INFORMATION:
Brodeur, Armand E., and James A. Monteleone. *Child Maltreatment: A Clinical Guide and Reference.* 2 vols. St. Louis: G. W. Medical Publishing, 1994. A complete and comprehensive guide to all aspects of child abuse. Contains numerous photographs and X rays that illustrate injuries sustained by abused children.
Gellert, George A. *Confronting Violence: Answers to Questions About the Epidemic Destroying America's Homes and Communities.* Boulder, Colo.: Westview Press, 1997. A comprehensive guide to all types of violence in society, including child abuse. The information is laid out in a logical format that is easy to read and follow.
Goulding, Regina A., and Richard C. Schwartz. *The Mosaic Mind: Empowering the Tormented Selves of Child Abuse Survivors.* New York: W. W. Norton, 1995.

A fascinating account of how a multiple personality disorder developed in a woman who had been sexually abused and how therapy attempted to help her overcome the trauma of her past.

Heger, Astrid, and S. Jean Emans. *Evaluation of the Sexually Abused Child.* New York: Oxford University Press, 1992. A medical textbook and photographic atlas that details the various aspects of the comprehensive evaluation of sexually abused children.

Reece, Robert M., ed. *Child Abuse: Medical Diagnosis and Management.* Philadelphia: Lea & Febiger, 1994. A basic reference book for anyone dealing with child abuse. The book details various aspects of abuse and is written in an authoritative and scholarly manner by many of the nation's experts on child abuse.

✧ CHILDBIRTH COMPLICATIONS

Type of issue: Children's health, women's health
Definition: The difficulties that can occur during childbirth, either for the mother or for the baby.

With medical monitoring and diagnostic tests, about 5 to 10 percent of pregnant women can be diagnosed as high-risk pregnancies, and appropriate precautions and preparations for possible complications can be made prior to labor. Yet up to 60 percent of complications of labor, childbirth, and the postpartum period (immediately after birth) occur in women with no prior indications of possible complications. Difficulties in childbirth can be placed into two general categories—problems with labor and problems with the child—and encompass a wide range of causes and possible treatments.

COMPLICATIONS OF LABOR

Cesarean birth (also called cesarean section, C-section, or a section) is the surgical removal of the baby from the mother. About one in ten infants is delivered by cesarean birth. In this procedure, one incision is made through the mother's abdomen and a second through her uterus. The baby is physically removed from the mother's uterus, and the incisions are closed. This type of surgery is very safe but carries with it the general risks of any major surgery and requires approximately five days of hospitalization. In some cases, diagnosed preexisting conditions suggest that a cesarean birth is necessary and can be planned; in the majority of cases, unexpected difficulties during labor dictate that an emergency cesarean section be performed.

Some conditions leave no question about the necessity of a cesarean section. These absolute indications include a variety of physical abnormalities. Placenta previa is a condition in which the placenta has implanted in the lower part of the uterus instead of the normal upper portion, thereby totally or partially blocking the cervix. The baby could not pass down the birth canal without dislodging or tearing the placenta, thereby interrupting its blood and oxygen supply. Placenta previa is frequently the cause of bleeding after the twentieth week of pregnancy, and it can be definitively diagnosed by ultrasound. For women with this

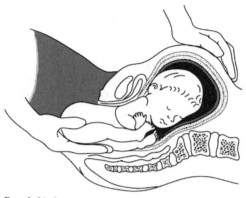

Breech birth, one of several complications that may occur during childbirth, is the emergence of the infant buttocks-first rather than head-first; such a birth is risky for the child, and often birth is accomplished by cesarean section, a surgical procedure to eliminate risk. (Hans & Cassidy, Inc.)

condition, bed rest is prescribed, and the baby will be delivered by cesarean birth at the thirty-seventh week of pregnancy.

Placental separation, also known as placenta abruptio, is the result of the placenta partially or completely separating from the uterus prior to the normal separation time after birth. This condition results in bleeding, with either mild or extreme blood loss depending on the severity of the separation. If severe, up to four pints of blood may be lost, and the mother is given a blood transfusion. If the pregnancy is near term, an emergency cesarean section is indicated to deliver the child.

Occasionally, as the baby begins traveling down the birth canal, the umbilical cord slips and lies ahead of the baby. This condition, called prolapsed cord, is very serious because the pressure of the baby against the cord during a vaginal delivery would compress the cord to the extent that the baby's blood and oxygen supply would be cut off. This condition necessitates an emergency cesarean section.

Some conditions that occur during labor are judged for their potential for causing harm to either the mother or the baby. The physician's decision to proceed with vaginal delivery will be based on the severity of the complication and consideration of the best option for the mother and baby. A few of the more common indicators for possible cesarean section which occur during labor include a fetal head size that is too large for the mother's birth canal; fetal distress, evidenced by insufficient oxygen supply reaching the baby; rupturing of the membranes without labor commencing or prolonged labor after membranes burst (usually twenty-four hours); and inelasticity of the pelvis in first-time mothers over forty years of age.

Other maternal conditions are diagnosed prior to the onset of labor, and the physician may or may not recommend a cesarean birth based on the severity of the complication. These include postmaturity, in which the onset of labor is at least two weeks overdue and degeneration of the placenta may compromise the health of the baby; maternal diseases, such as diabetes mellitus and toxemia, in which the stress of labor would be highly risky to the mother; and previous cesarean section.

Complications with the Baby

Premature labor can occur between twenty and thirty-six weeks gestation, and a premature infant is considered to be any infant whose birth weight is less than 5.5 pounds. Certain maternal illnesses or abnormalities of the placenta can lead to premature birth, but in 60 percent of the cases there is no identifiable cause. If labor begins six weeks or more prior to the due date, the best chance of infant survival is to be delivered and cared for at a hospital with a perinatal center and specialized intensive care for premature infants. Prior to twenty-four weeks development, a premature infant will not survive as a result of inadequate lung development. The survival rate of premature infants increases with age, weight, and body system maturity.

In about 4 percent of births, the baby is in the breech position—buttocks first or other body part preceding the head—rather than in the normal head-down position. Delivery in this position is complicated because the cervix will not dilate properly and the head may not be able to pass through the cervix. Other complications of breech position are prolapse or compression of the umbilical cord and trauma to the baby if delivered vaginally. Manual techniques may be used to rotate the baby into the correct position. Vaginal delivery may be attempted, frequently aided by gentle forceps removal of the baby. Breech babies are frequently born by cesarean section.

Cephalopelvic disproportion is a condition in which the baby's head is larger than the pelvic opening of the mother. This can only be determined after labor has begun, because the mother's muscles and joints expand to accommodate the baby's head. If at some point during labor the doctor determines that the baby will not fit through the mother's pelvic opening, a cesarean section will be performed.

—*Karen E. Kalumuck*

See also Amniocentesis; Birth defects; Diabetes mellitus; Genetic counseling; Miscarriage; Multiple births; Natural childbirth; Postpartum depression; Pregnancy among teenagers; Premature birth; Prenatal care; Women's health issues.

For Further Information:
Carlson, Karen J., Stephanie A. Eisenstat, and Terra Ziporyn. *The Harvard*

Guide to Women's Health. Cambridge, Mass.: Harvard University Press, 1996.

Gonik, Bernard, and Renee A. Bobrowski. *Medical Complications in Labor and Delivery.* Cambridge, Mass.: Blackwell Scientific, 1996.

Hotchner, Tracie. *Pregnancy and Childbirth.* Rev. ed. New York: Avon Books, 1997.

Sears, William, and Martha Sears. *The Birth Book.* Boston: Little, Brown, 1994.

Stoppard, Miriam. *Conception, Pregnancy, and Birth.* Rev. ed. London: Dorling Kindersley, 2000.

✧ CHILDHOOD INFECTIOUS DISEASES

Type of issue: Children's health, epidemics, public health
Definition: A group of diseases including diphtheria, tetanus, measles, polio, rubella (German measles), mumps, and pertussis (whooping cough).

Acute communicable diseases occur primarily in childhood because most adults have become immune to such diseases, either by having acquired them as children or by having been inoculated against them. For example, prior to the use of vaccine for measles—a highly contagious disease found in most of the world—the peak incidence of the disease was in five- to ten-year-olds. Most adults were immune. Before a vaccine was developed and used against measles, epidemics occurred at two- to four-year intervals in large cities. Today, most cases are found in nonimmunized preschool children or in teenagers or young adults who have received only one dose of the vaccine.

MEASLES

A person infected with red measles (also known as rubeola) becomes contagious about ten days after exposure to the disease virus, at which time the prodromal stage begins. Typically, the infected person experiences three days of slight to moderate fever, a runny nose, increasing cough, and conjunctivitis. During the prodromal stage, Koplik's spots appear inside the cheeks opposite the lower molars. These lesions—grayish white dots about the size of sand particles with a slightly reddish halo surrounding them that are occasionally hemorrhagic—are important in the diagnosis of measles.

After the prodrome, a rash appears, usually accompanied by an abrupt increase in temperature (sometimes as high as 104 or 105 degrees Fahrenheit). It begins in the form of small, faintly red spots and progresses to large, dusky red confluent areas, often slightly hemorrhagic. The rash frequently begins behind the ears but spreads rapidly over the entire face, neck, upper arms, and upper part of the chest within the first twenty-four hours. During the next twenty-four hours, it spreads over the back, abdomen, entire arms, and thighs. When it finally reaches the feet after the second or third day of the rash, it is already fading from the face. At this point, the fever is usually disappearing as well.

The chief complications of measles are middle-ear infections, pneumonia, and encephalitis (a severe infection of the brain). There is no correlation between the severity of the case of measles and the development of encephalitis, but the incidence of the infection of the brain runs to only one or two per every thousand cases. Measles can also exacerbate tuberculosis.

Rubella

The incubation period for rubella (German measles) lasts between fourteen and twenty-one days, and the disease occurs primarily in children between the ages of two and ten. Like the initial rash of measles, the initial rash of rubella usually starts behind the ears, but children with rubella normally have no symptoms save for the rash and a low-grade fever for one day. Adolescents may have a three-day prodromal period of malaise, runny nose, and mild conjunctivitis; adolescent girls may have arthritis in several joints that lasts for weeks. The red spots begin behind the ears and then spread to the face, neck, trunk, and extremities. This rash may coalesce and last up to five days. Temperature may be normal or slightly elevated.

Complications from rubella are relatively uncommon, but if pregnant women are not immune to the disease and are exposed to the rubella virus during early pregnancy, severe congenital anomalies may result. Because similar symptoms and rashes develop in many viral diseases, rubella is difficult to diagnose clinically. Except in known epidemics, laboratory confirmation is often necessary.

Mumps

The patient with mumps is likely to have fever, malaise, headache, and anorexia—all usually mild—but "neck swelling," a painful enlargement of the parotid gland near the ear, is the sign that often brings the child to a doctor. Maximum swelling peaks after one to three days and begins in one or both parotid glands, but it may involve other salivary glands. The swelling pushes the earlobe upward and outward and obscures the angle of the mandible. Drinking sour liquids such as lemon juice may increase the pain. The opening of the duct inside the cheek from the affected parotid gland may appear red and swollen.

The painful swelling usually dissipates by seven days. Abdominal pain may be caused by pancreatitis, a common complication but one that is usually mild. The most feared complication, sterility, is not as common as most believe. Orchitis rarely occurs in prepubertal boys and occurs in only 14 to 35 percent of older males. In 30 percent of patients with orchitis, both testes are involved, and a similar percentage of affected testes will atrophy. Surprisingly, impairment of fertility in males is only about 13 percent; absolute infertility is rare. Ovary involvement in women, with pelvic pain and tenderness, occurs in only about 7 percent of postpubertal women and with no evidence of impaired fertility.

Measles, rubella, and mumps are all viral illnesses, but *Hemophilus influenzae* type B is the most common cause of serious bacterial infection in the young child. It is the leading cause of bacterial meningitis in children between the ages of one month and four years, and it is the cause of many other serious, life-threatening bacterial infections in the young child. Bacterial meningitis, especially from *Hemophilus influenzae* and pneumococcus, is the major cause of acquired hearing impairment in childhood.

Polio

Poliomyelitis(polio), an acute viral infection, has a wide range of manifestations. The minor illness pattern accounts for 80 to 90 percent of clinical infections in children. Symptoms, usually mild in this form, include slight fever, malaise, headache, sore throat, and vomiting but do not involve the central nervous system. Major illness occurs primarily in older children and adults. It may begin with fever, severe headache, stiff neck and back, deep muscle pain, and abnormal sensations, such as of burning, pricking, tickling, or tingling. These symptoms of aseptic meningitis may go no further or may progress to the loss of tendon reflexes and asymmetric weakness or paralysis of muscle groups.

Fewer than 25 percent of paralytic polio patients suffer permanent disability. Most return in muscle function occurs within six months, but improvement may continue for two years. Twenty-five percent of paralytic patients have mild residual symptoms, and 50 percent recover completely. A long-term study of adults who suffered the disease has documented slowly progressive muscle weakness, especially in patients who experienced severe disabilities initially.

Tetanus, Diphtheria, and Whooping Cough

Tetanus is a bacterial disease which, once established in a wound of a patient without significant immunity, will build a substance that acts at the neuromuscular junction, the spinal cord, and the brain. Clinically, the patient experiences "lockjaw," a tetanic spasm causing the spine and extremities to bend with convexity forward; spasms of the facial muscles cause the famous "sardonic smile." Minimal stimulation of any muscle group may cause painful spasms.

Diphtheria is another bacterial disease that produces a virulent substance, but this one attacks heart muscle and nervous tissue. There is a severe mucopurulent discharge from the nose and an exudative pharyngitis (a sore throat accompanied by phlegm) with the formation of a pseudomembrane. Swelling just below the back of the throat may lead to stridor (noisy, high-pitched breathing) and to the dark bluish or purplish coloration of the skin and mucous membranes because of decreased oxygenation of the blood. The result may be heart failure and damaged nerves; respiratory insufficiency may be caused by diaphragmatic paralysis.

Clinically, pertussis (whooping cough) can be divided into three stages, each lasting about two weeks. Initial symptoms resembling the common cold are followed by the characteristic paroxysmal cough and then convalescence. In the middle stage, multiple, rapid coughs, which may last more than a minute, will be followed by a sudden inspiration of air and a characteristic "whoop." In the final stage, vomiting commonly follows coughing attacks. Almost any stimulus precipitates an attack. Seizures may occur as a result of hypoxia (inadequate oxygen supply) or brain damage. Pneumonia can develop, and even death may occur when the illness is severe.

CHICKENPOX AND HEPATITIS

Varicella (chickenpox) produces a generalized itchy, blisterlike rash with low-grade fever and few other symptoms. Minor complications, such as ear infections, occasionally occur, as does pneumonia, but serious complications such as infection in the brain are thankfully rare. It is a very inconvenient disease, however, requiring the infected person to be quarantined for about nine days or until the skin lesions have dried up completely.

Varicella, a herpes family virus, may lie dormant in nerve linings for years and suddenly emerge in the linear-grouped skin lesions identified as herpes zoster. These painful skin lesions follow the distribution of the affected nerve. Herpes zoster is commonly known as shingles.

HEPATITIS

Hepatitis type B is much more common in adults than in children, except in certain immigrant populations in which hepatitis B viral infections are endemic. High carrier rates appear in certain Asian and Pacific Islander groups and among some Inuits in Alaska, in whom perinatal transmission is the most common means of perpetuating the disease. Having this disease in childhood can cause problems later in life. An estimated five thousand deaths in the United States per year from cirrhosis or liver cancer occur as a result of hepatitis B. Carrier rates of between 5 and 10 percent result from disease acquired after the age of five, but between 80 and 90 percent will be carriers if they are infected at birth.

The serious problems of hepatitis B occur most often in chronic carriers. For example, 50 percent of carriers will ultimately develop liver cancer. The virus is fifty to one hundred times more infectious than human immunodeficiency virus (HIV), the virus that causes acquired immunodeficiency syndrome (AIDS). Health care workers are at high risk of contracting hepatitis B, but virtually everyone is at risk for contracting this disease because it is so contagious.

—Wayne R. McKinny, M.D.

See also AIDS and children; Antibiotic resistance; Children's health issues; Epidemics; Herpes; Immunizations for children; Influenza; Lice, mites, and ticks; Meningitis; Reye's syndrome; Tonsillectomy; Tuberculosis; Worms.

FOR FURTHER INFORMATION:

Behrman, Richard E., ed. *Nelson Textbook of Pediatrics.* 15th ed. Philadelphia: W. B. Saunders, 1996. This standard pediatrics textbook contains complete discussions of all common (and uncommon) causes of infectious disease in children. Many chapters are well written and easily understood by the nonspecialist.

Berkow, Robert, and Andrew J. Fletcher, eds. *The Merck Manual of Diagnosis and Therapy.* 17th ed. Rahway, N.J.: Merck Sharp & Dohme Research Laboratories, 1999. Published since 1899, this classic work is well indexed and easy to use. Discussions of the various infectious diseases of childhood are usually brief but thorough.

Burg, Fredric D., ed. *Treatment of Infants, Children, and Adolescents.* Philadelphia: W. B. Saunders, 1990. One can quickly find specific information about vaccine dosages and other valuable information in this text.

Korting, G. W. *Diseases of the Skin in Children and Adolescents.* Philadelphia: W. B. Saunders, 1970. An older textbook that contains color photographs of skin lesions in many childhood infectious diseases, matched by brilliant discussions of clinical patterns and signs.

Robbins, Stanley L., Ramzi S. Cotran, and Vinay Kumar, eds. *Robbins' Pathologic Basis of Disease.* 5th ed. Philadelphia: W. B. Saunders, 1999. An excellent textbook that combines the clinical and the pathological beautifully.

✦ CHILDREN'S HEALTH ISSUES

Type of issue: Children's health
Definition: The special health care needs of children and adolescents; at each stage of development, children experience different needs and have different abilities to be actively involved in good health practices.

The healthy growth and development of children are influenced by genetic and environmental elements. Yet, genetic and environmental elements can also contribute to unhealthy growth and development, as can be seen by infant mortality rates and the incidence of preventable diseases and abnormal development.

Health and Infant Mortality

Infant mortality in the United States has been declining, but it is still higher than in many other countries, including Japan, the Scandinavian countries, Great Britain, and Canada. In the United States there are nearly twice as many infant deaths among African Americans as among whites. Infant deaths among Hispanics approximately equal those among whites. Individual states vary greatly in their infant mortality rates. Teenage pregnancies and out-of-wedlock births are believed to be important factors in infant mortality, primarily because of associated risk factors such as poverty, substance abuse, or low levels of education. Preventable diseases such as tuberculosis and measles can contribute to infant mortality, but their effect can be decreased through access to primary health care. The same relationship exists for abnormal development, as seen in birth defects.

The causes of health problems or deaths in infants and older children are related to factors in society at large. These range from poor maternal health during pregnancy, to the decline in immunizations for some preventable diseases, to the presence and the use of health-threatening substances in the environment, to the lack of availability and use of health care, to the lack of family support resulting in accidents or death. Knowledge of these factors can affect the ability of parents and caregivers to provide an environment for infants and children that promotes healthy growth and development.

Prenatal Health

Sound prenatal health is an important factor in the development of healthy infants and children. The total dependence of unborn children on their mothers for nourishment and healthy development emphasizes the importance of a thoughtful approach to pregnancy at any age. Unplanned or unrecognized pregnancies can affect the health of infants and children if expectant mothers engage in activities that may prevent normal healthy development. Pregnancy in teenagers can create special problems, because growing mothers will compete with their fetuses for nutrients such as calcium, phosphorus, and iron. In addition, teenagers with low body weight are in danger of having infants with low birth weight, which is one of the leading causes of infant mortality. The thoughtful approach to pregnancy requires that mothers stop and think about what they are doing to themselves and how their behavior will affect their unborn children.

For example, foods and medicines ingested by mothers will be passed on to their unborn babies. Some substances pass quickly to fetuses while others pass on to them slowly. Still others concentrate in unborn children. The wrong drug or medicine during the first twelve weeks of pregnancy, when most birth defects are caused, could damage babies' development. Medical professionals generally agree that the use of drugs, alcohol, tobacco, and caffeine during pregnancy may have a harmful effect on fetuses, but they disagree on how much is too much. Expectant mothers can discuss these matters with health care providers to determine the appropriate approach to each individual pregnancy.

If women take drugs during pregnancy, either prescription or illicit drugs, their children can be born with drug dependencies or birth defects. Prenatal exposure to drugs such as cocaine and heroin has been associated with retarded growth, drug withdrawal, abnormal behavior, and drug dependency in infants. Prematurity and low birth weight have also been associated with drug exposure during pregnancy. Alcohol consumed during pregnancy is associated with fetal alcohol syndrome, which is characterized by a pattern of physical and mental defects. These include growth deficiencies, heart defects, and malformed facial features. Mental retardation is also associated with this syndrome. Fetal alcohol syndrome is considered to be an acute health problem, because it is associated with increased alcohol consumption in adolescents, who have a relatively high birth rate.

Smoking tobacco during pregnancy can cause nicotine and carbon monoxide to decrease the flow of blood and oxygen to unborn children. Infants of mothers who smoke may be born prematurely, have low birth weights, and be more susceptible to respiratory infections after birth. Caffeine in coffee, tea, chocolate, and soft drinks acts as a stimulant, but it builds up in concentrated amounts in the placenta. The effects of this are not completely known, but studies on animals have linked caffeine to bone deformities and the development of cleft palate.

Spina bifida is another condition that may be caused by unfavorable environmental patterns. This birth defect of the lower spinal cord develops shortly after conception and results in muscle paralysis, spine and limb deformities, and bowel and bladder problems. Spina bifida is believed to be caused by a combination of genetic and environmental factors, but the American Medical Association has noted that the children of women who use hot tubs are almost three times more likely to have this defect than the children of women who do not. Women who intend to become pregnant are thus encouraged to restrict their use of hot tubs and saunas.

PREVENTABLE DISEASE CONTROL

One of the major factors in the health of infants and children is access to immunizations. A vaccine, a substance made of dead or weakened bacteria or virus cells, is given either by injection (shot) or orally so that infants' and children's bodies may build defenses against preventable diseases. Immunizations cause the body to produce antibodies that fight against particular diseases and continue to protect against future exposures. Infants must be vaccinated against mumps, measles, polio, German measles, diphtheria, pertussis (whooping cough), tetanus, chickenpox, and Hib disease (associated with bacterial meningitis). In addition to protecting infants and children against specific diseases, immunizations help to ensure that they will not suffer from the side effects of these diseases, which can include hearing loss and damage to the nervous system or heart.

Older children may require booster shots for some diseases. The American Academy of Pediatrics has worked with the U.S. Centers for Disease Control (CDC) to establish a schedule for immunization of infants and children. Children's primary health care givers should be consulted on the appropriate schedule of immunizations. Regardless of the particular immunization schedule, it is important that children be immunized in order to prevent disease outbreak before they begin kindergarten at ages four to six and when they are in middle or junior high school at ages eleven to twelve. Primary health care givers should also be consulted about the possibility of adverse reactions to vaccines. The chance of adverse reactions is slight, but in some instances mild fever or soreness may be experienced. When compared with the greater danger posed by the diseases against which vaccines guard, such reactions are minor.

In addition to immunizations before starting school, children should be tested for tuberculosis. There has been a resurgence of tuberculosis in the United States, causing serious concern in child care or educational settings. This disease can cause lymph node infection, pulmonary complications, and possibly a form of meningitis. Because early symptoms resemble those associated with the common cold, tuberculosis has the potential to spread to other children or adults working with children.

EXPOSURE TO HEALTH-THREATENING SUBSTANCES

Many substances in the environment can pose a threat to the health of infants and children. Because of their less developed immune systems and small body size, children have lower resistance to toxic substances and may be at greater health risk than adults. Exposure can take different forms, such as inhalation of secondhand smoke or dust, absorption of chemicals that come in contact with the skin, or ingestion of solids or liquids. Secondhand smoke from cigarettes, pipes, or cigars can be released into the air from two sources. Mainstream smoke is first inhaled into a smoker's mouth and nasal passages before being exhaled. Sidestream smoke is more dangerous for nonsmokers, because it goes directly into the air from burning tobacco. It has higher concentrations of harmful compounds such as benzene and formaldehyde than mainstream smoke and has carbon monoxide levels that may be two to fifteen times higher than in mainstream smoke.

Studies have shown that secondhand smoke is detrimental to infants and children. Smoking by pregnant women may cause premature babies to be susceptible to respiratory distress syndrome. Babies of parents who smoke have a higher rate of lung diseases, such as bronchitis and pneumonia, in their first two years of life than babies of nonsmoking parents. Studies have also shown that babies of smokers may have problems with speech, intelligence, and attention span. Children ages five to nine years old have shown impaired lung function from secondhand smoke. Asthma attacks can be triggered by secondhand smoke. It is apparent that smokeless environments will give infants and children the best possible opportunity for healthy growth and development.

Infants and children are also at risk of exposure to toxic chemicals that may be used in households. Cleaning agents and insecticides may be absorbed through the skin if infants and children are accidentally exposed to them. The potential for absorption through the skin may be higher with those substances that contain organic solvents to maintain the chemicals' liquid form or to boost cleaning power. Acute exposure to toxic chemicals may have less severe results, such as nausea, dizziness, or fever, but chronic exposure could lead to the development of multiple chemical sensitivities or life-threatening diseases such as cancer. It is important to keep toxic chemicals out of the reach of children as well as to limit children's exposure to them. The use of more natural cleaning products and insecticides may help reduce the possible development of long-term health problems.

ENVIRONMENTAL HAZARDS

As infants and children develop, so does their tendency to put objects and substances into their mouths. Those objects that are small enough can pose a health threat if they are swallowed or lodged in the esophagus or lungs. Other substances that can be swallowed may pose a long-term health threat because of their chemical effects on the body. This is especially the case with lead, which may be present in paint and water pipes in older homes as well as in the soil in and around homes. Lead, whether swallowed or inhaled through dust, can build up in the blood and cause long-term effects such as learning disabilities, decreased growth, hyperactivity, impaired learning, and possibly brain damage. These effects can be reduced by medical treatment if lead poisoning is diagnosed early enough. Parents should have their children tested for lead poisoning if their homes contain paint that is more than thirty years old. Other ways to reduce the likelihood of lead exposure include keeping toys and pacifiers clean and preventing children from chewing on painted surfaces such as window sills, cribs, or playpens. Finally, parents should remember that good eating habits can help reduce the effects of lead; a diet with the appropriate amounts of iron and calcium will decrease the ability of the body to absorb lead.

—*Cherilyn Nelson*

See also Abortion among teenagers; AIDS and children; Alcoholism among teenagers; Asthma; Attention-deficit disorder (ADD); Autism; Birth defects; Breast-feeding; Burns and scalds; Child abuse; Childbirth complications; Childhood infectious diseases; Circumcision of boys; Circumcision of girls; Cleft lip and palate; Colic; Dental problems in children; Depression in children; Disabilities; Drowning; Drug abuse by teenagers; Exercise and children; Failure to thrive; Falls among children; Fetal alcohol syndrome; Hydrocephalus; Immunizations for children; Lead poisoning; Learning disabilities; Malnutrition among children; Münchausen syndrome by proxy; Nutrition and children; Obesity and children; Phenylketonuria (PKU); Physical fitness tests for children; Poisoning; Poisonous plants; Pregnancy among teenagers; Premature birth; Prenatal care; Reye's syndrome; Safety issues for children; Spina bifida; Sports injuries among children; Sudden infant death syndrome (SIDS); Suicide among children and teenagers; Sunburns; Tattoos and body piercing; Teething; Tobacco use by teenagers; Tonsillectomy; Well-baby examinations.

For Further Information:
Behrman, Richard E., ed. *Nelson Textbook of Pediatrics.* 14th ed. Philadelphia: W. B. Saunders, 1992. Standard pediatrics textbook that is written to be understood by nonspecialists and covers both common and uncommon causes of infectious disease in children.
Edelstein, Sari F. *The Healthy Young Child.* Minneapolis/St. Paul: West, 1995. Discusses infants from birth to one year old, toddlers and preschoolers from one to five years old, and elementary-age children from six to eight years old in terms of growth, development, physical activity, nutrition, safety, hygiene, and modern health issues.
Gravelle, Karen. *Understanding Birth Defects.* New York: Franklin Watts, 1990. Discusses the nature of birth defects, how to prevent them, and what to do for children who have them.
Reuben, Carolyn. *The Healthy Baby Book: A Parent's Guide to Preventing Birth Defects and Other Long-Term Medical Problems Before, During, and After Pregnancy.* New York: Jeremy P. Tarcher/Perigee, 1992. Straightforward guidebook on children's health written for parents.
Trahms, Christine M., and Peggy L. Pipes, eds. *Nutrition in Infancy and Childhood.* 6th ed. New York: McGraw-Hill, 1997. Comprehensive overview, written for both professionals and nonprofessionals, of the nutritional needs of both healthy and sick children from infancy through adolescence, the development of food habits, and the prevention of chronic diseases through dietary intervention.

✦ CHLORINATION

Type of issue: Environmental health, industrial practices, prevention, public health
Definition: The practice of disinfecting water by the addition of chlorine.

Although the chlorination of public water in the United States has helped reduce outbreaks of waterborne disease, it has raised concerns about the possible formation of chloro-organic compounds in treated water.

Drinking water, waste waters, and water in swimming pools are the most common water sources where chlorination is used to kill bacteria and prevent the spread of diseases. Viruses are generally more resistant to chlorination, but they can be eliminated by increasing the chlorine levels needed to kill bacteria. Common chlorinating agents include elemental chlorine gas and sodium or calcium hypochlorite. In water these substances generate hypochlorous acid, which is the chemical agent responsible for killing microorganisms by inactivating bacteria proteins or viral nucleoproteins.

Public drinking water was chlorinated in most large U.S. cities by 1914. The effectiveness of chlorination in reducing outbreaks of waterborne diseases in the early twentieth century was clearly illustrated by the drop in typhoid deaths: 36 per 100,000 in 1920 to 5 per 100,000 by 1928. Chlorination has remained the most economical method to purify public water, although it is not without potential risks. Chlorination has also been widely used to prevent the spread of bacteria in the food industry.

POTENTIAL HAZARDS OF CHLORINATION

In its elemental form, high concentrations of chlorine are very toxic, and solutions containing more than 1,000 milligrams per liter are lethal to humans. Chlorine has a characteristic odor that is detectable at levels of 2 to 3 milligrams per liter of water. Most public water supplies contain chlorine levels of 1 to 2 milligrams per liter, although the actual concentrations of water reaching consumer faucets fluctuates and is usually around 0.5 milligram per liter. Consumption of water containing 50 milligrams per liter has produced no immediate adverse effects.

The greatest environmental concern from chlorination is not usually from the chlorine itself, but from the potential toxic compounds that may form when chlorine reacts with organic compounds present in the water. Chlorine, which is an extremely reactive element, reacts with organic material associated with decaying vegetation (humic acids), forming chloro-organic compounds. Trihalo-methanes (THMs) are one of the most common chloro-organic compounds. At least a dozen THMs have been identified in drinking water since the 1970's, when health authorities came under pressure to issue standards for the identification and reduction of THM levels in drinking water.

Major concern has focused on levels of chloroform because of its known carcinogenic properties in animal studies. Once used in cough syrups, mouthwashes, and toothpastes, chloroform in consumer products is now severely restricted. A 1975 study of chloroform concentrations in drinking water found levels of more than 300 micrograms per liter in some water, with 10 percent of the water systems surveyed having levels of more than 105 micrograms per liter. In 1984, the World Health Organization used a guideline value of 30 micrograms per liter for chloroform in drinking water. Although there are risks associated with drinking chlorinated water, it has been estimated that the risk of death from cigarette smoking is two thousand times greater than that of drinking chloroform-contaminated water from most public sources. However, as water sources become more polluted and require higher levels of chlorination to maintain purity, continual monitoring of chloro-organic compounds will be needed.

—*Nicholas C. Thomas*

See also Environmental diseases; Epidemics; Fluoridation of water sources; Water quality.

FOR FURTHER INFORMATION:
Connell, Gerald F. *The Chlorination/Chloramination Handbook.* Denver: American Water Works Association, 1996.
De Zuane, John. *Handbook of Drinking Water Quality.* 2d ed. New York: Van Nostrand Reinhold, 1997.
Jolley, Robert L., and Lyman W. Condie. *Water Chlorination: Chemistry, Environmental Impact, and Health Effects.* Boca Raton, Fla.: Lewis, 1990.
White, George Clifford. *Handbook of Chlorination and Alternative Disinfectants.* 4th ed. New York: John Wiley & Sons, 1998.

✧ CHOKING

Type of issue: Children's health, public health
Definition: A condition in which the breathing passage (windpipe) is obstructed; it is one of the most common causes of death in young children.

A person who is choking may cough, turn red in the face, clutch his or her throat, or any combination of the above. If the choking person is coughing, it is probably best to do nothing; the coughing should naturally clear the airway. The true choking emergency occurs when a bit of food or other foreign object completely obstructs the breathing passage. In this case, there is little or no coughing—the person cannot make much sound. This silent choking calls for immediate action.

PERFORMING THE HEIMLICH MANEUVER

An individual witnessing a choking emergency should first call for emergency help and then perform the Heimlich maneuver. The choking person should never be slapped on the back. The Heimlich maneuver is best performed while the choking victim is standing or seated. If possible, the person performing the Heimlich maneuver should ask the victim to nod if he or she wishes the Heimlich maneuver to be performed. If the airway is totally blocked, the victim will not be able to speak and may even be unconscious.

The individual performing the Heimlich maneuver positions himself or herself behind the choking victim and places his or her arms around the victim's waist. Making a fist with one hand and grasping that fist with the other hand, the rescuer positions the thumb side of the fist toward the stomach of the victim—just above the navel and below the ribs. The person performing the maneuver pulls his or her fist upward into the abdomen of the victim with several quick thrusts. This action should expel the foreign object from the victim's throat, and he or she should begin coughing or return to normal breathing.

The Heimlich maneuver is not effective in dislodging fish bones and certain other obstructions. If the airway is still blocked after several Heimlich thrusts, a finger sweep should be tried to remove the obstruction. First the mouth of the victim must be opened: The chin is grasped, and the mouth is pulled open with one hand. With the index finger of the other hand, the rescuer sweeps through the victim's throat, pulling out any foreign material. One sweep should be made from left to right, and a second sweep from right to left. The Heimlich maneuver may then be repeated if necessary.

TREATING A CHOKING CHILD

Although it is possible for a child to choke when suffering from a disease such as croup, which involves swelling of the airways as a result of a viral infection, most children choke when foreign objects become lodged in the esophagus. Children frequently swallow and choke on coins, small batteries, balloons, marbles, small balls, and other toys. Almost any food can cause choking as well. Most experts agree that the most dangerous food items include hot dogs, carrots, grapes, cherries, raisins, nuts, popcorn, apples, pears, hard candy, celery, peanut butter, beans, chickpeas, marshmallows, and chunks of meat. A child who is eating may choke by suddenly inhaling while talking, laughing, or crying out in surprise. Parents can lessen the risk of choking by childproofing the environment, by closely monitoring play and other activities, by teaching safe eating habits, and by restricting the intake of dangerous foods.

A child who is choking but trying to cough up a swallowed object should be monitored. Intervention should take place only if the child is unable to make a sound, indicating that the airway is fully obstructed. At this point, the procedure for treatment varies. An infant under the age of one should be balanced facedown against an adult's forearm and given five quick and firm blows between the shoulder blades. If this does not dislodge the object, the infant should be turned face up and the adult should deliver five quick thrusts to the chest. Most experts agree that a child between one and three years of age should be placed on the back while an adult presses quickly and firmly upward and into the abdomen up to five times. The Heimlich maneuver can be performed on children over three. These procedures usually dislodge the object. If not, cardiopulmonary resuscitation (CPR) should be performed and help summoned.

—Steven A. Schonefeld; Cassandra Kircher

See also Children's health issues; First aid; Resuscitation; Safety issues for children; Safety issues for the elderly.

FOR FURTHER INFORMATION:

Anderson, Kenneth N., et al., eds. *Mosby's Medical, Nursing, and Allied Health Dictionary.* 5th ed. St. Louis: C. V. Mosby, 1998.

Castleman, Michael. "Emergency! Fifty-four Ways to Save Your Life." *Family Circle* 107, no. 4 (March 15, 1994): 37.

Heimlich, H. J., and E. A. Patrick. "The Heimlich Maneuver: The Best Technique for Saving Any Choking Victim's Life." *Postgraduate Medicine* 87, no. 6 (May 1, 1990): 38-48, 53.

Stern, Loraine. "Your Child's Health: Mom, I Can't Breathe!" *Woman's Day* 57, no. 6 (March 15, 1994): 18.

✧ CHOLESTEROL

Type of issue: Prevention, public health, social trends
Definition: A fatlike substance found in certain foods and manufactured in the liver.

The body needs cholesterol for a variety of purposes. It is a component of cell membranes, for example, and is needed for the production of bile and certain hormones (estrogen, testosterone, and adrenal hormones). It is a component of brain and nerve cells.

Cholesterol circulates in the blood attached to proteins called lipoproteins. Major lipoproteins include chylomicrons, which carry digested and absorbed dietary fats in the blood; very low-density lipoproteins (VLDLs); low-density lipoproteins (LDLs), which are also called "bad" cholesterol; and high-density lipoproteins (HDLs), also called "good" cholesterol because HDLs seem to have protective functions.

The liver manufactures about half of the cholesterol needed by the body; the rest comes from foods. Dietary sources of cholesterol include animal fats and oils such as egg yolk, whole milk, butter, cream, cheeses, ice cream, sour cream, lard, and meats, especially fatty meats. Dietary cholesterol raises LDLs and total cholesterol in the blood, but to a lesser extent than foods high in saturated fatty acids. Saturated fats are found in many of the same foods as cholesterol as well as in some vegetable oils, including coconut, palm, and palm kernel oils.

Despite the body's need for cholesterol, excessive amounts over long periods of time can accumulate in blood vessels, increasing the risk of atherosclerosis, coronary artery disease, or carotid artery disease. These increase the risk of heart attack or stroke. The American Heart Association recommends a blood cholesterol level of 200 milligrams per deciliter or less to lower the risk of heart disease. Elevated levels of LDLs increase the risk the most and should be below 130 milligrams per deciliter in the general population.

Blood cholesterol levels increase with age, especially LDL levels. Cholesterol levels are generally higher in men than in women until women reach the menopause, when their levels begin to increase. For both men and women, heart disease is the number one cause of death in the United States.

CHOLESTEROL AND NUTRITION

Both people with elevated blood cholesterol levels and the general population are advised to reduce their consumption of cholesterol (300 milligrams daily or less), of total fat (30 percent of dietary calories or less), of saturated fat (8 to 10 percent of total calories), and trans fats (or transfatty acids) in hydrogenated foods such as margarines and shortenings. One should choose lean cuts of meats with the fat trimmed, limit meat portions to 6 ounces daily, choose low-fat dairy products, use small amounts of monounsaturated vegetable oils such as olive and canola oils, and eat increased amounts of fruits, vegetables, and whole grains.

Reading the nutrition labels on foods to learn the grams of total fat, saturated fat, and cholesterol the foods contain is helpful in selecting appropriate foods. Increasing exercise, losing weight if overweight, and stopping smoking are also recommended for those with high levels of blood cholesterol. In addition, some people with high levels of blood cholesterol may need to take lipid-lowering drugs.

—Betsy B. Holli

See also Arteriosclerosis; Heart attacks; Heart disease; Heart disease and women; Malnutrition among the elderly; Nutrition and aging; Obesity; Obesity and aging; Smoking; Strokes.

For Further Information:
Dietschy, John M. "Physiology in Medicine: LDL Cholesterol: Its Regulation and Manipulation." *Hospital Practice* 25 (June 15, 1990): 67-78.
Grundy, Scott M. *Cholesterol and Atherosclerosis.* Philadelphia: J. B. Lippincott, 1990.
Nesto, N. W., and Lisa Christenson. *Cholesterol-Lowering Drugs: Everything You and Your Family Need to Know.* New York: William Morrow, 2000.
Yeagle, Philip L. *Understanding Your Cholesterol.* San Diego: Academic Press, 1991.

✧ Chronic fatigue syndrome

Type of issue: Public health, women's health
Definition: Chronic fatigue syndrome is a multifaceted disease state characterized by debilitating fatigue.

Chronic fatigue syndrome is a heterogenous disease state that has been difficult to define, diagnose, and treat because of poorly understood cause-and-effect relationships. The disease can be best described in terms of long-lasting and debilitating fatigue, the etiology of which has been linked to such external factors as microbial agents, stress, and lifestyle as well as such internal factors as genetic makeup and the body's immune response. The fact that it is a physical disease with psychological components has also caused confusion in the medical community.

Among the many names that have been used for the disease, the three that demonstrate the many factors that contribute to chronic fatigue syndrome are chronic Epstein-Barr virus syndrome, chronic fatigue immune dysfunction syndrome, and "Yuppie flu." Because of the marked immunological aspects of the disease and the fact that different viruses have been found in patients with chronic fatigue, the disease is referred to as chronic fatigue immune dysfunction syndrome by many involved in the study. The Centers for Disease Control (CDC) continues to refer to it as chronic fatigue syndrome (CFS).

Although the disease is not specific by race, sex, or age group, there is demographic evidence that young white females make up two-thirds of the known cases. It is estimated by the CDC that between 1 and 10 of every 10,000 people in the United States have CFS. The disease has also been identified as a problem in Europe and Australia.

ACUTE AND CHRONIC PHASES

CFS can manifest itself in acute and chronic phases, although some patients do not remember an acute phase presentation. Acute phase symptoms are general and flulike, with a low-grade fever, sore throat, headache, muscle pain, painful lymph nodes, and overall fatigue. Unlike with a bout of influenza, the symptoms do not subside with time, instead intensifying into a chronic phase. The fatigue can become disabling, with severe muscle and joint pain, swollen and painful lymph nodes, and the inability to develop proper sleep patterns. Some researchers blame psychological and emotional stress, with a viral infection having triggered the initial acute phase. Although the psychological description does not fit all cases, problems of concentration, attention, and depression have been implicated to the point that researchers recognize both psychological and physical components.

The working definition from both a research and a clinical perspective requires that the fatigue cause at least 50 percent incapacitation and last at least six months. The ineffectiveness of treatment, compounded by the inability to provide a concrete diagnosis, further complicates the psychological aspects of the disease for the patient.

ENVIRONMENTAL OR VIRAL AGENTS?

Although the environment provides an array of agents that could trigger the physical condition of CFS, the hypothesis for a viral cause is supported by the flulike symptoms, occasional clustering of cases, and the presence of antiviral antibodies in the patient's serum. The involvement of the Epstein-Barr virus in CFS seems likely because of its role as the etiological agent of mononucleosis and Burkitt's lymphoma, which are similar diseases. In both of these diseases, the Epstein-Barr virus has a unique and harmful effect on the immune system because it directly invades B lymphocytes, the antibody-producing cells of the body, using them to grow new virus particles while disrupting the proper functioning of the immune system. Like CFS, mononucleosis is characterized by flulike symptoms and fatigue, but the disease is self-limiting and the patient eventually recovers.

Despite this seeming difference in outcome, the Epstein-Barr virus can cause a chronic condition. The viruses that infect humans can become dormant within the cells that they infect. The nucleic acid of a virus can become incorporated into the DNA of its host cell, and the body no longer shows physical signs of their presence. A virus can become active at times of physical or emotional stress and can once again trigger the physical symptoms of disease. For example, herpes simplex virus 1 remains dormant in its host cell but periodically, in response to environmental factors, causes a cold sore lesion.

Some patients with CFS have also been infected with two retroviruses, human T cell lymphotropic virus type II (HTLV-II) and a Spumavirus. Both are related to the human immunodeficiency virus (HIV), the causative agent of acquired immunodeficiency syndrome (AIDS). Retrovirus genes are made of ribonucleic acid (RNA) rather than deoxyribonucleic acid (DNA), as are the genes of herpes-type viruses such as Epstein-Barr and herpes simplex virus 1. Retroviruses must convert their RNA into complementary DNA (cDNA) when they infect a host cell in order to incorporate their genes into the host cell genes. Although the two viruses are associated with some CFS patients, diagnostic tests developed to detect their presence have not confirmed that the CFS condition depends on their presence. This same finding is true of herpesvirus 6 and other viruses. Although viruses may play a role in CFS, they are not the only factors involved and are not substantive evidence to define a clinical or research case.

Immunological dysfunction has been observed in CFS patients because they demonstrate increased allergic sensitivity to skin tests when compared with normal individuals. Cells and cellular chemicals directly involved with protective immunity and the regulation of the immune response have been found in these patients in abnormal concentrations. For example, they have abnormal numbers of the natural killer cells and suppressor T cells that are essential to cell-mediated immunity. Cellular chemicals such as gamma interferon and interleuken II that regulate the activities of the cells in the cell-mediated and humeral immune responses are seen in abnormal concentrations in some CFS patients. Infectious agents, bacteria, viruses, yeasts, parasites, and even cancer cells are eliminated from the body when humeral and cell-mediated immune systems are operating properly. When the immune system is not working properly, however, not only is the body more susceptible to a variety of infectious agents but the immune system can actually begin to destroy normal body tissues, such as the thyroid gland and other vital organs. Such disease states are referred to as autoimmune diseases. Allergic reactions are also examples of uncontrolled immune responses. The component immune dysfunction of CFS is thought to be significant enough for some researchers to recommend that new and worsening allergies be added as minor criteria to the case definition for the disease.

The psychological and emotional aspects of CFS are also in question. Some studies indicate that the brain is physically affected by inflammation and hormonal changes. Other studies demonstrate that some of the known viral infective agents can have neurological effects. Psychiatric studies give ample evidence that depression, memory loss, and concentration are significant problems for some CFS patients. The extent to which stress is a factor in the disease is unknown.

Defining the Symptoms

In 1993, a meeting at the CDC attempted to evaluate what had been learned over the previous five-year period and to make recommendations regarding a case definition. It was suggested that the case definition format involve inclusion and exclusion criteria that would increase the number and range of cases being studied because of the heterogeneous nature of the disease. The cases should also be subcategorized to provide a homogeneity that would allow for subgroup identification and comparison. The inclusion evidence should be simple, with a descriptive interpretation of the fatigue being essential and having objective criteria to define a 50 percent reduction of physical activity. Symptoms that are specific to unexplained fatigue should be used, while the physical exam information should not be included. It was also suggested that exclusion of any cases should involve an in-depth history (both medical and psychiatric), a physical examination, and standardized testing that would involve medical, laboratory, and psychiatric information.

Because it appears that CFS overlaps with many other medical and psychiatric conditions that can be identified and treated, there is debate as to how to interpret CFS as it relates to patient care and research. Some believe that an in-depth history is fundamental to the understanding of CFS and that CFS could be the final pathway that occurs from a variety of biological and psychosocial insults to the body.

The minor criteria used to define CFS involve both symptom and physical criteria that have not been proved adequate to validate or define the condition. In fact, the conflicting data have only served to emphasize further the clinical heterogeneity of the disease and suggest a heterogeneity of cause. Suggestions have been made to drop the concept of minor criteria, use symptoms that are specific for the unexplained fatigue, and drop all physical examination criteria. The argument for eliminating physical criteria is that more specific criteria exist for a case definition. Because physical symptoms are inconsistent or periodic, it is believed that a documented patient history would provide more case-specific information.

Although symptom criteria have widespread support in the case definition of CFS, symptoms with the greatest sensitivity and specificity are also being debated. Night sweats, cough, gastrointestinal problems, and new and worsening allergies are not presently considered and are believed by some to be more specific than fever or chills and sore throat. Others have proposed that symptoms should be reduced to chills and fever, sore throat, neck or axilla adenopathy, and sudden onset of a main symptom complex. The most prevalent symptoms are believed to be muscle weakness and pain, problems in concentration, and sleep disturbance.

The importance of the psychiatric component in CFS continues to be a problem in case definition. Some believe that the neurological component is a major criterion in case definition and that behavior symptoms, including stress and psychiatric illness, must be emphasized in clinical diagnosis as well as in therapy. It has been recommended that objective neuropsychological testing be used to determine cognitive dysfunction and depression. There is agreement that CFS patients have impaired concentration and attention, but forgetfulness and memory problems are questioned. There is also evidence that the duration and severity of myalgia are closely associated with psychological distress and that psychotherapy improves physical symptoms. Finally, it has been argued that the psychiatric component of the case definition is essential because there is evidence that the disease directly affects the brain and that CFS can cause both isolation and limitation of the patient's normal lifestyle.

TESTING FOR THE DISEASE

Whatever the case definition, the second major criterion will be expressed in some form. Proper patient care necessitates extensive evaluation in order to identify the biological or psychological reasons for the problem. Proper CFS patient care demands the elimination of other serious disease possibilities that may appear superficially similar. Primary care physicians may find it difficult to make a diagnosis without a team of specialists in the areas of hematology, immunology, and psychiatry. Numerous laboratory tests must be made available. Although there are no specific recommended tests, those that must be performed should be tailored to specific patients and used by the team of specialists for their care.

The possibility of infectious disease, either as part of CFS (as in the case of certain viral agents) or as an autonomous infection having no relation to CFS, requires a variety of antibody tests to detect such viruses as Epstein-Barr or HIV. Skin tests such as the purified protein derivative (PPD) test for tuberculosis are used. Polymerase chain reaction and tissue culture for cytopathic effects have been developed to detect certain retroviruses for ultimate use in diagnosis at the clinical level.

The immune system is so intimately interactive with the entire body that most disease conditions are affected by or affect its function. The measure of its components provides a clue to the identity of the disease that is operating because they indicate whether normal protection activity or immune dysfunction (or a combination) is occurring in the patient.

The components of the immune system can be measured in numerous ways, from methodologies used in standard clinical laboratory procedures to research protocols used to study immune function and disease treatment. Tests are available that can measure total antibody concentration and the various subgroups IgG, IgM, IgA, IgE, IgD; cytokines such as interleuken II and gamma interferon; cellular components such as T cells and their subtypes (such as suppressor T cells and natural killer cells), and B cells.

Autoimmune diseases and allergies are immune dysfunction diseases in their own right. Because there is an immune dysfunction component to CFS, tests for these conditions are important considerations. An antinuclear antibody (ANA) test determines the presence of antibodies that attack the tissues of the patient, as in systemic lupus erythematosus. The type and extent of allergic reactions can be measured using the radioimmunosorbent (RIST) tests for total IgE concentration and radioallergosorbent (RAST) tests for IgE concentration for particular antigens.

Systemic disease states, including CFS, often involve generalized inflammation that is considered part of the body's protective response. While inflammation is important to the elimination of various infective agents, it is also involved in neurological and muscle tissue damage. C-reactive protein (CRP) and the erythrocyte sedimentation rate (ESR) tests measure the intensity of the inflammatory response. A variety of other tests provide information that indicates the extent of muscle, liver, thyroid, and other vital organ damage.

NO STANDARD TREATMENT

Although a diagnosis can be made for CFS, there is no standard treatment. Clinical treatment essentially takes the form of alleviating the symptoms. Antidepressants such as doxepin (Sinequan) are useful in the treatment of depression and are also used to control muscle pain, lethargy, and sleeping problems. Nonsteroidal anti-inflammatory drugs (NSAIDs) provide relief for headache and muscle pain. Two drugs that have demonstrated antiviral activities are acyclovir and ampligen; ampligen can also modulate the immune response.

An example of research to develop therapies that might alleviate other symptoms of CFS involves the treatment of a number of patients with dialyzable leukocyte extract and psychologic treatment in the form of cognitive-behavioral therapy. The patients' cell-mediated immune response after therapy was evaluated by peripheral blood T cell subset analysis and delayed hypersensitivity skin testing. Psychologic analysis was performed using numerous cognitive tests. Both therapies proved to be inconclusive.

Because of the systemic nature of the disease, including its psychoneurological component, consideration must be given to holistic medical treatment. Any treatment protocol must be able to address the interactive factors of CFS that are still being defined in terms of cause and effect. Some researchers believe that therapeutic treatment should comprise diet, exercise, vitamins, and homeopathic medicine. They further believe that psychoemotional treatment should allow patients to be responsible for their own recovery and help them to develop a personal lifestyle that provides general good health.

—Patrick J. DeLuca

See also Allergies; Environmental diseases; Influenza; Memory loss; Sleep disorders; Stress; Women's health issues.

FOR FURTHER INFORMATION:
Collinge, William. *Recovering from Chronic Fatigue Syndrome: A Guide to Self-*

Empowerment. New York: Body Press/Perigee, 1993. An excellent book written for the general public that speculates on the multifaceted nature of the disease. Offers information for those who have CFS, such as suggested diets and treatments. Also provides addresses for support groups.

National Institutes of Health. *Chronic Fatigue Syndrome: Information for Physicians*. Bethesda, Md.: Author, 1997. A brief, concise description of what is known about CFS. Although printed for physicians, this pamphlet can be read and understood by nonspecialists.

Stoff, Jesse A., and Charles Pellegrino. *Chronic Fatigue Syndrome*. Rev. ed. New York: HarperPerennial, 1992. An excellent book describing the biological aspects of the disease in layperson's terms. Essential reading for anyone suffering from the disease because of its diary-like accounts, anecdotal data, emphasis on holistic treatment, and inspirational tone.

Wessely, S., M. Hotopf, and M. Sharpe. *Chronic Fatigue and Its Syndromes*. Oxford, England: Oxford University Press, 1999. The authors consider chronic fatigue to be similar to any other illness in that its onset and course are influenced by physical, psychological, and social factors. Chapters review these topics as well as the history of chronic fatigue and neurasthenia and the influence of social circumstances.

Yehuda, Shlomo, and David I. Mostofsky, eds. *Chronic Fatigue Syndrome*. New York: Plenum Press, 1997. Provides an updated description of CFS, the medical conditions from which it must be distinguished, and current treatment approaches.

✦ CIRCUMCISION OF BOYS

Type of issue: Children's health, ethics, medical procedures, men's health
Definition: The removal of the foreskin (prepuce) covering the head of the penis.

Routine circumcision of the newborn male—in which the foreskin of the penis is stretched, clamped, and cut—is becoming an increasingly controversial procedure. Famed pediatrician Benjamin Spock once contended that circumcision is a good idea, especially if most of the boys in the neighborhood are circumcised; then a boy feels "regular." Yet many wonder if that is justification for circumcision. Allowing routine circumcision of newborns as a religious and cultural rite still leaves the debate over medical necessity. The United States is the only country in the world that circumcises a majority of newborn males without a religious reason. In fact, circumcision has been termed a "cultural surgery."

INDICATIONS AND CONTRAINDICATIONS

True medical indications for the surgery are seldom present at birth. Such conditions as infections of the head and/or shaft of the penis may be indications for circumcision; an inability to retract the foreskin in the newborn is not an indication. Some argue that circumcision should be delayed until the foreskin has become retractable, making an imprecise surgical procedure presumably less traumatic. In 96 percent of infant boys, however, the foreskin is not fully retractable; it is normally so tight and adherent that it cannot be pulled back and the penis cleaned. By age three, that percentage decreases to 10 percent.

There are other definite contraindications to newborn circumcision. Circumcising infants with abnormalities of the penal head or shaft makes treatment more difficult because the foreskin may later be needed for use in reconstruction. Prematurity, instability, or a bleeding problem also preclude early circumcision. The foreskin is a natural protective membrane, representing 50 to 80 percent of the skin system of the penis, having 240 feet of nerve fibers, more than 1,000 nerve endings, and 3 feet of veins, arteries, and capillaries. It keeps the sensitive head protected, facilitating intercourse, and prevents the surface of the glans from thickening and becoming desensitized. Also, within the inner surface of the foreskin are a series of tiny ridged bands that contribute significantly to stimulating the glans.

RISKS OF INFECTION AND CANCER

The two most persistent arguments for the operation, however, are the risks of infection and cancer in the uncircumcised. Without circumcision, smegma accumulates beneath the base of the covered head of the penis. This cheeselike material of dead skin cells and secretions of the sweat glands is thought to be a cause of cancer of the penis and prostate gland in uncircumcised men and cancer of the cervix in their female partners. Doctors who argue against circumcision, however, say that the presence of smegma in the uncircumcised is simply a sign of poor hygiene and that poor sexual hygiene, inadequate hygienic facilities, and sexually transmitted diseases cause an increased incidence of cancer in ethnic groups or populations that do not practice circumcision. Doctors who argue against circumcision also point out that complete circumcision is found as often in male partners of women without cancer of the cervix as in male partners of women who have cervical cancer. In Sweden, moreover—where newborn circumcision is not routinely practiced but where good hygiene is practiced—the rates of these cancers are essentially the same as those found in Israel, where ritual circumcision is practiced.

The increased incidence of urinary tract infections and sexually transmitted diseases (STDs) in uncircumcised males sufficiently argue for circumcision, say its proponents. They warn that the intact foreskin invites bacterial colonization, which leads to urethral infection ascending to the bladder that ultimately may spread upward to the kidneys and sometimes cause permanent kidney damage. On the other hand, no proof exists that uncircumcised male infants who sustain urinary tract infections will have future urologic problems. Furthermore, the operation is not a simple procedure and is not without peril. Penile amputation, life-threatening infections, and even death have been well documented.

Slightly increased rates of infection with sexually transmitted diseases in the uncircumcised argue the case for some proponents, but it is acquired immunodeficiency syndrome (AIDS) that they most fear. In Africa, where circumcision is seldom practiced, the acquisition of AIDS by heterosexual men from infected women during vaginal intercourse is the most common mode of transmission.

Proponents say that infection with human immunodeficiency virus (HIV), the virus that leads to AIDS, depends on a break or an abrasion of the skin to gain entry. The intact foreskin provides a site for transfer of infected cervical secretions. In Africa, doctors at the University of Nairobi noted a relationship of HIV infection to genital ulcers and lack of circumcision. Uncircumcised men had a history of genital ulcers more often than did the circumcised, and they were more often HIV-positive. They were also more frequently HIV-positive even if they did not have a history of genital ulcer disease.

POTENTIAL COMPLICATIONS

In 1989, the American Academy Pediatrics Task Force on Circumcision concluded that "newborn circumcision has potential medical benefits and advantages as well as disadvantages and risks. When circumcision is being considered, the benefits and risks should be explained to the parents and informed consent obtained." This neutral statement does not lessen the anxiety of parents who are trying to weigh the pros and cons of routine newborn circumcision, but examination of the evidence does allow parents to weigh the individual benefits and risks and see if the scale tips in either direction.

Worldwide studies of predominantly uncircumcised populations have shown a higher incidence of urinary tract infection in boys during the first few months of life, which is the reverse of what is found in older infants and children, where girls predominate. In 1986, Brooke Army Medical Center in Fort Sam Houston, Texas, took a closer look. The doctors found the incidence of urinary tract infection in circumcised infant males to be 0.11 percent but 1.12 percent in the uncircumcised. Even without proof that the uncircumcised male infants who get urinary tract infections will have future urologic problems, the proponents for the surgical procedure claim about a 1 percent advantage.

The evidence for an increase in sexually transmitted diseases (such as genital herpes, gonorrhea, and syphilis) among the uncircumcised is conflicting. Furthermore, apparent correlations between circumcision status and these diseases do not reflect confounding genetic and environmental variables. It is also difficult to factor in the risk from HIV infections. The studies from Africa do not look at any variables in the transmission of HIV except circumcision status and previous history of genital ulcers. The nutritional and economic status of the men was not examined, even though it is known that malnourishment suppresses the immune systems. Moreover, if everyone practiced "safe sex," the argument for circumcision would be moot.

Almost all the surgical complications of circumcision can be avoided if doctors performing the procedure adhere to strict asepsis, are properly trained and experienced in the procedure, remove the appropriate and correct amount of tissue, and provide adequate hemostasis. The variety of circumstances, populations, and physicians affects the incidence of complications. In the larger, teaching hospitals, often the newest physicians with the least experience or supervision perform the operation. As a result, complications may arise. Excessive bleeding is the most frequent complication. The incidence of bleeding after circumcision ranges from 0.1 percent to as high as 35 percent in some reports. Most of the episodes are minor and can be controlled by simple measures, such as compression and suturing, but some of these efforts can lead to diminished blood supply to the head and shaft of the penis with necrosis of the affected part. Chordee can result if improper technique or bad luck intervenes, and such penile deformity begets the risk of emotional distress. The urethral opening on the end of the penis can become infected or ulcerated when the glans is no longer protected by foreskin; such infection rarely occurs in the uncircumcised. Finally, any surgical procedure runs the risk of infection. These localized infections rarely spread to the blood, but death from sepsis and its sequelae has been documented.

Overall, the surgical complication rate after circumcision runs around 0.19 percent, which could be lowered with strict protocols, meticulous technique, strict asepsis, and well-trained, experienced physicians. Strict protocols, it is hoped, would ensure that absolute contraindications to the procedure—such as anomalies of the penis, prematurity, instability, or a bleeding disorder—were honored.

In part because of an additional cost that arises with anesthesia, the vast majority of infant circumcisions are performed without pain control. The surgery is painful, and yet some physicians claim that the minute that the operation ends, the circumcised baby no longer cries and frequently falls asleep. Continuing pain, therefore, is probably not present.

CHANGING ATTITUDES TOWARD ROUTINE CIRCUMCISION

Routine newborn circumcision originated in the United States in the 1860's, ostensibly as prophylaxis against disease. Some medical historians, however, believe that nonreligious circumcision was a deliberate surgical procedure to desensitize and debilitate the penis to prevent masturbation. Eventually, a general change in attitude occurred, notably in Great Britain and New Zealand, which virtually have abandoned routine circumcision. Rates of circumcision have also fallen dramatically in Canada, Australia, and even the United States. As recently as the mid-1970's, approximately 90 percent of U.S. male babies were circumcised. Not until 1971 did the American Academy of Pediatrics determine that circumcision is not medically valid. By 1995, the incidence of newborn circumcision had declined to 59 percent.

In 1971, the American Academy of Pediatrics' Committee on the Fetus and Newborn issued an advisory that said, "There are no valid medical indications for routine circumcision in the neonatal period." In 1978, when the American College of Obstetricians and Gynecologists affirmed this statement, the circumcision rate had already declined to an estimated 70 percent of newborn males, compared to previous rates of between 80 and 90 percent. In response to the critics who were worried about increased urinary tract infections in the uncircumcised, the 1989 American Academy of Pediatrics' Task Force on Circumcision concluded that "newborn circumcision has potential medical benefits and advantages as well as disadvantages and risks. When circumcision is being considered, the benefits and risks should be explained to the parents and informed consent obtained."

Undoubtedly, the future will bring improved surgical techniques. More emphasis will be placed on avoiding surgical complications by more rigid monitoring of the operation and who performs the procedure. It is unlikely that circumcision will disappear completely.

Organizations such as Doctors Opposing Circumcision and the National Organization to Halt the Abuse and Routine Mutilation of Males, however, are actively proposing an end to routine neonatal circumcision. Some nursing groups and concerned mothers have formed local groups to oppose circumcision. They argue that subjecting a baby to this procedure may impair mother-infant bonding. Another question posed by some physicians and parents is the ethics involved in the unnecessary removal of a functioning body organ, particularly without the patient's consent. Others claim that the baby's rights are being violated, noting that it is the child who must live with the outcome of the decision to perform a circumcision.

—*Wayne R. McKinny, M.D.; updated by John Alan Ross*

See also Children's health issues; Circumcision of girls; Ethics.

FOR FURTHER INFORMATION:
Behrman, Richard E., ed. *Nelson Textbook of Pediatrics.* 16th ed. Philadelphia:

W. B. Saunders, 2000. This standard pediatric textbook briefly covers the medical risks and benefits of routine newborn circumcision fairly and without bias or excessive medical jargon. Draws no conclusions.

Berkow, Robert, and Andrew J. Fletcher, eds. *The Merck Manual of Diagnosis and Therapy.* 17th ed. Rahway, N.J.: Merck Sharp & Dohme Research Laboratories, 1999. This classic textbook does say that circumcision "is rarely indicated medically." In contrast with longer review articles, however, *The Merck Manual* states that bleeding disorders in infants should include a history of the mother's taking medication for bleeding disturbances, such as anticoagulants or aspirin.

Bigelow, Jim. *The Joy of Uncircumcising!: Exploring Circumcision—History, Myths, Psychology, Restoration, Sexual Pleasure, and Human Rights.* Rev. ed. Aptos, Calif.: Hourglass, 1998. This book provides an alternative view of this controversial procedure.

King, L. R., ed. *Urologic Surgery in Neonates and Young Infants.* Philadelphia: W. B. Saunders, 1998. J. W. Duckett's contribution, "The Neonatal Circumcision Debate," is an excellent review of the controversies surrounding this operation. Although written for doctors, it will present minimal difficulty for laypersons.

Snyder, Howard M. "To Circumcise or Not." *Hospital Practice* 26 (January 15, 1991): 201-207. This widely available medical journal article examines in detail the medical evidence for and against circumcision. With a minimum of medical jargon, the author also states his own personal bias against the routine use of the procedure.

✧ CIRCUMCISION OF GIRLS

Type of issue: Children's health, ethics, medical procedures, women's health
Definition: The partial or complete surgical removal of the clitoris, labia minora, and labia majora for cultural reasons.

The 1989-1990 Demographic Health Survey of Circumcision stated that circumcision is performed annually on an estimated 80 to 114 million women; 85 percent of these procedures involve clitoridectomy, while approximately 15 percent involve infibulation. Certain contemporary cultures of Africa, the Middle East, and parts of Yemen, India, and Malaysia continue these practices. Contemporary Middle Eastern countries practicing female circumcision and genital mutilation are Jordan, Iraq, the two Yemens, Syria, and southern Algeria. In Africa, it is practiced in the majority of the countries, including Egypt, Ivory Coast, Kenya, Mali, Mozambique, Sudan, and Upper Volta. It has been estimated that 99 percent of northern Sudanese women, aged fifteen to forty-nine, are circumcised. In and around

Alexandria, Egypt, 99 percent of rural and lower income urban women are circumcised.

Types of Female Circumcision

Cross-culturally, there are essentially four types of female genital circumcision and female genital mutilation. Circumcision or sunna circumcision is removal of the prepuce or hood of the clitoris, with the body of the clitoris remaining intact. Sunna means "tradition" in Arabic. Excision circumcision or clitoridectomy is the removal of the entire clitoris (both prepuce and glans) and all or part of the adjacent labia majora and the labia minora. Intermediate circumcision is the removal of the clitoris, all or part of the labia minora, and sometimes part of the labia majora. Infibulation or pharaonic circumcision is the removal of the clitoris, the labia minora, and much of the labia majora; on occasion, the remaining sides of the vulva are stitched together to close up the vagina, except for a small opening maintained for the passage of blood and urine.

All types of female genital mutilation frequently create severe, long-term effects, such as pelvic infections that usually lead to infertility; chronic recurrent urinary tract infections; painful intercourse; obstetrical complications; and, in some cases, surgically induced scars that can cause tearing of the tissue, and even hemorrhaging, during childbirth. In fact, it is not unusual for women who have been infibulated to require surgical enlargement of the vagina on their wedding night or when delivering children. Unfortunately, babies born to infibulated women frequently suffer brain damage because of oxygen deprivation (hypoxia) caused by a prolonged and obstructed delivery. The baby may die during the painful birthing process because of a damaged birth canal. Other physical and psychological difficulties for the circumcised woman may be sexual dysfunction, delayed menarche, and genital malformation.

Cultural Contexts

From a cultural perspective, there are numerous reasons for these surgical procedures. It is a rite of passage and proof of adulthood. It raises a woman's status in her community, because of both the added purity that circumcision brings and the bravery that initiates are called upon to demonstrate. It is also thought to confer maturity and inculcate positive character traits, such as the ability to endure pain and to be submissive. In some cultures, the circumcision ritual is a positive one in which the girl is the center of attention and receives presents and moral instruction from her elders. It creates a bond between the generations, as all women in the society must undergo the procedure and thus have shared an important experience.

It is thought that a girl who has been circumcised will not have her conscience troubled by lustful thoughts or sensations or by physical tempta-tions such as masturbation. Therefore, there is less risk of premarital rela-tionships that can end in the stigma and social difficulties of illegitimate birth. The bond between husband and wife may be closer because one or both of them will never have had sex with anyone else. The relationship may be motivated by love rather than lust because there will be no physical drive for the wife, only an emotional one. There is little incentive for extramarital sex for the wife; hence, the marriage may be more secure. Children may be better cared for because the husband can be more confident that they are his. Generally, a girl who is not circumcised is considered "unclean" by local villagers and therefore unmarriageable. In some societies, a girl who is not circumcised is believed to be dangerous, even deadly, if her clitoris touches a man's penis.

Unfortunately, female genital circumcision and female genital mutilation surgeries are invariably conducted in unsanitary conditions in which a midwife or close female relative uses unsterile sharp instruments, such as pieces of glass, razor blades, kitchen knives, or scissors. The induction of tetanus, septicemia, hemorrhaging, and even shock are not uncommon. Human immunodeficiency virus (HIV) can be transmitted. No anesthesia is used. These procedures usually are experienced by the child at approxi-mately three years of age, although the actual age depends upon the customs of the particular society or village. In order to minimize the risk of the transmission of viruses, countries such as Egypt have made it illegal for female genital mutilation to be practiced by anyone other than trained doctors and nurses in hospitals.

FEMALE CIRCUMCISION AS A VIOLATION OF HUMAN RIGHTS

Because of the high number of female genital mutilations and the deaths that this procedure has caused, it is now prohibited in Great Britain, France, Sweden, Switzerland, and some countries of Africa, such as Egypt, Kenya, and Senegal. The National Organization of Circumcision Information Re-source Centers (NOCIRC) is opposed to the procedures, as well as to male circumcision. The United Nations Children's Fund (UNICEF) and the World Health Organization (WHO) consider female genital mutilation to be a violation of human rights, recommending its eradication. In the United States, former Congresswoman Patricia Schroeder introduced a bill that would outlaw female genital mutilation. The bill, called the Federal Prohi-bition of Female Genital Mutilation of 1995, was passed in 1996. The Canadian Criminal Code was enacted to protect children who are ordinarily residents in Canada from being removed from the country and subjected to female genital mutilation.

Both female genital circumcision and female genital mutilation perpetu-ate customs that seek to control female bodies and sexuality. It is hoped that with increasing legislation and attitude changes regarding bioethical issues, fewer girls and young women will undergo these mutilating surgical procedures. One problem in this campaign is the conflict between cultural self-determination and basic human rights. Feminists, physicians, and ethicists must work respectfully with, and not independently of, local resources for cultural self-examination and change.

—*John Alan Ross*

See also Circumcision of boys; Ethics; Health equity for women; Infertility in women; Menstruation; Sexual dysfunction.

FOR FURTHER INFORMATION:

Elchala, U., B. Ben-Ami, R. Gillis, and A. Brezezinski. "Ritualistic Female Genital Mutilation: Current Status and Future Outlook." *Obstetrical and Gynecological Survey* 52, no. 10 (1997): 643-653.

Gollaher, David L. *Circumcision: A History of the World's Most Controversial Surgery.* New York: Basic Books, 2000.

James, Stephen A. "Reconciling International Human Rights and Cultural Relativism: The Case of Female Circumcision." *Bioethics* 8, no. 1 (1994): 1-26.

Kluge, E. W. "Female Genital Mutilation: Cultural Values and Ethics." *Journal of Obstetrics and Gynecology* 16, no. 2 (1997): 71.

Walker, Alice, and Pratibha Parmar. *Warrior Marks: Female Genital Mutilation and the Sexual Blinding of Women.* New York: Harcourt Brace, 1993.

❖ CLEFT LIP AND PALATE

Type of issue: Children's health

Definition: A fissure in the midline of the palate so that the two sides fail to fuse during embryonic development; in some cases, the fissure may extend through both hard and soft palates into the nasal cavities.

Cleft palate is a congenital defect characterized by a fissure along the midline of the palate. It occurs when the two sides fail to fuse during embryonic development. The gap may be complete, extending through the hard and soft palates into the nasal cavities, or may be partial or incomplete. It is often associated with cleft lip or "hare lip." About one child in eight hundred live births is affected with some degree of clefting, and clefting is the most common of the craniofacial abnormalities.

DEVELOPMENT OF CLEFT PALATE IN THE FETUS

Cleft palate is not generally a genetic disorder; rather, it is a result of defective cell migration. Embryonically, in the first month, the mouth and nose form one cavity destined to be separated by the hard and soft palates. In addition, there is no upper lip. Most of the upper jaw is lacking; only the part near the ears is present. In the next weeks, the upper lip and jaw are formed from structures growing in from the sides, fusing at the midline with a third portion growing downward from the nasal region. The palates develop in much the same way. The fusion of all these structures begins with the lip and moves posteriorly toward, then includes, the soft palate. The two cavities are separated by the palates by the end of the third month of gestation.

If, as embryonic development occurs, the cells that should grow together to form the lips and palate fail to move in the correct direction, the job is left unfinished. Clefting of the palate generally occurs between the thirty-fifth and thirty-seventh days of gestation. Fortunately, it is an isolated defect not usually associated with other disabilities or with mental retardation.

If the interference in normal growth and fusion begins early and lasts throughout the fusion period, the cleft that results will affect one or both sides of the top lip and may continue back through the upper jaw, the upper gum ridge, and both palates. If the disturbance lasts only part of the time that development is occurring, only the lip may be cleft, and the palate may be unaffected. If the problem begins a little into the fusion process, the lip is normally formed, but the palate is cleft. The cleft may divide only the soft palate or both the soft and the hard palate. Even the uvula may be affected; it can be split, unusually short, or even absent.

About 80 percent of cases of cleft lip are unilateral; of these, 70 percent occur on the left side. Of cleft palate cases, 25 percent are bilateral. The mildest manifestations of congenital cleft are mild scarring and/or notching of the upper lip. Beyond this, clefting is described by degrees. The first degree is incomplete, which is a small cleft in the uvula. The second degree is also incomplete, through the soft palate and into the hard palate. Another type of "second-degree incomplete" is a horseshoe type, in which there is a bilateral cleft proceeding almost to the front. Third-degree bilateral is a cleft through both palates but bilaterally through the gums; it results in a separate area of the alveolus where the teeth will erupt, and the teeth will show up in a very small segment. When the teeth appear, they may not be normally aligned. In addition to the lip, gum, and palate deviations, abnormalities of the nose may also occur.

Cleft palate may be inherited, probably as a result of the interaction of several genes. In addition, the effect of some environmental factors that affect embryonic development may be linked to this condition. They might include mechanical disturbances such as an enlarged tongue, which prevents the fusion of the palate and lip. Other disturbances may be caused by toxins introduced by the mother (drugs such as cortisone or alcohol) and defective blood. Other associated factors include deficiencies of vitamins or minerals in the mother's diet, radiation from X rays, and infectious diseases such as German measles. No definite cause has been identified, nor does it appear that one cause alone can be implicated. It is likely that there is an interplay between mutant genes, chromosomal abnormalities, and environmental factors.

PROBLEMS DUE TO CLEFT PALATE

Problems begin at birth for the infant born with a cleft palate. The most immediate problem is feeding the baby. If the cleft is small and the lip unaffected, nursing may proceed fairly easily. If the cleft is too large, however, the baby cannot build up enough suction to nurse efficiently. To remedy this, the hole in the nipple of the bottle can be enlarged, or a plastic obturator can be fitted to the bottle.

Babies with cleft palate apparently are more susceptible to colds than other children. Since there is an open connection between the nose and mouth, an infection that starts in either location will easily and quickly spread to the other. Frequently, the infection will spread to the middle ear via the Eustachian tube.

Other problems associated with cleft palate are those related to dentition. In some children there may be extra teeth, while in others the cleft may prevent the formation of tooth buds so that teeth are missing. Teeth that are present may be malformed; those malformations include injury during development, fusion of teeth to form one large tooth, teeth lacking enamel, and teeth that have too little calcium in the enamel. If later in development and growth the teeth are misaligned, orthodontia may be undertaken. Another possible problem met by patients with a cleft palate is maxillary (upper-jaw) arch collapse; this condition is also remedied with orthodontic treatment.

SURGICAL REPAIR

One of the first questions a parent of a child with a cleft palate will pose regards surgical repair. The purpose of surgically closing the cleft is not simply to close the hole—although that goal is important. The major purpose is to achieve a functional palate. Whether this can be accomplished depends on the size and shape of the cleft, the thickness of the available tissue, and other factors. When the child is scheduled for surgery, it is a tangible sign that the condition is correctable. When the lip is successfully closed, it is positive affirmation that a professional team can help the family. The goals of both the team and the family are extremely similar: Both want the patient to look as normal as possible and to have a functional palate.

Cleft lip surgery is performed when the healthy baby weighs at least seven pounds; it is done under a general anesthetic. If the cleft is unilateral, one operation can accomplish the closure, but a bilateral cleft lip is often repaired in two steps at least a month apart. When the lip is repaired, normal lip pressure is restored, which may help in closing the cleft in the gum ridge. It may also reduce the gap in the hard palate, if one is present. Successive operations may be suggested when, even years after surgery, scars develop on the lip.

Surgery to close clefts of the hard and soft palate is typically done when the baby is at least nine months of age, unless there is a medical reason not to do so. Different surgeons prefer different times for this surgery. The surgeon attempts to accomplish three goals in the repair procedure. The surgeon will first try to ensure that the palate is long enough so that function and movement will result (this is essential for proper speech patterns). Second, the musculature around the Eustachian tube should work properly in order to cut down the incidence of ear infections. Finally, the surgery should promote the development of the facial bones and, as much as possible, normal teeth. This goal aids in eating and appearance. All this may be accomplished in one operation, if the cleft is not too severe. For a cleft that requires more procedures, the surgeries are usually spaced at least six months apart so that complete healing can occur. This schedule decreases the potential for severe scarring.

Successful repair greatly improves speech and appearance, and the physiology of the oral and nasal cavities is also improved. Additional surgery may be necessary to improve appearance, breathing, and the function of the palate. Sometimes the palate may partially reopen, and surgery is needed to reclose it.

POSTSURGICAL TREATMENT

When the baby leaves the operating room, there are stitches in the repaired area. Sometimes a special device called a Logan's bow is taped to the baby's cheeks; this device not only protects the stitches but also relieves some of the tension on them. In addition, the baby's arms may be restrained in order to keep the baby's hands away from the affected area. A parent of a child that has just undergone cleft palate repair should not panic at the sight of bleeding from the mouth. To curb it, gauze may be packed into the repaired area and remain about five days after surgery. As mucus and other body fluids accumulate in the area, they may be suctioned out.

During the initial recovery, the child is kept in a moist, oxygen-rich environment (an oxygen tent) until respiration is normal. The patient will be observed for signs of airway obstruction or excessive bleeding. Feeding is done by syringe, eyedropper, or special nipples. Clear liquids and juices only are allowed. The child sits in a high chair to drink, when possible. After feeding, the mouth should be rinsed well with water to help keep the stitches clean and uncrusted. Peroxide mixed with the water may help, as well as ointment. Intake and output of fluids are measured. Hospitalization may last for about a week, or however long is dictated by speed of healing. At the end of this week, stitches are removed and the suture line covered and protected by a strip of paper tape.

An alternative to surgery is the use of an artificial palate known as an obturator. It is specially constructed by a dentist to fit into the child's mouth. The appliance, or prosthesis, is carefully constructed to fit precisely and snugly, but it must be easily removable. There must be enough space at the back so the child can breathe through the nose. While speaking, the muscles move back over this opening so that speech is relatively unaffected.

Speech Therapy

Speech problems are likely the most residual of the problems in the cleft palate patient. The speech of the untreated, and sometimes the treated, cleft palate patient is very nasal. If the soft palate is too short, the closure of the palate may leave a space between the nose and the throat, allowing air to escape through the nose. There is little penetrating quality to the patient's voice, and it does not carry well. Some cleft palate speakers are difficult to understand because there are several faults in articulation. Certainly not all cleft lip or palate patients, however, will develop communication problems; modern surgical procedures help ensure that most children will develop acceptable speech and language without necessitating the help of a speech therapist.

Psychological and Emotional Responses

The problems accompanying clefting may alter family morale and climate, increasing the complexity of the problem. A team of specialists usually works together to help the patient and the family cope with these problems. This team may include a pediatrician, a speech pathologist, a plastic surgeon, an orthodontist, a psychiatrist, a social worker, an otologist, an audiologist, and perhaps others. The formation and cooperation of a team of professionals and the emotional support that they provide for an affected family hopefully will enable that family to perceive the baby more positively, to focus on the child's potential rather than on the disability.

The cooperating team should monitor feeding problems, family and friends' reactions to the baby's appearance, how parents encourage the child to talk or how they respond to poor speech, and whether the parents are realistic about the long-term outcome for their child. The grief, guilt, and shock that the parents often feel can be positively altered by how the professional team tackles the problem and by communication with the parents. Usually the team does not begin functioning in the baby's life until he or she is about a month old. Some parents have confronted their feelings, while others are still struggling with the negative feeling that the birth brought to bear. Therefore, the first visit that the parents have with the team is important, because it establishes the foundation of a support system which should last for years.

—Iona C. Baldridge

See also Birth defects; Children's health issues; Disabilities; Speech disorders.

FOR FURTHER INFORMATION:

Batshaw, Mark L. *Children with Disabilities*. Baltimore: Paul H. Brookes, 1997. This book first takes the reader through the basics of genetics. Based on this information, diagnoses and descriptions of birth defects are made relative to the various organ systems. Concludes by examining the emotional aspects of living with a handicapped child.

Clifford, Edward. *The Cleft Palate Experience*. Springfield, Ill.: Charles C Thomas, 1987. This author writes from the perspective of a cleft palate team participant and incorporates the value of the team in his chapters. Much space is given to the child's development of a positive self-image and the parents' role, from birth, in forming this image.

Dronamraju, Krishna R. *Cleft Lip and Palate*. Springfield, Ill.: Charles C Thomas, 1986. A compilation of research emphasizing population genetics, dental genetics, evolution, teratology, reproductive biology, and epidemiology. The purpose is to provide a basis for genetic counseling. An extensive bibliography is included.

Lorente, Christine, et al. "Tobacco and Alcohol Use During Pregnancy and Risk of Oral Clefts." *American Journal of Public Health* 90, no. 3 (March, 2000): 415-419. This study examines the relationship between maternal tobacco and alcohol consumption during the first trimester of pregnancy and oral clefts. Multivariate analyses showed an increased risk of cleft lip with or without cleft palate associated with smoking and an increased risk of cleft palate associated with alcohol consumption.

Stengelhofen, Jackie, ed. *Cleft Palate*. Edinburgh, Scotland: Churchill Livingstone, 1989. Explores the various communication problems met by those with a cleft palate. An appeal to the entire team of professionals treating the patient and their partnership with parents. Case histories are discussed.

✧ Colic

Type of issue: Children's health

Definition: As a general term, a paroxysm of acute abdominal pain caused by spasm, obstruction, or twisting of a hollow abdominal organ. As a specific entity, infantile colic is a group of behaviors displayed by young infants including crying, facial grimacing, drawing-up of the legs over the abdomen, and clenching of the fists.

As a general term, colic can arise from any site in the abdomen. For example, cramplike pain caused by a stone obstructing the bile ducts or a stone obstructing the urinary tract are known as biliary colic and renal colic, respectively. More specifically, the term "colic," when unmodified, generally refers to infantile colic.

The crying of colicky infants tends to be more prominent in the evening, although they cry more than other infants at other times of day. The "rule of threes" of infantile colic holds that infants with colic cry for more than three hours per day for more than three days per week for more than three weeks. The associated gestures suggest to some that the infant is experiencing abdominal pain and is responsible for the use of the term "colic" to describe the condition.

Possible Causes

Several causes of infantile colic have been postulated, but conclusive evidence is lacking for any of them. This combination of behaviors has been interpreted as abdominal pain, leading to the idea that cramping somewhere in the intestine is the cause. Neurobehavioral explanations have been offered. The most common is that colic represents a state of agitation that may not require a noxious stimulus for agitation and crying to continue. Rarely is colic the result of organic disease, and the prevailing opinion is that it is a variant of normal infant behavior. It appears to be unrelated to caregiving style or intensity. Other proposed mechanisms include difficult temperament, sleep disturbance, diarrhea, child abuse, and irritable bowel syndrome. Some theories ascribe colic to hypersensitivity to dietary protein—usually proteins derived from cow's milk, which can be secreted in breast milk—thus explaining the occurrence of colic in breast-fed infants. Intestinal gas, either from air swallowed during feeding or from fermentation of incompletely absorbed carbohydrates in the colon, has also been implicated. Parents of colicky infants frequently describe flatulence as an associated symptom.

TREATING COLIC

The medical treatment of the infant with colic begins with a thorough medical history and a careful physical examination. While the likelihood of finding a cause of the infant's symptoms are slight, the thoroughness of this approach provides an effective basis for reassurance and demonstrates that the parents' complaint is taken seriously.

Infantile colic virtually always resolves spontaneously, leaving the infant healthy and thriving. The essentials of therapy are demystification, reassurance, and support for the haggard and anxious parents. Demystification is the explanation of the source of the infant's distress, which alleviates the anxiety attendant on diagnostic hypotheses that occur to or are suggested to the parents. It is important for pediatricians to deal with the anxiety aroused by the infant's symptoms with reassurance, pointing out that the baby will be fine; the only risk of lasting damage is to the parents.

Quick, superficial attempts to solve the problem with formula changes or medications, particularly when not accompanied by patient demystification and reassurance, reinforce the parents' suspicion that there is something wrong with the child, ultimately increasing parental perception of the child's vulnerability. The results of studies in the medical literature investigating the usefulness of switching formulas and using agents such as simethicone to deal with intestinal gas are mixed. Dicyclomine, an anticholinergic medication used in the past, should not be given to infants under six months of age because of the possibility that it will interfere with the baby's breathing.

More frequent, smaller feedings may help, as may increased carrying (called "walking the floor") and rocking. One theory holds that mimicking the environment in the womb is reassuring—closeness to a warm person with a detectable heartbeat, swaddling (wrapping the baby in a blanket to restrict movement of the extremities), and rhythmic stimulation provided by background music and car or stroller rides. One commonly used method involves placing the baby in an infant seat on top of a running washer or dryer, thus exposing the infant to constant vibration. Care must be taken to stay with the baby or to secure the infant seat to prevent injury resulting from a fall off the appliance. Most colicky infants have excessive gas, and "gas pains" have long been suspected as responsible for colic. Since virtually all the gas in the intestine is swallowed air, minimizing air swallowing and maximizing burping after feedings are important measures in reducing colic. The use of cereal to ease the infant's hunger and decrease the vigor with which he or she sucks on the nipple results in less air being swallowed. Unfortunately, many parents are advised to put the cereal in the bottle; this increases the negative pressure required to suck the slurry of milk and cereal and increases the amount of air swallowed.

—Wallace A. Gleason, Jr., M.D.

See also Children's health issues; Lactose intolerance.

FOR FURTHER INFORMATION:

Balon, Angie Juszczyk. "Management of Infantile Colic." *American Family Physician* 55, no. 1 (January, 1997): 235-242, 245-246.

Berkowitz, C. D. "Management of the Colicky Infant." *Comprehensive Therapy* 23, no. 4 (April, 1997): 277-280.

Lehtonen, L. A., and P. T. Rautava. "Infantile Colic: Natural History and Treatment." *Current Problems in Pediatrics* 26, no. 3 (March, 1996): 79-85.

Sferra, T. J., and L. A. Heitlinger. "Gastrointestinal Gas Formation and Infantile Colic." *Pediatric Clinics of North America* 43, no. 2 (April, 1996): 489-510.

Waltman, Alicia Brooks. "The Crying Game." *Parenting* 14, no. 3 (April, 2000): 128-132. Waltman offers information about the latest research on colic and the best ways to soothe a crying baby. For many babies, a surefire soother is a breast or a bottle.

❖ COLON CANCER

Type of issue: Public health
Definition: Cancer occurring in the large intestine, which is the second deadliest type of this disease.

With an estimated 60,000 deaths per year in the United States, cancer of the colon and rectum (also called large bowel or colorectal cancer) is the second most deadly cancer, ranking only behind lung cancer. About 90 percent of colorectal cancers arise from the glandular epithelium lining the inner surface of the large bowel and are termed adenocarcinomas. The cells of this layer are constantly being replaced by new cells. This fairly rapid cell division, along with the relatively hostile environment within the bowel, promotes internal cellular errors that lead to the formation of aberrant cells. These cells can become disordered and produce abnormal growths or tumors. Often, colorectal tumors protrude into the lumen (the spaces within the bowel), forming growths called polyps. Some polyps are benign and do not spread to other parts of the body, but they may still disturb normal bowel functions. Other polyps become malignant by forming more aggressive cell types, which allows them to grow larger and spread to other organs. The cancer can grow through the layers of the colon wall and extend into the body cavity and nearby organs such as the urinary bladder. Cancer cells can also break away from the main tumor and spread (metastasize) through the blood or lymphatic vessels to other organs, such as the lungs or liver. If not controlled, the spreading cancer eventually causes death by impairment of organ and system functions.

The risk of colorectal cancer is increased by certain hereditary and environmental factors. The dietary intake of fat and fiber also influences colorectal cancer risk. Researchers believe that fiber reduces the exposure of colon cells to cancer-causing chemicals (carcinogens) by diluting them and causing them to move more rapidly through the colon. Fats may promote colorectal cancer by triggering the excess secretion of bile, which is known to be carcinogenic in animals. In addition, fat may be converted to carcinogens by bacteria that live in the colon. Diets high in protein or low in fruit and vegetables may also elevate the risk. The tendency to develop colorectal polyps and cancer can be inherited; this genetic predisposition may be responsible for about 5 to 7 percent of all colorectal cancers. One example is an inherited disorder called familial adenomatous polyposis (FAP), in which multiple polyps develop in the colon; it often leads to colorectal cancer. Some of the defective genes that cause this and other types of colorectal cancers have been identified and are being studied to determine their role. The interplay between the various oncogenes (mutated cell division and growth genes) and tumor suppressor genes (cell division and growth inhibitor genes) has been determined. Whether inherited or caused by carcinogens, damage to these specific genetic regions disrupts the delicate balance that regulates orderly and perfectly timed cell reproduction and development, producing cancer cells. Irritable bowel syndrome (IBS) and exposure to certain occupational carcinogens are also known to increase the risk.

TREATING COLON CANCER

The chances for survival are greatly increased when colorectal cancer is detected and treated at an early stage. Early detection in the general population is possible with the use of three common medical tests: digital rectal examination, in which the physician checks the inner surface of the rectal wall with gloved finger for abnormal growths; fecal occult blood test, in which a stool sample is tested for hidden blood that may have emanated from a cancerous growth; and sigmoidoscopy, in which the physician examines the rectal and lower colon inner lining with a narrow tubular optical instrument inserted through the anus. If cancer is suspected, further tests will be done to arrive at a diagnosis. These tests may include a computed tomography (CT) scan, double-contrast barium enema X-ray series, and colonoscopy. The CT scan and contrast X rays reveal abnormal growths, and colonoscopy is similar to sigmoidoscopy but uses a longer, flexible tube in order to inspect the entire colon. During sigmoidoscopy and colonoscopy, the physician can remove polyps and obtain tissue samples for biopsy. Microscopic examination of the tissue samples by a pathologist can determine the stage or extent of growth of the cancer. This is important because it helps determine the type of treatment. In one type of staging, the following criteria are used: stage 0 (cancer confined to epithelium lining of the bowel), stage 1 (cancer confined to the bowel wall), stage 2 (cancer penetrating through all layers of the bowel wall and possibly invading adjacent tissues), stage 3 (cancer invading lymph nodes and/or adjacent tissues), and stage 4 (cancer spreading to distant sites, forming metastases).

Surgery is the primary treatment for colorectal cancer. Very small tumors in stage 0 can be removed surgically with the colonoscope. Tumors in more advanced stages require abdominal surgery in which the tumor is removed along with a portion of the bowel and possibly some lymph nodes. For cases in which the bowel cannot be reconnected, an opening is created through the abdominal wall (colostomy). This is usually a temporary procedure, and the hole will be closed when the bowel can be rejoined. Some advanced cancers cannot be cured by surgery alone. Adjuvant therapies—chemotherapy, radiation therapy, and biological therapy—may be used in combination with surgery. Chemotherapy drugs kill spreading cancer cells. The most common is 5-fluorouracil (5-FU), a chemical that interferes with the production of deoxyribonucleic acid (DNA) in dividing cells. 5-FU is more effective when given together with leucovorin (a compound similar to folic acid) and levamisole (an immune system stimulant). Levamisole and other treatments that reinforce the immune system are forms of biological therapy. Radiation therapy, given either before or after surgery, is helpful in killing undetected cancer cells near the site of the tumor.

A Disease of Developed Societies

More than 150,000 new cases of colorectal cancer are diagnosed in the United States each year, or roughly 15 percent of all cancers. The incidence of colorectal cancer is lower among females than males and rises dramatically after the age of fifty. Colorectal cancer is more common in developed countries such as the United States and in densely populated, industrialized regions. American mortality rates from colorectal cancer are higher in the Northeast and north-central regions of the country than in the South and Southwest. Populations moving from low-risk parts of the world, such as Asia or Africa, to high-risk areas, such as the United States or Europe, take on the higher risk within a generation or two, and vice versa.

—*Rodney C. Mowbray; updated by Connie Rizzo, M.D.*

See also Cancer; Chemotherapy; Nutrition and aging; Radiation.

For Further Information:

De Vita, Vincent T., Jr., Samuel Hellman, and Steven A. Rosenberg, eds. *Cancer: Principles and Practice of Oncology.* 5th ed. Philadelphia: J. B. Lippincott, 1997.

Miles, Andrew, David Cunningham, and Daniel Haller, eds. *The Effective Management of Colorectal Cancer.* London: Aesculapius, 2000.

Miskovitz, Paul, and Marian Betancourt. *What to Do If You Get Colon Cancer: A Specialist Helps You Take Charge and Make Informed Choices*. New York: Wiley, 1997.

Murphy, G., L. Morris, and D. Lange. *Informed Decisions: The Complete Book of Cancer Diagnosis, Treatment, and Recovery*. New York: Viking Press, 1997.

Taylor, Irving, Stanley M. Goldberg, and Julio Garcia-Aguilar. *Colorectal Cancer*. Oxford, England: Oxford University Press, 1999.

✧ CONDOMS

Type of issue: Men's health, public health, women's health

Definition: The most commonly used form of barrier contraceptive; when used properly, they can prevent the sexual transmission of disease, as well as pregnancy.

Condoms are included, along with the diaphragm, cervical cap, and contraceptive sponge, in the category of birth control devices called barrier methods; these devices reduce the probability of pregnancy by blocking the transmission of semen into the cervix, thus preventing sperm from reaching the egg. Because they prevent the exchange of body fluids, condoms also prevent the transmission of the viruses, bacteria, and other microorganisms that cause sexually transmitted diseases such as syphilis, chlamydia, genital warts, and acquired immunodeficiency syndrome (AIDS).

Male condoms have been in existence for hundreds of years; made of animal or artificial membranes, they are put, like a sheath, over the erect penis. Female condoms are a relatively recent invention; also called the vaginal pouch, they are bag-shaped membranes inserted in the vagina.

When used consistently and correctly, condoms are a highly effective method of preventing pregnancy and the transmission of sexual diseases. Correct usage means making sure the product has not passed its shelf life (it should be dated); has not been stored at high temperatures (including in a pocket or a wallet pressed close to the body); is used in conjunction with a spermicide (sold separately or included with the condom); is put on properly and at the proper time (not too tightly and before any fluid is present on the tip of the penis); and is not removed or allowed to slip off until after intercourse is completed. Unfortunately, many users do not follow all these rules or do not use condoms for every episode of intercourse. As a result, the actual failure rate for condom use is about 20 percent (measured in the percentage of couples per year using condoms as their only method of birth control who experience an unwanted pregnancy), compared to laboratory failure rates of only 1 to 2 percent. Human error and inconsistency also increase the actual rates of disease transmission above the near-zero measures of microbial passage through condom membranes as studied in the laboratory.

Male condoms are relatively inexpensive and are easy to obtain, but many men do not like them because they reduce stimulation of the penis. This fact has resulted in many unwanted pregnancies and sexual diseases among women who do not have access to other forms of birth control and who have been unsuccessful in persuading their partners to use condoms. Because female condoms do not cause as much reduction in penile stimulation as do male condoms and because they cause very little change in female sensations, a woman is more likely to convince a male partner that the couple should use a female condom. Thus, the introduction of this option gives women more control over their health and reproductive choices.

Controversy exists, however, regarding whether teenagers should be given easy access to condoms to protect against STDs and unwanted pregnancies. Advocates argue that condom availability, perhaps even in schools, would save many lives and promote health. Critics claim that providing condoms or other forms of contraception sends the wrong message about the appropriateness of sexual activity among minors.

—Linda Mealey

See also Abortion among teenagers; AIDS; AIDS and women; Birth control and family planning; Herpes; Morning-after pill; Pregnancy among teenagers; Sexually transmitted diseases (STDs).

FOR FURTHER INFORMATION:

Covington, Timothy R., and J. Frank McClendon. *Sex Care: The Complete Guide to Safe and Healthy Sex.* New York: Pocket Books, 1987. Detailed information on how to use contraceptives. Sexually transmitted diseases and other reproductive health problems are also covered.

Green, Shirley. *The Curious History of Contraception.* London: Ebury Press, 1971. A lighthearted account of contraceptive history, this book makes entertaining reading, with ample coverage of some of the more outlandish methods of contraception that people have used.

Harlap, Susan, Kathryn Kost, and Jacqueline Darroch Forrest. *Preventing Pregnancy, Protecting Health: A New Look at Birth Control Choices in the United States.* New York: Alan Guttmacher Institute, 1991. This well-researched book presents information on the health impact of different forms of contraception, such as sexually transmitted diseases, cancer, and later infertility. Highly recommended.

Hatcher, Robert A., et al. *Contraceptive Technology.* 17th ed. New York: Irvington, 1998. This frequently revised book offers a thorough and readable discussion of most aspects of contraception.

✦ Cosmetic surgery and aging

Type of issue: Elder health, medical procedures, social trends
Definition: Plastic surgery intended to minimize the visible effects of aging, giving the person a more youthful, rested appearance.

Plastic surgery can be divided into two basic types: reconstructive and cosmetic. Reconstructive surgery is done to restore function to a damaged body part, as with congenital abnormalities or traumatic lesions. Cosmetic surgery is done to remove blemishes or change contours. In some instances, such as traumatic injuries or cancer surgeries, plastic surgery may be used both to restore function and to remove blemishes or change contours. This entry focuses on cosmetic surgery that is done to counteract some of the effects of the aging process.

Types of Cosmetic Surgeries

Cosmetic surgery may be requested to counteract the normal changes of the skin that appear with aging. The area around the eye is the first to show signs of aging. The procedure that removes excess skin and fatty tissue from eyelids and eye area is called blepharoplasty. Areas involved can include one or both eyes and either upper or lower lids, or both. Incisions are made in the eyelid fold and extend out toward the smile lines.

A later sign of aging is the gradual stretching downward of the cheeks and deep wrinkling of the forehead. Face lifts (rhytidectomy) and brow lifts are procedures to address these issues. Rhytidectomy tightens the skin of the face and neck. The face and neck are often done together because aging changes occur in both at the same time. A brow lift relieves sagging eyebrows and a wrinkling forehead. Tightness occurs after these procedures because skin and sometimes underlying tissue and muscles are moved. Extra skin is cut off. Incisions are made in existing creases and in the hairline around ears.

While there are many reasons for hair loss—severe infection, thyroid disease, some medications, chemotherapy—the main reason is

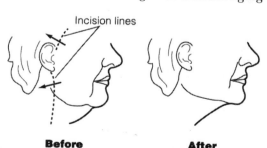

Before   **After**

A "face lift" is the term used for the excision and pulling upward of sagging skin on the face. This cosmetic procedure can smooth wrinkles and provide a more attractive profile, but there are drawbacks: The patient's appearance may be changed too dramatically, and the procedure must be repeated periodically to maintain the desired results. (Hans & Cassidy, Inc.)

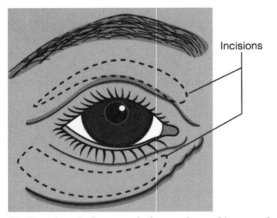

Incisions

Blepharoplasty is the removal of excess, baggy skin around the eyes. (Hans & Cassidy, Inc.)

heredity. Hair loss can begin in the twenties or thirties. It occurs both in men and women, but women seldom go bald. There are many treatments: systemic steroids or hormones, ointments, and antibiotics. Hair transplantation is another method. The older type of hair transplantation takes grafts from the back and side of the scalp and places them in the bald areas. Several sessions are usually required. A disadvantage of this method is that it often gives the appearance of "doll's hair." A newer method is microtransplantation, or minigrafts, which takes a few hairs with each graft. The result is a more natural look.

The surgeries outlined here are only a few of the numerous procedures that are offered. Many of the cosmetic surgeries can be done in an outpatient setting, while others can be done only in a hospital. The surgical time can last from thirty minutes to four or five hours. All procedures will produce some degree of swelling and bruising—which can last for several weeks.

Opinions About Cosmetic Surgery

There are two basic camps regarding cosmetic surgery: those who think that it is a waste of money and those who believe that it is the best thing offered. Those in the first group believe no cream, drug, or surgery can stop or reverse the aging process. They are quick to point out that cosmetic surgery is temporary and that the aging process continues, which means that wrinkles and sags will reappear. The money wasted on attempts to defy reality could be better used to meet more basic needs. Many also argue that American society tends to take the "quick fix" approach and jump at medication or surgeries to solve their problems. This group of people is more likely to avoid the sun, maintain proper nutrition, and not smoke as more natural methods to slow the signs of aging.

Members of the other group acknowledge that cosmetic surgery does not stop the aging process but seem pleased at the temporary reversal of the process. These people believe there is a positive impact on their daily life. Studies have demonstrated that there is an increase in self-esteem, more self-confidence, more satisfaction with appearance, and less depression after a person undergoes cosmetic surgery.

ISSUES TO CONSIDER

Before cosmetic surgery is performed, several issues need to be addressed. The first is the general health of the person considering surgery. With age and the natural decline of some body functions, there can be a greater likelihood of adverse reactions to anesthesia and a delay in healing.

The desired results of the surgery need to be reviewed. Cosmetic surgery will not yield a "model-like" appearance. People with unrealistic expectations will not be satisfied with the results. It is important to remember that the results of surgery are not seen immediately. There can be extreme bruising and swelling for several weeks after most surgeries. It may take up to a year for healing to be complete.

While cosmetic surgery is not the fountain of youth, it can be an effective method to aid people in looking their best.

—*Jennifer J. Hostutler*

See also Aging; Cosmetic surgery and women; Hair loss and baldness; Liposuction; Obesity and aging; Skin disorders with aging; Weight changes with aging.

FOR FURTHER INFORMATION:
Henry, Kimberly A., and Penny S. Heckaman. *The Plastic Surgery Sourcebook.* Los Angeles: Lowell House, 1997.
Marfuggi, Richard A. *Plastic Surgery: What You Need to Know Before, During, and After.* New York: Berkeley, 1998.
Perry, Arthur W., and Robin K. Levinson. *A Complete Question and Answer Guide.* New York: Avon Books, 1997.
Sarnoff, Deborah S., and Joan Swirsky. *Beauty and the Beam: Your Complete Guide to Cosmetic Laser Surgery.* New York: St. Martins Griffin, 1998.
Wyer, E. Bingo. *The Unofficial Guide to Cosmetic Surgery.* New York: Simon & Schuster/Macmillan, 1999.

✧ COSMETIC SURGERY AND WOMEN

Type of issue: Medical procedures, social trends, women's health
Definition: The use of surgical techniques to reshape parts of a woman's body.

The term "plastic surgery" comes from the Latin *plasticere*, meaning "to mold"; the terms "plastic surgery" and "cosmetic surgery" have often been used interchangeably, although "cosmetic" implies procedures performed purely for aesthetic purposes. While cosmetic surgery could conceivably be performed on any part of the female body, the most common procedures are face and neck lifts, blepharoplasty (upper and lower eyelid tucks), breast enhancement and reduction, abdominoplasty (tummy tucks), and rhino-plasty (nose reshaping). Others include collagen injections, dermabrasion, chemical peels, cheek implants, and liposuction.

A face and neck lift once simply pulled the skin and did not last more than five years, but new techniques involve changes in fat, tissue, and muscles, with results lasting between five and ten years. The surgeon makes cuts along the hairline above, in front of, and behind the ear and then removes fat deposits in the neck, frees up deep layers of tissues in the face, and pulls muscle layers in the face and neck so that they can be stitched behind the ears. Upper eyelid surgery removes loose skin, stretched muscle, and excess fat to correct droopy lids, while lower eyelid surgery smoothes out bulges, removes bags, and tightens the skin.

Augmentation mammoplasty, or breast enlargement, has received the most publicity in recent years because the most common technique involves silicone implants. The implants may consist of semisolid, soft silicone in a solid silicone envelope or silicone covered with polyurethane; the latter is less common than it once was because of resulting infections and the difficulty involved in removing them. Implants may also consist of a water-filled silicone envelope or a double-walled envelope. Breast enlargement surgery involves placing the implants either on top of or under the pectoral muscles.

Reduction mammoplasty, or breast reduction surgery, is performed when overly large breasts cause medical problems and discomfort. Reduction can relieve backaches, shoulder aches, and breast crease irritation. In this pro-cedure, excess breast tissue is removed, and the nipple is repositioned and sewn into the skin. Other stitches close the skin under the nipple, and another closes the gap between the skin and the breast crease.

Techniques have improved in all areas of plastic surgery—for example, lasers can destroy spidery blood vessels, and endoscopic techniques can replace traditional incisions in face lifts—and the process has been stream-lined. Surgery may be performed in a doctor's office rather than in a hospital, and, depending on the procedure, patients may have a choice between regional and general anesthesia. They may be able to go home shortly after surgery.

RISKS AND CONTROVERSY

Most types of plastic surgery are major operations, and all cost considerable money. Depending on the procedure, the doctor, and the location, the costs range from a few thousand dollars to eight or ten thousand dollars. Medical insurance will not pay for cosmetic surgery. Recovery time may be a few days or a few weeks, or tissues may take several months to heal completely.

In addition, physical risks accompany any surgery, and plastic surgery is no exception. In *The Complete Book of Cosmetic Surgery* (1988), Elizabeth

Morgan argues that after a face lift, minor surgery may be needed to correct scarring, nerves may be numb or bruised, and further surgery may be needed to stop bleeding. With breast enlargement surgery, the breasts may become permanently numb, the implants may leak and require removal, and infections (though unlikely) may occur. With breast reduction surgery, scar surgery or steroid injections may be needed, nipple feeling may not return, and the nipple may blister and become scarred or discolored.

Many women object to such procedures because of the societal view that youth and beauty are paramount and that those women who fall short of perfection should alter themselves surgically. This view is reinforced in magazines, which are filled with pencil-thin models with perfect features and in businesses, where attractive women are often promoted more quickly than less attractive women. Many women are driven to plastic surgery by their own desires to correct what may or may not be actual flaws, others by the urging of parents or partners. Naomi Wolf, author of *The Beauty Myth* (1991), writes of a woman whose boyfriend rewarded her with breast implants for finishing her Ph.D. and of the trend in which some wealthy parents give their graduating daughters breast implants while their graduating sons receive trips to Europe. She complains, too, that women are not given enough information about the risks of surgery and are told there will be "some discomfort" rather than pain after the surgery. Wolf claims that such surgery is painful. In an apparent contradiction, women who had undergone such procedures, interviewed for an article in *Hemisphere* magazine, spoke of discomfort rather than of pain. Yet the article also quotes a plastic surgeon who says that women are accustomed to inconveniencing themselves in the pursuit of improving their looks, which is one reason that they make such good patients.

—Kate L. Peirce

See also Breast surgery; Cosmetic surgery and aging; Hair loss and baldness; Liposuction; Tattoos and body piercing; Women's health issues.

FOR FURTHER INFORMATION:
Adams, Jan R. *Everything Women of Color Should Know About Cosmetic Surgery.* New York: St. Martin's Press, 2000.
Chapkis, Wendy. *Beauty Secrets: Women and the Politics of Appearance.* Boston: South End Press, 1986.
Davis, Kathy. *Reshaping the Female Body: The Dilemma of Cosmetic Surgery.* New York: Routledge, 1995.
Sapiro, Virginia. *Women in American Society.* 4th ed. Mountain View, Calif.: Mayfield, 1998.
Wolf, Naomi. *The Beauty Myth.* New York: William Morrow, 1991.

✧ Death and dying

Type of issue: Ethics, mental health, public health, social trends
Definition: The process and result of a major, irreversible failure in bodily
  systems.

Medicine determines that death has occurred by assessing bodily functions
in either of two areas. Persons with irreversible cessation of respiration and
circulation are dead; persons with irreversible cessation of ascertainable
brain functions are also dead. There are standard procedures used to
diagnose death, including simple observation, brain-stem reflex studies, and
the use of confirmatory testing such as electrocardiography (ECG or EKG),
electroencephalography (EEG), and arterial blood gas analysis (ABG). The
particular circumstances—anticipated or unanticipated, observed or unob-
served, the patient's age, drug or metabolic intoxication, or suspicion of
hypothermia—will favor some procedures over others, but in all cases both
cessation of functions and their irreversibility are required before death can
be declared.

A Physical and Psychological Process

Between 60 and 75 percent of all people die from chronic terminal conditions. Therefore, except in sudden death (as in a fatal accident) or when
there is no evidence of consciousness (as in a head injury which destroys
cerebral, thinking functions while leaving brain-stem, reflexive functions
intact), dying is both a physical and a psychological process. In most cases,
dying takes time, and the time allows patients to react to the reality of their
own passing. Often, they react by becoming vigilant about bodily symptoms
and any changes in them. They also anticipate changes that have yet to
occur. For example, long before the terminal stages of illness become
manifest, dying patients commonly fear physical pain, shortness of breath,
invasive procedures, loneliness, becoming a burden to loved ones, losing
decision-making authority, and facing the unknown of death itself.

Medicine has come to acknowledge that physicians should understand
what it means to die. Indeed, while all persons should understand what their
own deaths will mean, physicians must additionally understand how their
dying patients find this meaning. Physicians who see death as the final
calamity coming at the end of life, and thus primarily as something that only
geriatric medicine has to face, are mistaken. Independent of beliefs about
"life after life," the life process on this planet inexorably comes to an end for
everyone, whether as a result of accident, injury, or progressive deterioration.

QUALITY OF DEATH

In 1969, psychiatrist Elisabeth Kübler-Ross published the landmark *On Death and Dying*, based on her work with two hundred terminally ill patients. In it, she provided a framework which explained how people cope with and adapt to the profound and terrible news that their illness is going to kill them. Although other physicians, psychologists, and thanatologists have shortened, expanded, and adapted her five stages of the dying process, neither the actual number of stages nor what they are specifically called is as important as the information and insight that any stage theory of dying yields. As with any human process, dying is complex, multifaceted, multidimensional, and polymorphic.

DENIAL, ANGER, AND BARGAINING

Denial is Kübler-Ross's first stage, but it is also linked to shock and isolation. Whether the news is told outright or gradual self-realization occurs, most people react to the knowledge of their impending death with existential shock. Broadly considered, denial is a complex cognitive-emotional capacity which enables temporary postponement of active, acute, but in some way detrimental, recognition of reality. In the dying process, this putting off of the truth prevents a person from being overwhelmed while promoting psychological survival. Denial plays an important stabilizing role, holding back more than could be otherwise managed while allowing the individual to marshal psychological resources and reserves. It enables patients to consider the possibility, even the inevitability, of death and then to put the consideration away so that they can pursue life in the ways that are still available. In this way, denial is truly a mechanism of defense.

Many other researchers, along with Kübler-Ross, report anger as the second stage of dying. The stage is also linked to rage, fury, envy, resentment, and loathing. Patients then begin to replace denial with attempts to understand what is happening to and inside them. When they do, they often ask, "Why me?" Though logically an unanswerable question, the logic of the question is clear. People, to remain human, must try to make intelligible their experiences and reality. The asking of this question is an important feature of the way in which all dying persons adapt to and cope with the reality of death.

People react with anger when they lose something of value; they react with greater anger when something of value is taken away from them by someone or something. Rage and fury, in fact, are often more accurate descriptions of people's reactions to the loss of their own life than anger. Anger is a difficult stage for professionals and loved ones, more so when the anger and rage are displaced and projected randomly into any corner and crevice of the patient's world. An unfortunate result is that caretakers often experience the anger as personal, and the caretakers' own feelings of guilt, shame, grief, and rejection can contribute to lessening contact with the dying person, which increases his or her sense of isolation.

Bargaining is Kübler-Ross's third stage, but it is also the one about which she wrote the least and the one that other thanatologists are most likely to leave unrepresented in their own models and stages of how people cope with dying. Nevertheless, it is a common phenomenon wherein dying people fall back on their faith, belief systems, or sense of the transcendent and the spiritual and try to make a deal—with God, life, fate, a higher power, or the composite of all the randomly colliding atoms in the universe. They ask for more time to help family members reconcile or to achieve something of importance. They may ask if they can simply attend their child's wedding or graduation or if they can see their first grandchild born. Then they will be ready to die; they will go willingly. Often, they mean that they will die without fighting death, if death can only be delayed or will delay itself. Some get what they want; others do not.

DEPRESSION AND ACCEPTANCE

The depression can take many forms, for indeed there are always many losses, and each loss individually or several losses collectively might need to be experienced and worked through. For example, dying parents might ask themselves who will take care of the children, get them through school, walk them down the aisle, or guide them through life. Children, even adult children who are parents themselves, may ask whether they can cope without their own parents. They wonder who will support and anchor them in times of distress, who will (or could) love, nurture, and nourish them the way that their parents did. Depression accompanies the realization that each role, each function, will never be performed again. Both the dying and those who love them mourn.

Much of the depression takes the form of anticipatory grieving, which often occurs both in the dying and in those who will be affected most by their death. It is a part of the dying process experienced by the living, both terminal and nonterminal. Patients, family, and friends can psychologically anticipate what it will be like when the death does occur and what life will, and will not, be like afterward. The grieving begins while there is still life left to live.

Bereavement specialists generally agree that anticipatory grieving, when it occurs, seems to help people cope with what is a terrible and frightening loss. It is an adaptive psychological mechanism wherein emotional, mental, and existential stability is painfully maintained. When depression develops, not only in reaction to death but also in preparation for it, it seems to be a necessary part of how those who are left behind cope in order to survive the loss themselves. Those who advocate or advise cheering up or looking on the bright side are either unrealistic or unable to tolerate the sadness in themselves or others. The dying are in the process of losing everything and everyone they love. Cheering up does not help them; the advice to "be strong" only helps the "helpers" deny the truth of the dying experience.

Both preparatory and reactive depression are often accompanied by unrealistic self-recrimination, shame, and guilt in the dying person. Those who are dying may judge themselves harshly and criticize themselves for the wrongs that they committed and for the good that they did not accomplish. They may judge themselves to be unattractive, unappealing, and repulsive because of how the illness and its treatment have made them appear. These feelings and states of minds, which have nothing to do with the reality of the situation, are often amenable to the interventions of understanding and caring people. Disfigured breasts do not make a woman less a woman; the removal of the testes does not make a man less a man. Financial and other obligations can be restructured and reassigned. Being forgiven and forgiving can help finish what was left undone.

Kübler-Ross's fifth stage, acceptance, is an intellectual and emotional coming to terms with death's reality, permanence, and inevitability. Ironically, it is manifested by diminished emotionality and interests and increased fatigue and inner (many would say spiritual) self-focus. It is a time without depression or anger. Envy of the healthy, the fear of losing all, and bargaining for another day or week are also absent. This final stage is often misunderstood. Some see it either as resignation and giving up or as achieving a happy serenity. Some think that acceptance is the goal of dying well and that all people are supposed to go through this stage. None of these viewpoints is accurate. Acceptance, when it does occur, comes from within the dying person. It is marked more by an emotional void and psychological detachment from people and things once held important and necessary and by an interest in some transcendental value (for the atheist) or his or her God (for the theist). It has little to do with what others believe is important or "should" be done. It is when dying people become more intimate with themselves and appreciate their separateness from others more than at any other time.

Accepting Death as Natural

All patients die—a fact that the actual practice of clinical Western medicine has too often discounted. Dealing with death is difficult in life, and it is difficult in medicine. As the ultimate outcome of all medical interventions, however, it is unavoidable. Dealing with the dying and those who care about them is also difficult. Patients ask questions that cannot be answered; families in despair and anger seek to find cause and sometimes lay blame. It takes courage to be with individuals as they face their deaths, struggling to find meaning in the time that they have left. It takes special courage simply to witness this struggle in a profession which prides itself on how well it intervenes. Working with death also reminds professionals of their own inevitable death. Facing that fact inwardly, spiritually, and existentially also requires courage.

Cure and treatment become care and management in the dying. They should live relatively pain-free, be supported in accomplishing their goals, be respected, be involved in decision making as appropriate, be encouraged to function as fully as their illness allows, and be provided with others to whom control can comfortably and confidently be passed. The lack of a cure and the certainty of the end can intimidate health care providers, family members, and close friends. They may dread genuine encounters with those whose days are knowingly numbered. Yet the dying have the same rights to be helped as any of the living, and how a society assists them bears directly on the meaning that its members are willing to attach to their own lives.

Today, largely in response to what dying patients have told researchers, medicine recognizes its role to assist these patients in working toward an appropriate death. Caretakers must determine the optimum treatments, interventions, and conditions which will enable such a death to occur. For each terminally ill person, these should be unique and specific. Caretakers should respond to the patient's needs and priorities, at the patient's own pace and as much as possible following the patient's lead. For some dying patients, the goal is to remain as pain-free as is feasible and to feel as well as possible. For others, finishing whatever unfinished business remains becomes the priority. Making amends, forgiving and being forgiven, resolving old conflicts, and reconciling with self and others may be the most therapeutic and healing of interventions. Those who are to be bereaved fear the death of those they love. The dying fear the separation from all they know and love, but they fear as well the loss of autonomy, letting family and friends down, the pain and invasion of further treatment, disfigurement, dementia, loneliness, the unknown, becoming a burden, and the loss of dignity.

—*Paul Moglia*

See also Abortion; Abortion among teenagers; Aging; AIDS; AIDS and children; AIDS and women; Depression; Depression in children; Depression in the elderly; Ethics; Euthanasia; Hippocratic oath; Hospice; Hospitalization of the elderly; Law and medicine; Living wills; Stress; Sudden infant death syndrome (SIDS); Suicide; Suicide among children and teenagers; Suicide among the elderly; Terminal illnesses.

FOR FURTHER INFORMATION:
Becker, Ernest. *The Denial of Death.* New York: Free Press, 1997. Written by an anthropologist and philosopher, this is an erudite and insightful analysis and synthesis of the role that the fear of death plays in motivating human activity, society, and individual actions. A profound work.
Cook, Alicia Skinner, and Daniel S. Dworkin. *Helping the Bereaved: Therapeutic*

Interventions for Children, Adolescents, and Adults. New York: Basic Books, 1992. Although not a self-help book, this work is useful to professionals and nonprofessionals alike as a review of the state of the art in grief therapy. Practical and readable. Of special interest for those becoming involved in grief counseling.

Corr, Charles A., Clyde M. Nabe, and Donna M. Corr. *Death and Dying, Life and Living.* 3d ed. Belmont, Calif.: Wadsworth, 1999. This book provides perspective on common issues associated with death and dying for family members and others affected by life-threatening circumstances.

Kübler-Ross, Elisabeth, ed. *Death: The Final Stage of Growth.* Reprint. New York: Simon & Schuster, 1986. A psychiatrist by training, Kübler-Ross brings together other researchers' views of how death provides the key to how human beings make meaning in their own personal worlds. The author, who is regarded as the pioneer in death and dying studies, addresses practical concerns over how people express grief and accept the death of those close to them, and how they might prepare for their own inevitable ends.

Kushner, Harold. *When Bad Things Happen to Good People.* New York: Summit, 1985. The first of Rabbi Kushner's works on finding meaning in one's life, it was originally his personal response to make intelligible the death of his own child. It has become a highly regarded reference for those who struggle with the meaning of pain, suffering, and death in their lives. Highly recommended.

✦ DEMENTIA

Type of issue: Elder health, mental health

Definition: A generally irreversible decline in intellectual ability resulting from a variety of causes; differs from mental retardation, in which the affected person never reaches an expected level of mental growth.

Dementia affects about four million people in the United States and is a major cause of disability in old age. Its prevalence increases with age. Dementia is characterized by a permanent memory deficit affecting recent memory in particular and of sufficient severity to interfere with the patient's ability to take part in professional and social activities. Although the aging process is associated with a gradual loss of brain cells, dementia is not part of the aging process. It also is not synonymous with benign senescent forgetfulness, which is very common in old age and affects recent memory. Although the latter is a source of frustration, it does not significantly interfere with the individual's professional and social activities because it tends to affect only trivial matters (or what the individual considers trivial).

Furthermore, patients with benign forgetfulness usually can remember what was forgotten by utilizing a number of subterfuges, such as writing lists or notes to themselves and leaving them in conspicuous places. Individuals with benign forgetfulness also are acutely aware of their memory deficit, while those with dementia—except in the early stages of the disease—have no insight into their memory deficit and often blame others for their problems.

In addition to the memory deficit interfering with the patient's daily activities, patients with dementia have evidence of impaired abstract thinking, impaired judgment, or other disturbances of higher cortical functions such as aphasia (the inability to use or comprehend language), apraxia (the inability to execute complex, coordinated movements), or agnosia (the inability to recognize familiar objects).

CAUSES OF DEMENTIA

Dementia may result from damage to the cerebral cortex (the outer layer of the brain), as in Alzheimer's disease, or from damage to the subcortical structures (the structures below the cortex), such as white matter, the thalamus, or the basal ganglia. Although memory is impaired in both cortical and subcortical dementias, the associated features are different. In cortical dementias, for example, cognitive functions such as the ability to understand speech and to talk and the ability to perform mathematical calculations are severely impaired. In subcortical dementias, on the other hand, there is evidence of disturbances of arousal, motivation, and mood, in addition to a significant slowing of cognition and of information processing.

Alzheimer's disease, the most common cause of presenile dementia, is characterized by progressive disorientation, memory loss, speech disturbances, and personality disorders. Pick's disease is another cortical dementia, but unlike Alzheimer's disease, it is rare, tends to affect younger patients, and is more common in women. In the early stages of Pick's disease, changes in personality, disinhibition, inappropriate social and sexual conduct, and lack of foresight may be evident—features that are not common in Alzheimer's disease. Patients also may become euphoric or apathetic. Poverty of speech is often present and gradually progresses to mutism, although speech comprehension is usually spared. Pick's disease is characterized by cortical atrophy localized to the frontal and temporal lobes.

Vascular dementia is the second most common cause of dementia in patients over the age of sixty-five and is responsible for 8 percent to 20 percent of all dementia cases. It is caused by interference with the blood flow to the brain. Although the overall prevalence of vascular dementia is decreasing, there are some geographical variations, with the prevalence being higher in countries with a high incidence of cardiovascular and cerebrovascular diseases, such as Finland and Japan. About 20 percent of patients with dementia have both Alzheimer's disease and vascular dementia. Several types of vascular dementia have been identified.

Multiple infarct dementia (MID) is the most common type of vascular dementia. As its name implies, it is the result of multiple, discrete cerebral infarcts (strokes) that have destroyed enough brain tissue to interfere with the patient's higher mental functions. The onset of MID is usually sudden and is associated with neurological deficit, such as the paralysis or weakness of an arm or leg or the inability to speak. The disease characteristically progresses in steps: With each stroke experienced, the patient's condition suddenly deteriorates and then stabilizes or even improves slightly until another stroke occurs. In about 20 percent of patients with MID, however, the disease displays an insidious onset and causes gradual deterioration. Most patients also show evidence of arteriosclerosis and other factors predisposing them to the development of strokes, such as hypertension, cigarette smoking, high blood cholesterol, diabetes mellitus, narrowing of one or both carotid arteries, or cardiac disorders, especially atrial fibrillation (an irregular heartbeat). Somatic complaints, mood changes, depression, and nocturnal confusion tend to be more common in vascular dementias, although there is relative preservation of the patient's personality. In such cases, magnetic resonance imaging (MRI) or a computed tomography (CT) scan of the brain often shows evidence of multiple strokes.

Strokes are not always associated with clinical evidence of neurological deficits, since the stroke may affect a "silent" area of the brain or may be so small that its immediate impact is not noticeable. Nevertheless, when several of these small strokes have occurred, the resulting loss of brain tissue may interfere with the patient's cognitive functions. This is, in fact, the basis of the lacunar dementias. The infarcted tissue is absorbed into the rest of the brain, leaving a small cavity or lacuna. Brain-imaging techniques and especially MRI are useful in detecting these lacunae.

TREATING DEMENTIA

It is estimated that dementia affects about 0.4 percent of the population aged sixty to sixty-four years and 0.9, 1.8, 3.6, 10.5, and 23.8 percent of the population aged sixty-five to sixty-nine, seventy to seventy-four, seventy-five to seventy-nine, eighty to eighty-four, and eighty-five to ninety-three years, respectively. Different surveys may yield different results, depending on the criteria used to define dementia.

For physicians, an important aspect of diagnosing patients with dementia is detecting potentially reversible causes which may be responsible for the impaired mental functions. A detailed history followed by a meticulous and thorough clinical examination and a few selected laboratory tests are usually sufficient to reach a diagnosis. Various investigators have estimated that reversible causes of dementia can be identified in 10 percent to 20 percent of patients with dementia. Recommended investigations include brain imaging (CT scanning or MRI), a complete blood count, and tests of erythrocyte sedimentation rate, blood glucose, serum electrolytes, serum calcium, liver function, thyroid function, and serum B_{12} and folate. Some investigators also recommend routine testing for syphilis. Other tests, such as those for the detection of HIV infection, cerebrospinal fluid examination, neuropsychological testing, drug and toxin screen, serum copper and ceruloplasmin analysis, carotid and cerebral angiography, and electroencephalography, are performed when appropriate.

It is of paramount importance for health care providers to adopt a positive attitude when managing patients with dementia. Although at present little can be done to treat and reverse dementia, it is important to identify the cause of the dementia. In some cases, it may be possible to prevent the disease from progressing. For example, if the dementia is the result of hypertension, adequate control of this condition may prevent further brain damage. Moreover, the prevalence of vascular dementia is decreasing in countries where efforts to reduce cardiovascular and cerebrovascular diseases have been successful. Similarly, if the dementia is the result of repeated emboli (blood clots reaching the brain) complicating atrial fibrillation, then anticoagulants or aspirin may be recommended.

Dealing with the Diagnosis

The casual observer of the dementing process is often overwhelmed with concern for the patient, but it is the family that truly suffers. The patients themselves experience no physical pain or distress, and except in the very early stages of the disease, they are oblivious to their plight as a result of their loss of insight. Health care professionals therefore are alert to the stress imposed on the caregivers by dealing with loved ones with dementia. Adequate support from agencies available in the community is essential.

When a diagnosis of dementia is made, the physician discusses a number of ethical, financial, and legal issues with the family, and also the patient if it is believed that he or she can understand the implications of this discussion. Families are encouraged to make a list of all the patient's assets, including insurance policies, and to discuss this information with an attorney in order to protect the patient's and the family's assets. If the patient is still competent, it is recommended that he or she select a trusted person to have durable power of attorney. Unlike the regular power of attorney, the former does not become invalidated when the patient becomes mentally incompetent and continues to be in effect regardless of the degree of mental impairment of the person who executed it. Because durable power of attorney cannot be easily reversed once the person is incompetent, great care should be taken when selecting a person, and the specific powers granted should be clearly specified. It is also important for the patient to make his or her desires known concerning advance directives and the use of life support systems.

Courts may appoint a guardian or conservator to have charge and custody of the patient's property (including real estate and money) when no responsible family members or friends are willing or available to serve as guardian. Courts supervise the actions of the guardian, who is expected to report all the patient's income and expenditures to the court once a year. The court may also charge the guardian to ensure that the patient is adequately housed, fed, and clothed and receiving appropriate medical care.

Long-Term Prognoses

Dementia is a very serious and common condition, especially among the older population. Dementia permanently robs patients of their minds and prevents them from functioning adequately in their environment by impairing memory and interfering with the ability to make rational decisions. It therefore deprives patients of their dignity and independence.

Because dementia is mostly irreversible, cannot be adequately treated at present, and is associated with a fairly long survival period, it has a significant impact not only on the patient's life but also on the patient's family and caregivers and on society in general. The expense of long-term care for patients with dementia, whether at home or in institutions, is staggering. Every effort, therefore, is made to reach an accurate diagnosis and especially to detect any other condition that may worsen the patient's underlying dementia. Finally, health care professionals do not treat the patient in isolation but also concern themselves with the impact of the illness on the patient's caregivers and family.

—Ronald C. Hamdy, M.D., Louis A. Cancellaro, M.D.,
and Larry Hudgins, M.D.

See also Aging; Alzheimer's disease; Arteriosclerosis; Hypertension; Malnutrition among the elderly; Medications and the elderly; Memory loss; Nursing and convalescent homes; Nutrition and aging; Parkinson's disease; Reaction time and aging; Safety issues for the elderly; Sleep changes with aging; Strokes.

For Further Information:

Coons, Dorothy H., ed. *Specialized Dementia Care Units*. Baltimore: The Johns Hopkins University Press, 1991. A collection of articles reviewing the benefits and disadvantages of caring for patients with dementia in specialized care units. Several problems encountered when running such units are addressed.

Hamdy, Ronald C., J. M. Turnbull, L. D. Norman, and M. M. Lancaster, eds. *Alzheimer's Disease: A Handbook for Caregivers.* 3d ed. St. Louis: Mosby Year Book, 1998. A comprehensive discussion of the symptoms and characteristic features of Alzheimer's disease and other dementias. Abnormal brain structure and function in these patients are discussed, and the normal effects of aging are reviewed. Gives caregivers practical advice concerning the encouragement of patients with dementia.

Kovach, Christine, ed. *Late Stage Dementia Care: A Basic Guide.* Washington, D.C.: Taylor & Francis, 1997. Provides information on assessment and treatment management for individuals experiencing dementia. A valuable source for caregivers and family members of those affected.

U.S. Congress. Office of Technology Assessment. *Confused Minds, Burdened Families: Finding Help for People with Alzheimer's and Other Dementias.* Washington, D.C.: Government Printing Office, 1990. A report from the Office of Technology Assessment analyzing the problems of locating and arranging services for people with dementia in the United States. Also presents a framework for an effective system to provide appropriate services and discusses congressional policy options for establishing such a system.

West, Robin L., and Jan D. Sinnott, eds. *Everyday Memory and Aging.* New York: Springer-Verlag, 1992. A review of issues relating to memory research and methodology, especially as they apply to aging.

✦ Dental problems in children

Type of issue: Children's health, public health
Definition: Structures in the mouth that assist in the processing of food prior to swallowing and the diseases that can affect them.

A tooth is composed of three parts: the crown, pulp, and root. The crown of the tooth is the portion exposed above the gums. Its surface is made of a hard, crystalline material called enamel. The rest of the crown is a substance known as dentin. At the center is pulp, which contains nerves and blood vessels. The root joins the crown to the jawbone. The outer surface of the root is a thin layer of cementum, with dentin underneath.

Humans normally have twenty baby (deciduous or primary) teeth and thirty-two adult (permanent) teeth. The baby teeth begin to erupt through the gums in infancy. Most adult teeth develop below these baby teeth; as they grow, they push on the roots of the baby teeth, which are shed throughout childhood and into adolescence. The shape and size of permanent teeth are related to their functions. The four front incisors cut food like scissors. The four cuspids, or canines, are pointed; their primary function is to grasp and tear food. The eight premolars are used for tearing and also to crush and grind food. The twelve molars grind food into even smaller portions. The third molars, commonly called wisdom teeth, are the last to develop, often appearing during adolescence. If the wisdom teeth are unable to erupt normally, then they may have to be removed.

Teething

Teething in infants is the time of primary incisor eruption, usually occurring between four and ten months of age. Symptoms associated with teething can include irritability, increased crying, restlessness, disturbed sleep, drooling, and decreased appetite but increased thirst. The gum around the erupting tooth is red, swollen, and tender. Sometimes, fever and/or diarrhea develops. Teething infants often like to put their fingers into their mouths. Some infants gain their baby teeth without any symptoms.

A child who is teething may be given smooth, clean, hard, chewable objects on which to bite, such as water-filled "teethers" cooled in a refrigerator before use. To relieve pain, topical anesthetics can be applied, such as oral sugar-free choline salicylate dental gel, to be used every three to four hours. Parents should be informed that teething is normal and will resolve in time. If fever is persistent, the child should be treated by a pediatrician.

Among some children, eruption cysts are observed as a complication of tooth eruption. An eruption cyst may develop a few weeks before the eruption of a primary or permanent tooth, often seen in the primary second molar or the first permanent molar regions. An eruption cyst appears as a bluish-purple elevated area of tissue, filled with fluid and blood. Sometimes, an eruption cyst is surrounded by inflammation.

Usually within a few days the tooth breaks through the tissue, and the eruption cyst resolves itself. This process can be assisted with the usual teething aids, such as "teethers." In rare cases, it may be necessary to open the cyst surgically. Under local anesthesia, the tissue of the cyst is cut away and the crown of the underlying tooth is exposed.

Marginal Gingivitis

Marginal gingivitis is a common periodontal disorder, or gum disease, in children of all ages. A published survey showed a rate of 87 percent of children having such a condition. It is more frequently seen in Asians and Africans than in Caucasians. The causes of this condition may be local oral or systemic factors. The major local oral cause is that the mouth contains a large number and variety of bacteria. Together with food, the bacteria form plaque. In the plaque, the bacteria create toxins, which irritate the gums. With poor oral hygiene, the plaque is not removed and hardens into calculus, which is occasionally seen in young children. Mouth breathing, tooth eruption, and other oral diseases may also increase the occurrence of marginal gingivitis. Systemic factors include diabetes mellitus, hematological disorders, vitamin C deficiency, and Down syndrome.

Children with marginal gingivitis have an appearance of inflammatory gums that are red, tender, swollen, and bleed easily. The affected regions can be small or large, but the most commonly affected regions are the anterior segments. After the age of six, the risk of developing marginal gingivitis increases, reaching a peak at puberty (eleven years in girls and thirteen years in boys), which may be related to hormonal changes. Gingivitis leading to irreversible periodontal changes is rare in young children. However, after puberty, teenagers are more likely to have periodontal pockets and alveolar bone loss.

Children should start brushing their teeth thoroughly twice a day with a fluoride toothpaste as soon as the primary teeth erupt. The toothbrush should be soft-bristled and replaced every three months. Use of dental floss may be started when the child can cooperate. From the age of six months, dental checkups every six months are necessary. The most common procedure performed for the treatment of gingivitis is cleaning and polishing. The frequency or need for semiannual prophylaxis for this age group is a topic of controversy. Frequent prophylaxis is beneficial to tissues, but the cost-benefit ratio may not justify providing such services to children at the community level.

Developmental Defects

Developmental defects associated with the teeth and oral structures may be caused by hereditary factors, infection, or metabolic disturbances during pregnancy or infancy. Congenital absence of teeth can be seen as anodontia or hypodontia. Anodontia implies complete failure of the development of the teeth. This condition may be related to a severe form of ectodermal dysplasia. In addition to the absence of all teeth, children with ectodermal dysplasia also have dry skin without sweat glands, thin hair and eyebrows, and a deficiency in salivary flow. Other ectodermal dysplasia features include protuberant lips, a saddle-nose appearance, and defects of the fingernails.

Hypodontia represents a deficiency in tooth number or a developmental absence of some of the teeth. Familial heredity is commonly observed for the occurrence of hypodontia. This condition may also be associated with ectodermal dysplasia. The teeth that develop may be malformed. Hypodontia can occur for both the primary teeth and permanent teeth; those who have primary teeth with hypodontia are more likely to have permanent teeth with the same condition. In some cases, an excess number of teeth exists, which is described as hyperdontia or supernumerary teeth. Hyperdontia can occur in both the primary and permanent teeth and is often found in the incisor, premolar, and occasionally molar regions. Boys are affected twice as frequently as girls.

Amelogenesis imperfecta affects the enamel of both the primary and permanent teeth. The cause of amelogenesis imperfecta is generally accepted as a hereditary defect. However, some reports have indicated that a few children have had this condition without any hereditary background. There are three common types of amelogenesis imperfecta: hypoplastic, hypocalcified, and hypomatured. In the hypoplastic type, the enamel of the teeth is thin. The affected teeth appear small with open contacts. In the hypocalcified type, the enamel of the teeth is soft and fragile caused by poor calcification. The enamel of the affected teeth is easily fractured and the underlying dentin is exposed. Thus, children with hypocalcified enamel show an unaesthetic appearance. In the hypomatured type, the teeth have normal enamel thickness but a low value of mineral content. The enamel of the affected teeth chips away easily from the dentin. In the areas of the affected teeth where dentin is exposed, cavities can develop, but it is not always true that hypoplastic teeth are more susceptible to dental caries than normal teeth.

The causes of environmental enamel hypoplasia are associated with varied environmental factors. Nutritional deficiencies, especially in vitamins A, C, and D and in calcium and phosphorus, can cause enamel hypoplasia. Research has shown that children with brain injuries and renal disease are more likely to have enamel hypoplasia than normal children are. There is also an observed correlation between enamel defects and the presence of severe allergies. The fetus of a lead-poisoned or rubella-infected mother has an increased risk of developing enamel hypoplasia. Other causes include severe infection, fevers, congenital syphilis, use of certain drugs, and excess fluoride. However, it is not always possible to identify environmental causes of enamel hypoplasia.

Dentinogenesis imperfecta is an inherited dentin defect originating during the histodifferentiation stage of tooth development. This anomaly includes a defect of the predentin matrix that results in amorphic, disorganized, and atubular circumpulpal dentin. For both the primary and permanent teeth, dentinogenesis imperfecta is characterized by a reddish brown to gray opalescent color. There are three types of dentinogenesis imperfecta. Type I occurs with osteogenesis imperfecta, which is an inherited defect in collagen formation resulting in osteoporotic brittle bones, bowing of the limbs, bitemporal bossing, and blue sclera. Type I dentinogenesis imperfecta affects the primary teeth more than the permanent teeth. The affected teeth show an amber translucent color, periapical radiolucencies, bulbous crowns, obliteration of pulp chambers, and root fractures. Type II is known as hereditary opalescent dentin. The symptoms of this type are similar to that of type I, but type II affects the primary and the permanent teeth equally, although these two types are separate entities.

Type III has the features described with a predominance of bell-shaped crowns, particularly seen in the permanent teeth. Affected teeth often have a shell-like appearance and multiple pulp exposures. Type III dentinogenesis imperfecta rarely occurs, and it has been suggested as a different expression of the same type II gene.

Extremely high levels of fluoride ingested during the tooth formation stage can affect the ameloblasts. The appearance of fluorosis varies greatly, showing white or brown patches of discoloration on the affected teeth. Brown pigmentation is often seen in the maxillary anterior teeth.

Children who have taken antibiotic tetracycline during the period of calcification of the primary or permanent teeth can have severe tooth discoloration. Tetracycline is bound to calcium and deposited in growing teeth (as well as bones). Affected teeth show bands of discoloration, ranging from gray to dark orange-brown. Research has indicated that when tetracycline is given in concentrations of 21 to 26 milligrams per kilogram or greater over a period as short as three days, both the primary and permanent teeth can be seriously affected.

Tooth Decay

Dental caries are the most common dental disorder. This condition affects both the primary and permanent teeth. The development of dental caries involves many factors, including bacteria, food, saliva, and poor oral hygiene. The predisposing risk factors for tooth decay include a frequent high sugar consumption in the diet, poor oral hygiene, lack of fluoride, and decreased flow of saliva. Dental caries are caused by acid produced from the action of bacteria on food, especially carbohydrates such as sugar. The caries-causing bacteria form a sticky film, called plaque, on tooth surfaces, and proliferate within plaque to produce both acid and enzymes. The acid and enzymes break down the calcified substances of the teeth, resulting in demineralization of the enamel surface. Sweets and other carbohydrate foods provide the caries-causing bacteria an excellent culture medium to produce such action. Saliva of healthy people contains immunoglobulins and other antibacterial substances, which can limit the activity of caries-causing bacterial. Thus, when the flow of saliva decreases, the risk of developing dental caries increases. A person's susceptibility to dental caries is also determined by some other factors, such as heredity and tooth shape.

As the acid produced by bacteria dissolves the tooth enamel, a cavity is formed. In the primary teeth, the sequence of caries follows a specific pattern: mandibular molars, maxillary molars, and maxillary anterior teeth. The second primary molars are much more susceptible to caries than the first primary molars, which erupt earlier. This difference in caries susceptibility between molars may be due to the differences of the occlusal surface. For the permanent teeth, caries are more likely to be seen in the mandibular molars and maxillary molars. However, the maxillary lateral incisors often erupt with a defect in the lingual surface in many children. If caries occur in this area of the maxillary molars, the progression of the decay can be rapid, even involve the pulp before the awareness of the presence of the cavity.

A lesion develops in the enamel initially, causing a cavity. If untreated, it will spread to the dentin, and sometimes, to an adjacent tooth, or to the pulp. Eventually, the infection will result in necrosis and abscess formation. The rate of caries progression is more rapid in the primary teeth than in the permanent teeth. Children with dental decay may feel pain, food impaction, and a sharp edge of tooth. However, these symptoms do not necessarily show themselves in all patients. Changes have been noticed for both the symptoms and the incidence of dental caries in the past decades. These changes are associated with the use of fluoride through fluoride toothpastes, dietary supplementation, and water supply augmentation. With the use of fluoride, the incidence rate of dental caries in adolescents decreased 50 percent. The progression of dental caries has become slower, and the changes in tooth structure usually are not observed in a short period of time.

Before examination of dental caries, teeth should be dried well and viewed with a bright light. Fissures may be tested gently with a probe. Cavities may be detected by a fiber-optic light terminal placed against one wall of the tooth. Through this light, the cavity may be observed by the lack of light conduction.

Rampant caries is a dental condition in which the child suffers from an acute onset of destructive lesions involving most of the erupted teeth, progressing rapidly to pulp. This condition can even affect those teeth usually regarded as immune to ordinary decay. Rampant caries is usually diagnosed when ten or more new lesions develop per year. Although it has been observed in all ages, young teenagers are most susceptible to rampant caries. The risk factors for rampant caries are similar to that of ordinary caries, but the mechanism of this condition is obscure. There is some evidence suggesting that emotional disturbances might be the cause in some children with rampant caries. These emotional disturbances could be stress, depression, anxiety, fear, dissatisfaction, and tension.

Nursing caries is a condition seen in children with prolonged bottle feeding, beyond the time when most children are weaned from the bottle. Nursing caries occur among children aged two to four years old. These children often have been put to bed with a nursing bottle containing milk, formula, or juice. When the child falls asleep, the liquid from the nursing bottle remains in the mouth, especially pooling around the maxillary anterior teeth. Thus, there is a specific pattern for nursing caries: early caries development of the maxillary anterior teeth, the maxillary and mandibular first primary molars, and the mandibular canines. Nursing caries usually do not affect mandibular incisors.

Treating Children's Teeth

For children with anodontia, the dental deficiencies can be overcome by the construction of dentures. The dentures should be constructed at an early age (two to three years old), and need to be remade from time to time to ensure facial growth. Children with a number of missing primary teeth (hypodontia) can have partial dentures constructed at an early age. A partial denture also needs to be adjusted and remade from time to time to allow the eruption of permanent teeth. Hyperdontia tends to cause orthodontic problems with adverse effects on adjacent teeth; thus, it often requires early extraction. Children with any problems related to tooth number need to have regular and closely monitored dental care.

The treatment of amelogenesis imperfecta depends on the severity of the condition and the demands of aesthetic appearance. Porcelain jacket crowns can be used, as the dentin structure is normal. For some children with the hypoplastic and hypomatured types, bonded veneer restorations may provide a conservative alternative for the management of aesthetic appearance. Another reported successful treatment includes porcelain laminate veneer restorations.

The treatment for hypoplastic teeth depends on the size of the affected areas. Small caries and precaries areas can be restored with amalgam, resin, or glass ionomer. The restoration is generally confined to the area of involvement of the teeth. Large areas of defective enamel and exposed dentin, which can be seen in both hypoplastic primary and permanent teeth, may become sensitive as soon as they erupt; however, the possibility of good restoration at this stage is rare. To reduce the sensitivity of the tooth, the topical application of fluoride is found useful, and can be repeated as often as necessary.

The treatment of dentinogenesis imperfecta is quite difficult for both the primary and permanent teeth. The placement of stainless steel crowns on the primary posterior teeth may be used as a means of preventing gross abrasion of the tooth structure. Some approaches may be used to restore the teeth to functional and aesthetic standards, such as metal-ceramic restorations for the premolar teeth and those anterior to them and full cast crowns on the molars. For some patients, full coverage restorations may not be necessary; veneer restorations on anterior teeth can be helpful. In the case of teeth that have periapical rarefaction and root fracture, the affected teeth should be removed. However, the extraction of such teeth can be difficult because of the brittleness of the dentin.

Correcting Tooth Color

Several methods are available for the color correction of fluorosis. One technique is the use of 18 percent hydrochloric acid on the affected enamel surfaces. After careful isolation of tooth or teeth with the rubber dam and proper preparations for safe use, the caustic agent, a slurry of fine pumice and hydrochloric acid, is applied under pressure, and abraded with a wooden stick. After each five seconds of such application, the slurry should be rinsed away with water. This procedure should be repeated till the desired color change has occurred. After a final rinsing, 1.1 percent neutral sodium fluoride gel is applied to the area for three minutes. Then, a fine fluoridated prophylaxis paste is applied with a rotating rubber cup. The final step is polishing the enamel with an aluminum oxide disk.

Tetracycline should not be given to children under twelve years of age or to pregnant women. Observations have shown that the sensitive period for tetracycline induced discoloration for the primary teeth covers the four-month-old fetus to the three-month-old baby for maxillary and mandibular incisors, and the five-month-old fetus to the nine-month-old infant for maxillary and mandibular canines. The sensitive period for permanent maxillary and mandibular incisors and canines is from three months to seven years of age. Techniques are available for bleaching the teeth stained by tetracycline.

TREATING CAVITIES

The treatment for dental caries varies depending on the extent of the decay. Restorations (fillings) are commonly done on living teeth. Under local anesthesia, decay is first completely removed; the resulting hole is then shaped and filled with material. Different filling materials are chosen to ideally match the tooth tissue in resistance, strength, and color. If the pulp is involved by the caries, and pulpitis (inflammation of the pulp) is observed, root canal therapy is often required. Root canal therapy is a multiphase procedure, including removing all traces of pulp tissue from the pulp chamber and the canals, cleaning out all bacteria, shaping the canals, and filling with filling material. A seal is placed to avoid reinfection. The tooth needs to be restored and protected after root canal therapy. For those permanently dead teeth where root canal therapy is not feasible, extraction is necessary. For children who have a primary tooth extracted and whose permanent tooth does not erupt for six or more months, space maintainers should be considered. A fixed bridge, a partial denture, or an implant supported prosthesis can be used to replace the extracted tooth.

When rampant caries are diagnosed, the treatment of all cavities should be initiated immediately. As this condition develops rapidly, a plan of restoring one tooth at a time is impossible to achieve a full restoration. A more appropriate approach is the technique of gross excavation, gross caries removal, which can usually be accomplished in one appointment, except for some occasions where a second or third appointment is necessary for a large number of extensive caries. Following gross excavation there should be a systematic therapy for rampant caries, including taking a medical and dental history, completing tests to determine the cause of the condition, and treatment of relevant medical and dental conditions.

Parents should be educated about the cause of nursing caries. Infants should be held while bottle feeding, and should never be allowed to nap or sleep with the bottle propped in the mouth. Children need to begin brushing with a fluoride-enhanced paste once any teeth have erupted. Multiple vitamins containing fluoride can also be prescribed for a child by a pediatrician.

—*Kimberly Y. Z. Forrest*

See also Children's health issues; Dental problems in the elderly; Fluoridation of water sources; Fluoride treatments in dentistry; Teething.

For Further Information:

McDonald, Ralph E., and David R. Avery. *Dentistry for the Child and Adolescent.* 6th ed. St. Louis: C. V. Mosby, 1994. This book is designed to help dental students provide efficient and superior comprehensive oral health care for infants, children, and teenagers. The newest edition provides current diagnostic and treatment recommendations for pediatric dental diseases based on research, clinical experience, and current literature.

Parkin, Stanley F. *Notes on Paediatric Dentistry.* Boston: Wright, 1991. This book provides the main core subject matter of dental diseases in children. Each disease is discussed in a simple and clear context.

Pinkham, J. R., ed. *Pediatric Dentistry: Infancy Through Adolescence.* 2d ed. Philadelphia: W. B. Saunders, 1994. This book initiates some basic information on pediatric dental problems pertinent to all age levels; the text is then divided into four large sections by developmental age. Dental diseases associated with specific age groups are described in detail.

Taintor, Jerry F., and Mary Jane Taintor. *The Complete Guide to Better Dental Care.* Reprint. New York: Checkmark Books, 1999.

✧ Dental problems in the elderly

Type of issue: Elder health, public health
Definition: Treatment and prevention of diseases of the mouth, teeth, and gums.

As the geriatric population increases in the United States, the provision of dental services for the elderly will have to expand to provide adequate regular dental follow-ups. This population will also need to be educated about how to care for their teeth, gums, and dentures in order to maintain good dental health and retain their natural teeth as long as possible.

Normal Age-Related Changes

Approximately 90 percent of the elderly have some form of mouth disorder. Normal age-related changes of the mouth have a minimal effect on overall functioning. Muscle weakening and decreased bone density in the jaw, decreased elasticity in the gums and cheeks, reduced secretion of saliva, and increased alkalinity in saliva make chewing foods more difficult. Thinning and staining of tooth enamel leads to chipping of teeth. The soft dentin in the teeth slowly and gradually dissolves as a result of exposure to the acid in saliva. Receding gums encourage the trapping of food in crevices between teeth and gums and in tooth borders. This accumulation of food and debris can promote gum irritation and tooth decay if proper dental hygiene, such as brushing and flossing, is not followed.

Disorders of the Teeth

Being toothless (edentulous) is not a normal part of aging. The major causes of tooth loss in adults are tooth decay and periodontal disease. Lack of water fluoridation, limited access to dental care, and inadequate dental hygiene are also causes of tooth loss in adults. Today, there are fewer cases of adults who are edentulous, owing to increased availability of preventive dental care and early diagnosis and intervention to prevent disease that causes tooth loss. Treatment for tooth loss includes bridges that replace one or more teeth and anchor onto teeth on either side of the bridge, partial dentures to replace missing teeth, full dentures to cover the entire gum of missing teeth, and dental implants to replace individual teeth by anchoring a post in the jaw and placing an artificial tooth over it.

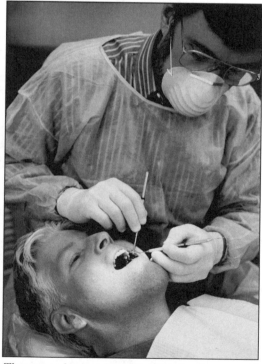

The wear-and-tear and potential for injury increase with age, making regular dental checkups crucial. (Photo-Disc)

Cavities (caries) are the major cause of all tooth loss

in the United States. Because older adults have receding gums, most caries in older adults form at the gum line and the roots of teeth. Caries are areas in a tooth in which enamel has thinned (demineralized), causing weak areas in tooth enamel that eventually decay. This decay is a result of the acid in saliva, which increases during eating. Fluoride helps to slow enamel demineralization. Fluoride is present in many water supplies, toothpaste, and mouth rinses. Brushing the teeth at least twice daily and flossing between teeth help to prevent enamel demineralization.

An abscessed tooth is an inflammation and infection in the pulp of a tooth. It most frequently results from a cavity that exposes the tooth pulp to bacteria. The major symptom is a constant, severe pain in the affected tooth. The pain increases when the tooth is exposed to heat and cold. Treatment includes drainage of the abscess by a dentist. If the pulp of the tooth is severely infected, a root canal may be the only means to save the tooth. A root canal is a procedure in which the diseased pulp is removed and the remaining space is filled with a compound that will maintain the integrity of the tooth.

A fractured tooth is one that has cracked from trauma, poor health, or demineralized enamel. If the fracture is severe, a crown may be placed over the tooth to protect, strengthen, and prevent tooth loss.

Malocclusion occurs when the teeth do not align in the mouth properly. This condition causes uneven wear on the teeth. Over time, it can create dental problems that require dental procedures to correct the damage that is caused. Common malocclusions are an overbite, in which the upper teeth greatly overhang the lower teeth, and an underbite, in which the lower teeth jut out beyond the upper teeth.

When the gums recede or teeth are chipped or fractured, the dentin of the teeth allows the nerves to be exposed to irritants that cause pain or discomfort. The result is sensitive teeth. Frequently, these irritants are heat, cold, and sweet or sour foods and drinks. Using toothpaste for sensitive teeth and a soft toothbrush may help to relieve discomfort.

Age-related color changes that occur in the teeth are normal. Years of exposure to coffee, tea, colas, fruit juices, and smoking gradually and steadily stain the teeth, causing color changes from whiter to more yellow. Professional bleaching by a dentist can help to restore some of the whiteness of teeth.

DISORDERS OF THE GUMS

Periodontal disease, also called gum disease or pyorrhea, is a major cause of tooth loss in older adults. It results from an inflammatory process caused by the accumulation of plaque and tartar that destroys the bones supporting the teeth. Plaque is composed of sticky components of bacteria and saliva that adhere to the gum line and the crevices of the teeth. It forms constantly and must be brushed away to prevent tartar. Tartar is the hardened mineral deposits that are formed from plaque that is not removed. The accumulation of plaque and tartar may be the result of food impurities, malnutrition, vitamin deficiencies, endocrine disorders, certain medications, breathing through the mouth, poor dental hygiene, poor-fitting dentures, and inadequate access to dental care. The incidence of periodontal disease increases with age because of a reduction in saliva. Saliva aids in rinsing food particles from the teeth and gums and prevents plaque from forming.

There are early and late stages in periodontal disease. Gingivitis is the earliest and least-invasive stage; it involves only the gums surrounding the teeth. The major cause of gingivitis is poor dental hygiene. Gingivitis produces bleeding, tender gums. Periodontitis is a more severe stage of periodontal disease in which the gums recede and separate from the teeth and the bone depletes. If this condition is left untreated, the gums recede and bone depletes even further. Food becomes trapped in the pockets that form between the gums and teeth; the resulting infection causes the teeth to loosen and fall out.

Tobacco use also leads to periodontal disease, ulcerative gingivitis, tooth staining, delayed healing, and precancerous mouth tissue. Regular brushing of the teeth, gums, and tongue helps to fight periodontal disease.

Receding gums shrink away from the gum line and expose the root of the tooth, which is normally covered. Improper tooth brushing techniques, firm-bristle toothbrushes, and periodontal disease cause the gums to shrink away from the gum line. Once the gums shrink, they do not grow back, even when there is an improvement in tooth brushing techniques and soft-bristle toothbrushes are used. Exposing the root of the tooth increases the chances for periodontal disease.

Overgrowth of gum tissue (gingival hyperplasia) can result from irritation caused by plaque from poor dental hygiene or from physical or chemical irritant to the gums. Medications such as phenytoin and cyclosporine commonly cause gingival hyperplasia.

Dentures

Many older adults have the misconception that wearing dentures indicates that they no longer need to make regular visits to the dentist. This misconception causes many to experience dental problems that could be prevented. If identified in early stages of development, many dental problems are treatable or preventable. Denture wearers have 50 percent of the chewing and biting ability of those who have their natural teeth. Dentures that do not fit well can cause pain or discomfort that causes even more difficulty in chewing foods. Poor-fitting dentures may also cause speech problems because of the inability to enunciate words clearly. Poor-fitting dentures are an indication that a dentist visit is needed. Over time, the bone in the mouth that supports the dentures shrinks. Adjustments must be made to ensure that the denture fits properly and comfortably and to prevent additional dental problems.

—Sharon W. Stark

See also Aging; Cancer; Dental problems in children; Malnutrition among the elderly; Nutrition and aging.

For Further Information:
Academy of General Dentistry. *AGD Impact* 13 (August/September, 1998).
Epidemiology and Oral Disease Prevention Program. National Institute of Dental Research. *Oral Health of the United States Adults: The National Survey of Oral Health in U.S. Employed Adults and Seniors, 1985-1986—National Findings.* NIH Publication no. 87-2868. Bethesda, Md.: U.S. Department of Health and Human Services, Public Service, National Institutes of Health, 1987.
Little, James W., and Donald A. Falace, eds. *Dental Management of the Medically Compromised Patient.* 5th ed. St. Louis: Mosby Year Book, 1996.

✧ Depression

Type of issue: Mental health
Definition: The single most common psychiatric disorder, caused by biological and/or psychological factors; approximately 15 percent of cases result in suicide.

The term "depression" is used to describe a fleeting mood, an outward physical appearance of sadness, or a diagnosable clinical disorder. It is estimated that 13 million Americans suffer from a clinically diagnosed depression, a mood disorder that often affects personal, vocational, social, and health functioning. The *Diagnostic and Statistical Manual of Mental Disorders* (4th ed., 1994, DSM-IV) of the American Psychiatric Association delineates a number of mood disorders that subsume the various types of clinical depression.

Major Depressive Disorder

A major depressive episode is a syndrome of symptoms, present during a two-week period and representing a change from previous functioning. The symptoms include at least five of the following: depressed or irritable mood, diminished interest in previously pleasurable activities, significant weight loss or weight gain, insomnia or hypersomnia, physical excitation or slowness, loss of energy, feelings of worthlessness or guilt, indecisiveness or a diminished ability to concentrate, and recurrent thoughts of death. The clinical depression cannot be initiated or maintained by another illness or condition, and it cannot be a normal reaction to the death of a loved one (some symptoms of depression are a normal part of the grief reaction).

In major depressive disorder, the patient experiences a major depressive episode and does not have a history of mania or hypomania. Major depressive disorder is often first recognized in the patient's late twenties, while a major depressive episode can occur at any age, including infancy. Women are twice as likely to suffer from the disorder than are men.

There are several potential causes of major depressive disorder. Genetic studies suggest a familial link with higher rates of clinical depression in first-degree relatives. There also appears to be a relationship between clinical depression and levels of the brain's neurochemicals, specifically serotonin and norepinephrine. It is important to keep in mind, however, that 20 to 30 percent of adults will experience depression in their lifetime. Common causes of clinical depression include psychosocial stressors, such as the death of a loved one or the loss of a job, or any of a number of personal stressors; it is unclear why some people respond to a specific psychosocial stressor with a clinical depression and others do not. Finally, certain prescription medications have been noted to cause clinical depression. These drugs include muscle relaxants, heart medications, hypertensive medications, ulcer medications, oral contraceptives, and steroids. Thus there are many causes of clinical depression, and no single cause is sufficient to explain all clinical depressions.

BIPOLAR DISORDERS

Another category of depressive disorder is bipolar disorders, which affect approximately 1 to 2 percent of the population. Bipolar I disorder is characterized by one or more manic episodes along with persisting symptoms of depression. A manic episode is defined as a distinct period of abnormally and persistently elevated, expansive, or irritable mood. Three of the following symptoms must occur during the period of mood disturbance: inflated self-esteem, decreased need for sleep, unusual talkativeness or pressure to keep talking, racing thoughts, distractibility, excessive goal-oriented activities (especially in work, school, or social areas), and reckless activities with a high potential for negative consequences (such as buying sprees or risky business ventures). For a diagnosis of bipolar disorder, the symptoms must be sufficiently severe to cause impairment in functioning and/or concern regarding the person's danger to himself/herself or to others, must not be superimposed on another psychotic disorder, and must not be initiated or maintained by another illness or condition. Bipolar II disorder is characterized by a history of a major depressive episode and current symptoms of mania.

Patients with bipolar disorder will display cycles in which they experience a manic episode followed by a short episode of a major depressive episode, or vice versa. These cycles are often separated by a period of normal mood. Occasionally, two or more cycles can occur in a year without a period of remission between them, in what is referred to as rapid cycling. The two mood disorders can also occur simultaneously in a single episode. Bipolar disorder is often first recognized in adolescence or in the patient's early twenties; it is not unusual, however, for the initial recognition to occur later in life. Bipolar disorder is equally common in both males and females.

Genetic patterns are strongly involved in bipolar disorder. Brain chemicals (particularly dopamine, acetylcholine, GABA, and serotonin), hormones, drug reactions, and life stressors have all been linked to its development. Of particular interest are findings which suggest that, for some patients with bipolar disorder, changes in the seasons affect the frequency and severity of the disorder. These meteorological effects, while not well understood, have been observed in relation to other disorders of mood.

CYCLOTHYMIA AND DYSTHYMIA

Cyclothymia is another cyclic mood disorder related to depression; it has a reported lifetime prevalence of approximately 1 to 2 percent. This chronic mood disorder is characterized by manic symptoms without marked social or occupational impairment ("hypomanic" episodes) and symptoms of major depressive episode that do not meet the clinical criteria (less than five of the nine symptoms described above). These symptoms must be present for at least two years, and if the patient has periods without symptoms, these periods cannot be longer than two months. Cyclothymia cannot be superimposed on another psychotic disorder and cannot be initiated or maintained by another illness or condition. This mood disorder has its onset in adolescence and early adulthood and is equally common in men and women. It is a particularly persistent and chronic disorder with an identified familial pattern.

Dysthymia is another chronic mood disorder affecting approximately 2 to 4 percent of the population. Dysthymia is characterized by at least a two-year history of depressed mood and at least two of the following symptoms: poor appetite, insomnia or hypersomnia, low energy or fatigue, low self-esteem, poor concentration or decision making, or feelings of hopelessness. There cannot be evidence of a major depressive episode during the first two years of the dysthymia or a history of manic episodes or hypomanic episodes. The patient cannot be without the symptoms for more than two months at a time, the disorder cannot be superimposed on another psychotic disorder, and it cannot be initiated or maintained by another illness or condition. Dysthymia appears to begin at an earlier age, as young as childhood, with symptoms typically evident by young adulthood. Dysthymia is more common in adult females, equally common in both sexes of children, and with a greater prevalence in families. The causes of dysthymia are believed to be similar to those listed for major depressive disorder.

PHARMACOLOGICAL TREATMENTS

Once a clinical depression (or a subclinical depression) is identified, there are at least four general classes of treatment options available. These options are dependent on the subtype and severity of the depression and include psychopharmacology (drug therapy), individual and group psychotherapy, light therapy, family therapy, electroconvulsive therapy (ECT), and other less traditional treatments. These treatment options can be provided to the patient as part of an outpatient program or, in certain severe cases of clinical depression in which the person is a danger to himself/herself or others, as part of a hospitalization.

Three primary types of medications are used in the treatment of clinical depression: cyclic antidepressants, monoamine oxidase inhibitors (MAOIs), and lithium salts. These medications are considered equally effective in decreasing the symptoms of depression, which begin to resolve in three to four weeks after initiating treatment. The health care professional will select an antidepressant based on side effects, dosing convenience (once daily versus three times a day), and cost.

The cyclic antidepressants are the largest class of antidepressant medications. As the name implies, the chemical makeup of the medication contains chemical rings, or "cycles." There are unicyclic (buproprion and fluoxetine, or Prozac), bicyclic (sertraline and trazodone), tricyclic (amitriptyline, desipramine, and nortriptyline), and tetracyclic (maprotiline) antidepressants. These antidepressants function to either block the reuptake of neurotransmitters by the neurons, allowing more of the neurotransmitter to be available at a receptor site, or increase the amount of neurotransmitter produced. The side effects associated with the cyclic antidepressants—dry mouth, blurred vision, constipation, urinary difficulties, palpitations, and sleep disturbance—vary and can be quite problematic. Some of these antidepressants have deadly toxic effects at high levels, so they are not prescribed to patients who are at risk of suicide.

Monoamine oxidase inhibitors (isocarboxazid, phenelzine, and tranylcypromine) are the second class of antidepressants. They function by slowing the production of the enzyme monoamine oxidase. This enzyme is responsible for breaking down the neurotransmitters norepinephrine and serotonin, which are believed to be responsible for depression. By slowing the decomposition of these transmitters, more of them are available to the receptors for a longer period of time. Restlessness, dizziness, weight gain, insomnia, and sexual dysfunction are common side effects of the MAO inhibitors. MAO inhibitors are most notable because of the dangerous adverse reaction (severely high blood pressure) that can occur if the patient consumes large quantities of foods high in tyramine (such as aged cheeses, fermented sausages, red wine, foods with a heavy yeast content, and pickled fish). Because of this potentially dangerous reaction, MAO inhibitors are not usually the first choice of medication and are more commonly reserved for depressed patients who do not respond to the cyclic antidepressants.

A third class of medication used in the treatment of depressive disorders consists of the mood stabilizers, the most notable being lithium carbonate, which is used primarily for bipolar disorder. Lithium is a chemical salt that is believed to effect mood stabilization by influencing the production, storage, release, and reuptake of certain neurotransmitters. It is particularly useful in stabilizing and preventing manic episodes and preventing depressive episodes in patients with bipolar disorder.

Another drug occasionally used in the treatment of depression is alprazolam, a muscle relaxant benzodiazepine commonly used in the treatment of anxiety. Alprazolam is believed to affect the nervous system by decreasing the sensitivity of neuronal receptors believed to be involved in depression. While this may in fact occur, the more likely explanation for its positive effect for some patients is that it reduces the anxiety or irritability often coexisting with depression in certain patients.

Psychotherapy, Shock Therapy, and Psychosurgery

Psychotherapy refers to a number of different treatment techniques used to deal with the psychosocial contributors and consequences of clinical depression.

Psychotherapy is a common supplement to drug therapy. In psychotherapy, the patients develop knowledge and insight into the causes and treatment for their clinical depression. In cognitive psychotherapy, cure comes from assisting patients in modifying maladaptive, irrational, or automatic beliefs that can lead to clinical depression. In behavioral psychotherapy, patients modify their environment such that social or personal rewards are more forthcoming. This process might involve being more assertive, reducing isolation by becoming more socially active, increasing physical activities or exercise, or learning relaxation techniques. Research on the effectiveness of these and other psychotherapy techniques indicates that psychotherapy is as effective as certain antidepressants for many patients and, in combination with certain medications, is more effective than either treatment alone.

Electroconvulsive (or "shock") therapy is the single most effective treatment for severe and persistent depression. If the clinically depressed patient fails to respond to medications or psychotherapy and the depression is life-threatening, electroconvulsive therapy is considered. It is also considered if the patient cannot physically tolerate antidepressants, as with elders who have other medical conditions. This therapy involves inducing a seizure in the patient by administering an electrical current to specific parts of the brain. The therapy is quite sophisticated and safe, involving little risk to the patient. Patients undergo six to twelve treatments over a two-day to five-day period. Some temporary memory impairment is a common side effect of this treatment.

A variant of clinical depression is known as seasonal affective disorder (SAD). Patients with this illness demonstrate a pattern of clinical depression during the winter, when there is a reduction in the amount of daylight hours. For these patients, phototherapy has proven effective. Phototherapy, or light therapy, involves exposing patients to bright light (greater than or equal to 2,500 lux) for two hours daily during the depression episode. The manner in which this treatment approach modifies the depression is unclear and awaits further research.

Psychosurgery, the final treatment option, is quite rare. It refers to surgical removal or destruction of certain portions of the brain believed to be responsible for causing severe depression. Psychosurgery is used only after all treatment options have failed and the clinical depression is life-threatening. Approximately 50 percent of patients who undergo psychosurgery benefit from the procedure.

RATES AND RISKS OF DEPRESSION

The rates of clinical depression have increased since the early twentieth century, while the age of onset of clinical depression has decreased. Women appear to be at least twice as likely as men to suffer from clinical depression, and people who are happily married have a lower risk for clinical depression than those who are separated, divorced, or dissatisfied in their marital relationship. These data, along with recurrence rates of 50 to 70 percent, indicate the importance of this psychiatric disorder.

While most psychiatric disorders are nonfatal, clinical depression can lead to death. Of the approximately 30,000 suicide deaths per year in the United States, 40 to 80 percent are believed to be related to depression. Approximately 15 percent of patients with major depressive disorder will die by suicide. There are, however, other costs of clinical depression. In the United States, billions of dollars are spent on clinical depression, divided among the following areas: treatment, suicide, and absenteeism (the largest). Clinical depression obviously has a significant economic impact on a society.

—Oliver Oyama; updated by Nancy A. Piotrowski

See also Addiction; Alcoholism; Alcoholism among teenagers; Alcoholism among the elderly; Child abuse; Death and dying; Dementia; Depression in children; Depression in the elderly; Domestic violence; Drug use among teenagers; Eating disorders; Elder abuse; Light therapy; Postpartum depression; Seasonal affective disorder (SAD); Sleep disorders; Stress; Suicide;

Suicide among children and teenagers; Suicide among the elderly; Terminal illnesses.

For Further Information:

American Psychiatric Association. *Diagnostic and Statistical Manual of Mental Disorders: DSM-IV-TR.* Rev. 4th ed. Washington, D.C.: Author, 2000. This reference book lists the clinical criteria for psychiatric disorders, including the mood disorders that incorporate the depressions.

DePaulo, J. Raymond, Jr., and Keith R. Ablow. *How to Cope with Depression: A Complete Guide for You and Your Family.* New York: McGraw-Hill, 1989. Written for patients diagnosed with depression and for their families and friends. The authors use case histories of patients seen at The Johns Hopkins University Hospital to highlight their clinical information. Includes a nice section on bipolar (manic-depressive) disorder.

Greist, John H., and James W. Jefferson. *Depression and Its Treatment.* Rev. ed. Washington, D.C.: American Psychiatric Press, 1992. A patient's guide to depression. The authors describe mood disorders and the identification of depression, and they review the various treatments that are available. The appendices offer a listing of national organizations concerned with depression and an excellent reading list.

Matson, Johnny L. *Treating Depression in Children and Adolescents.* New York: Pergamon Press, 1989. This book, written by one of the leaders in the scientific study of depression, presents a guide to the evaluation and treatment of depression in children and adolescents. The author describes the assessment and treatment approaches that are unique for this nonadult population.

Roesch, Roberta. *The Encyclopedia of Depression.* 2d. Ed. New York: Facts on File, 2000. This volume was written for both a lay and a professional audience. Covers all aspects of depression, including bereavement, grief, and mourning. The appendices include references, self-help groups, national associations, and institutes.

✧ Depression in children

Type of issue: Children's health, mental health
Definition: A mood disorder in which children are unhappy, irritable, demoralized, self-derogatory, and bored.

Depressed children feel worthless and hopeless. They fail to enjoy their usual activities. They may be unpopular, withdrawn from normal social interactions, and either agitated or lethargic. They cry easily and eat and sleep poorly. Cognitively, they have poor concentration, slowed thinking, guilt, and recurrent thoughts of death or suicide. Their syndrome seriously impairs their well-being and everyday functioning.

Depression is not simply an immediate reaction to a recent event but a long-term syndrome that has lasted for some time. Many features of childhood depression match those of depression in adulthood, although the features of childhood depression are often mixed with a broader array of behaviors.

How Common Is Childhood Depression?

The prevalence of depression in childhood is controversial. Some experts believe that symptoms of depression are rare in infants and preschool children. Others, in contrast, believe that depression is quite common, perhaps affecting 2 percent of the general child population and 15 to 20 percent of youngsters referred to clinics. Recorded statistics, however, may be lower because childhood depression can be obscured by other complaints and because young children have trouble talking about feelings of despair. Most experts agree that depression probably occurs less frequently in early childhood than in adolescence, when feelings of hopelessness and low self-esteem, and the incidence of suicide attempts, increase sharply. Episodes of major depression usually end after seven to nine months, but they may recur.

Depression occurs at different rates for boys and girls. In childhood, depression is as common among boys as girls. In adolescence and adulthood, the ratio changes, with more girls and women reporting depression than boys and men. Children who have major depressive episodes sometimes experience no psychological problems as adults. Depressive disorders show the greatest continuity between childhood and adulthood when they first occur before puberty and are accompanied by other problems.

Several factors probably contribute to childhood depression. First, depression seems to have a genetic component. Children with depressed parents are more likely to become depressed themselves. Researchers have also identified possible biochemical markers (lower levels of neurotransmitters and unusual reactions to drugs) in depressed children and teenagers, as well as in depressed adults. Second, depression seems to have a social support component. Depressed children may lack familial support for their psychological needs or may be insecurely attached to their parents. Parents of depressed children are often less warm, more controlling, and more punitive than parents of normal children. Third, severe environmental stress may contribute to depression. Children who are depressed are more likely than nondepressed children to live in poverty, to experience school problems, to come into contact with the police, and to have parents with alcohol problems. Thus, in addition to a genetic vulnerability, depressed children have problems at home, at school, and in their neighborhoods.

TREATING DEPRESSION

A major problem in determining depression in children is the lack of practical, valid assessment instruments. Depression in adults is usually diagnosed from the sufferer's own description of the symptoms. Young children, however, may be unable to describe their own pessimism, sadness, sense of failure, or other unhappy feelings. One common self-report measure of depression in children is the Children's Depression Inventory, created by Maria Kovacs in 1992. It consists of twenty-seven items about depressive symptoms—for example, "I feel like crying every day," "I feel like crying many days," or "I feel like crying once in a while"—that describe the child's mood in the previous two weeks.

A warm, caring relationship with a parent or another adult acts as a protective factor against depression. Young adults who lost a parent before the age of sixteen experience more depression and suicide attempts than those adults who came from intact families. Consistent nurturance from another adult, however, can lessen these negative reactions.

—Lillian M. Range

See also Alcoholism among teenagers; Child abuse; Children's health issues; Drug abuse by teenagers; Suicide among children and teenagers.

FOR FURTHER INFORMATION:
Axline, Virginia Mae. *Dibs, in Search of Self: Personality Development in Play Therapy.* Boston: Houghton Mifflin, 1964. A case history of a withdrawn five-year-old boy and his struggle for identity through play therapy.
Kovacs, Maria. *The Children's Depression Inventory.* New York: Multi-Health Systems, 1992. A commonly used measure of depression in children.
Matson, Johnny L. *Treating Depression in Children and Adolescents.* New York: Pergamon Press, 1989. This book, written by one of the leaders in the scientific study of depression, presents a guide to the evaluation and treatment of depression in children and adolescents. The author describes the assessment and treatment approaches that are unique for this nonadult population.
Ollendick, Thomas H., and Michel Hersen, eds. *Handbook of Child Psychopathology.* 3d ed. New York: Plenum Press, 1998. In short, to-the-point chapters, this book covers all major topics from assessment to prevention and treatment. Most chapters about specific disorders end with a description of one case that illustrates the main points. Easy, interesting reading.
Walker, C. Eugene, and Michael C. Roberts, eds. *Handbook of Clinical Child Psychology.* 2d ed. New York: John Wiley & Sons, 1992. An excellent reference work on nearly every aspect of child disorders and therapies.

✦ DEPRESSION IN THE ELDERLY

Type of issue: Elder health, mental health
Definition: A morbid sadness, dejection, or melancholy; more generally, a loss of affect or functionality.

Community surveys have reported depressive symptoms in 30 percent to as many as 65 percent of people over the age of sixty. Depressions severe enough to warrant psychiatric intervention are generally estimated to affect 10 to 15 percent of the geriatric population, and depressive disorders are estimated to account for nearly one-half of the admissions of older adults to acute-care psychiatric hospitals in the United States.

DEMOGRAPHIC ASPECTS

Strong associations have been found between geriatric depression and a number of demographic variables. Many of these variables involve decreases or losses in social, physical, and financial resources. Geriatric depression has been found to increase as financial status, the quality of interpersonal relationships, and general health decreases. Additional factors frequently associated with geriatric depression include marital discord, marital separation or divorce, living alone, lack of children (childlessness), the lack of a confiding relationship, decreases in social support, deaths of relatives and friends, physical disabilities affecting employment, high levels of stress, physical pain, chronic medical conditions, and lower levels of attained education.

Considered together, these factors suggest that quality-of-life issues are crucial in understanding the onset, severity, and chronicity of geriatric depression. These factors do not cause geriatric depression per se but, in general, make the older individual much more vulnerable to its occurrence. On an individual basis, the effects of any one of these factors may be significantly mitigated by the attitude and psychological resources of a given individual. Specifically, greater overall coping with social, medical, and environmental stressors seems to be related to a given individual's overall mental health before the onset of the stressors. Those older individuals who manifest more extensive psychological strengths and a greater repertoire of social and interpersonal skills tend to succumb to stressors much less frequently than individuals with histories of poor coping or impaired social functioning.

PSYCHOLOGICAL ASPECTS

Susceptibility to geriatric depression has been linked to a number of psychological variables. Extensive research has focused on the areas of self-esteem, engagement in general life activities, and learned helplessness. Lowered self-esteem has been consistently associated with geriatric depression. Many elderly feel stigmatized or marginalized, especially after leaving positions of importance or prominence. The elderly in Western societies lack the high levels of respect and reverence shown toward the elderly of Eastern societies and many tribal cultures. Poor adjustment to retirement can often result in newly acquired feelings of inferiority or uselessness. Low self-esteem in elderly individuals has also been associated with overall poor coping following the death of a spouse. In addition to its association with geriatric depression, low self-esteem has been linked with greater levels of reported pain, lower levels of self-reported health, higher levels of physical disability, and increased anxiety.

Investigation into the relationship between geriatric depression and "engagement" has produced fairly consistent results. Engagement theory conceptualizes geriatric depression as resulting from an overall "disengagement" from general life activities, especially social activities, recreational activities, volunteer work, and meaningful interactions within the larger community. According to this theory, many older individuals "withdraw inside themselves," increasingly narrowing their personal worlds and levels of activity, eventually reaching a psychological state of stagnation and boredom resulting in depression. Depressed geriatric individuals do report a greater use of avoidance coping behaviors than their nondepressed peers. However, older individuals who engage in volunteer work have been found to manifest higher levels of life satisfaction, stronger desires to live, and overall fewer symptoms of anxiety and bodily complaints. In addition, nursing home residents who volunteer in a range of activities within their facilities have been found to manifest significant reductions in perceived hopelessness and depression. Overall, general activity and age-appropriate work appear to result in greater social contacts, reduced boredom, and increased sense of usefulness and satisfaction.

A theoretical framework that has been quite influential in explaining the cognitive, motivational, and psychological deficits associated with depression is the learned helplessness model proposed by Martin Seligman. According to this model, depression is often the result of a perceived condition of "independence" between one's actions and the results of one's actions. A "helpless" individual is one who increasingly sees aspects of life as uncontrollable. It is this very feature of uncontrollability that, over time, leads to the perception of personal helplessness; the perception of helplessness, in turn, leads to depression. A factor that has been thought to encourage perceptions of noncontrol and helplessness in the aged is the widespread stereotyping of this population as infirm and fragile. It has been found that nurses who view their aged patients as dependent reinforce helplessness and "sick role" behaviors. It has also been found that residents from private retirement homes who were given control of both the frequency and duration of the visits they received were consistently superior on measures of physical and psychological well-being to residents who had not been given this control.

MEDICAL ISSUES

Given the psychological, cultural, and medical issues frequently faced by the elderly, the phenomenon of depression is highly complicated and frequently not detected. Adding to this complication is the phenomenon of pseudodementia, in which an elderly individual is incorrectly evaluated as manifesting severe cognitive impairments while the true diagnosis of depression is missed.

The relatively extensive number of medical issues faced by the elderly often focuses the attention of medical professionals and the elderly themselves on bodily and pain-oriented complaints. What is often missed is a coexisting depression that preceded the onset of medical issues or occurred during the onset of medical issues but is unrelated to medical issues; a coexisting depression that is the elderly individual's reaction to medical issues; or both. Nondetection of geriatric depression may also result from the hesitation of many elderly individuals to discuss psychological or emotional issues. The stigma sometimes associated with psychological issues is often a forceful factor in the elderly individual's tendency to minimize them in favor of a wholly medical or pain-oriented presentation of symptoms. A medical or mental health professional who accepts this presentation without inquiring about issues related to emotional well-being may fail to uncover a coexisting depression underlying medical issues or even a depression unaccompanied by true medical difficulties.

Another phenomenon involving the nondetection of geriatric depression is pseudodementia, in which the elderly individual is diagnosed as manifesting significant deficits in memory and intellectual processing typical of true dementia victims. This misdiagnosis can result from the unrecognized fact that depressions of all kinds, affecting individuals of all age groups, typically involve temporary deficits in memory processing, concentration, and general intellectual functioning; the fact that temporary deficits in memory and cognitive functioning are often brought on by prescriptions of drug dosages beyond the delicate physiological needs of the elderly; or the inaccurate assumption that severe memory and intellectual deficits are a normal part of aging.

—John Monopoli

See also Aging; Alcoholism among the elderly; Death and dying; Dementia; Depression; Depression in children; Disabilities; Light therapy; Medications and the elderly; Memory loss; Overmedication; Stress; Suicide among the elderly; Terminal illnesses.

FOR FURTHER INFORMATION:

Billig, Nathan. *To Be Old and Sad: Understanding Depression in the Elderly.* Lexington, Mass.: Lexington Books, 1987.

Birren, James E., R. Bruce Sloane, and Gene D. Cohen, eds. *Handbook of Mental Health and Aging.* 2d ed. San Diego: Academic Press, 1992.

Brink, Terry L. *Clinical Gerontology: A Guide to Assessment and Intervention.* New York: Haworth Press, 1986.

Gallagher, Dolores, and Larry W. Thompson. *Depression in the Elderly: A Behavioral Treatment Manual.* Los Angeles: University of Southern California, Ethel Percy Andrus Gerontology Center, 1981.

Knight, Bob G. *Psychotherapy with Older Adults.* Thousand Oaks, Calif.: Sage Publications, 1996.

✧ DIABETES MELLITUS

Type of issue: Public health, social trends

Definition: A hormonal disorder in which the pancreas is not able to produce sufficient insulin to process and maintain proper blood sugar levels; if left untreated, it leads to secondary complications such as blindness, dementia, and eventually death.

Diabetes mellitus is by far the most common of all endocrine (hormonal) disorders. The disease has been depicted as a state of starvation in the midst of plenty. Although there is plenty of sugar in the blood, without insulin it does not reach the cells that need it for energy. Glucose, the simplest form of sugar, is the primary source of energy for many vital functions. Deprived of glucose, cells starve and tissues begin to degenerate. The unused glucose builds up in the bloodstream, which leads to a series of secondary complications.

EFFECTS OF INSULIN INSUFFICIENCY

The acute symptoms of diabetes mellitus are all attributable to inadequate insulin action. The immediate consequence of an insulin insufficiency is a marked decrease in the ability of both muscle and adipose (fat) tissue to remove glucose from the blood. In the presence of inadequate insulin action, a second problem manifests itself. People with diabetes continue to make the hormone glucagon. Glucagon, which raises the level of blood sugar, can be considered insulin's biological opposite. Like insulin, glucagon is released from the pancreatic islets. The release of glucagon is normally inhibited by insulin; therefore, in the absence of insulin, glucagon action elevates concentrations of glucose. For this reason, diabetes may be considered a "two-hormone disease." With a reduction in the conversion of glucose into its storage forms of glycogen in liver and muscle and lipids in adipose cells, concentrations of glucose in the blood steadily increase (hyperglycemia). When the amount of glucose in the blood exceeds the capacity of the kidney to reabsorb this nutrient, glucose begins to spill into the urine (glucosuria). Glucose in the urine then drags additional body water along with it so that the volume of urine dramatically increases. In the absence of adequate fluid intake, the loss of body water and accompanying electrolytes (sodium) leads to dehydration and, ultimately, death caused by the failure of the peripheral circulatory system.

Insulin deficiency also results in a decrease in the synthesis of triglycerides (storage forms of fatty acids) and stimulates the breakdown of fats in adipose tissue. Although glucose cannot enter the cells and be used as an energy source, the body can use its supply of lipids from the fat cells as an alternate source of energy. Fatty acids increase in the blood, causing hyperlipidemia. With large amounts of circulating free fatty acids available for processing by the liver, the production and release of ketone bodies (breakdown products of fatty acids) into the circulation are accelerated, causing both ketonemia and an increase in the acidity of the blood. Since the ketone levels soon also exceed the capacity of the kidney to reabsorb them, ketone bodies soon appear in the urine (ketonuria).

Insulin deficiency and glucagon excess also cause pronounced effects on protein metabolism and result in an overall increase in the breakdown of proteins and a reduction in the uptake of amino acid precursors into muscle protein. This leads to the wasting and weakening of skeletal muscles and, in children who are diabetics, results in a reduction in overall growth. Unfortunately, the increased level of amino acids in the blood provides an additional source of material for glucose production (gluconeogenesis) by the liver. All these acute metabolic changes in carbohydrates, lipids, and protein metabolism can be prevented or reversed by the administration of insulin.

TYPES OF DIABETES

There are two distinct types of diabetes mellitus. Type I, or insulin-dependent diabetes mellitus (IDDM), is an absolute deficiency of insulin that accounts for approximately 10 percent of all cases of diabetes. Until the discovery of insulin, people stricken with Type I diabetes faced certain death within about a year of diagnosis. In Type II or non-insulin-dependent diabetes mellitus (NIDDM), insulin secretion may be normal or even increased, but the target cells for insulin are less responsive than normal (insulin resistance); therefore, insulin is not as effective in lowering blood glucose concentrations. Although either type can be manifested at any age, Type I diabetes has a greater prevalence in children, whereas the incidence of Type II diabetes increases markedly after the age of forty and is the most common type of diabetes. Genetic and environmental factors are important in the expression of both types of diabetes mellitus.

Type I diabetes is an autoimmune process that involves the selective destruction of the insulin-producing beta cells in the islets of Langerhans (insulitis). The triggering event that initiates this process in genetically susceptible persons may be a virus or, more likely, the presence of toxins in the diet. The body's own T lymphocytes progressively attack the beta cells but leave the other hormone-producing cell types intact. T lymphocytes are white blood cells that normally attack virus-invaded cells and cancer cells. For up to ten years, there remains a sufficient number of insulin-producing cells to respond effectively to a glucose load, but when approximately 80 percent of the beta cells are destroyed, there is insufficient insulin release in response to a meal and the deadly spiral of the consequences of diabetes mellitus is triggered. Insulin injection can halt this lethal process and prevent it from recurring but cannot mimic the normal pattern of insulin release from the pancreas. It is interesting that not everyone who has insulitis actually progresses to experience overt symptoms of the disease, although it is known that the incidence of Type I diabetes around the world is on the increase.

Type II diabetes is normally associated with obesity and lack of exercise as well as with genetic predisposition. Family studies have shown that as many as 25 to 35 percent of persons with Type II diabetes have a sibling or parent with the disease. The risk of diabetes doubles if both parents are affected. Because there is a reduction in the sensitivity of the target cells to insulin, people with Type II diabetes must secrete more insulin to maintain blood glucose at normal levels. Because insulin is a storage, or anabolic, hormone, this increased secretion further contributes to obesity. In response to the elevated insulin concentrations, the number of insulin receptors on the target cell gradually decreases, which triggers an even greater secretion of insulin. In this way, the excess glucose is stored despite the decreased availability of insulin binding sites on the cell. Over time, the demands for insulin eventually exceed even the reserve capacity of the "genetically weakened" beta cells, and symptoms of insulin deficiency develop as the plasma glucose concentrations remain high for increasingly larger periods of time. Because the symptoms of Type II diabetes are usually less severe than those of Type I diabetes, many persons have the disease but remain unaware of it. Unfortunately, once the diagnosis of diabetes is made in these individuals, they also exhibit symptoms of long-term complications that include atherosclerosis and nerve damage. Hence, Type II diabetes has been called the "silent killer."

Insulin Treatments for Type I Diabetes

Insulin is the only treatment available for Type I diabetes, and in many cases it is used to treat individuals with Type II diabetes. Insulin is available in many formulations, which differ in respect to the time of onset of action, activity, and duration of action. Insulin preparations are classified as fast-acting, intermediate-acting, and long-acting; the effects of fast-acting insulin last for thirty minutes to twenty-four hours, while those of long-acting preparations last from four to thirty-six hours. Some of the factors that affect the rate of insulin absorption include the site of injection, the patient's age and health status, and the patient's level of physical activity. For a person with diabetes, however, insulin is a reprieve, not a cure.

Because of the complications that arise from chronic exposure to glucose, it is recommended that glucose concentrations in the blood be maintained as close to physiologically normal levels as possible. For this reason, it is preferable to administer multiple doses of insulin during the day. By monitoring plasma glucose concentrations, the diabetic person can adjust the dosage of insulin administered and thus mimic normal concentrations of glucose relatively closely. Basal concentrations of plasma insulin can also be maintained throughout the day by means of electromechanical insulin delivery systems. Whether internal or external, such insulin pumps can be programmed to deliver a constant infusion of insulin at a rate designed to meet minimum requirements. The infusion can then be supplemented by a bolus injection prior to a meal. Increasingly sophisticated systems automatically monitor blood glucose concentrations and adjust the delivery rate of insulin accordingly. These alternative delivery systems are intended to prevent the development of long-term tissue complications.

COMPLICATIONS OF DIABETES

A number of chronic complications account for the shorter life expectancy of diabetics, including atherosclerotic changes throughout the entire vascular system. The thickening of basement membranes that surround the capillaries can affect their ability to exchange nutrients. Cardiovascular lesions are the most common cause of premature death in diabetic persons. Kidney disease, which is commonly found in longtime diabetics, can ultimately lead to kidney failure. For these persons, expensive medical care, including dialysis and the possibility of a kidney transplant, overshadows their lives. Diabetes is the leading cause of new blindness in the United States. In addition, diabetes leads to a gradual decline in the ability of nerves to conduct sensory information to the brain. For example, the feet of some diabetics feel more like stumps of wood than living tissue. Consequently, weight is not distributed properly; in concert with the reduction in blood flow, this problem can lead to pressure ulcers. If not properly cared for, areas of the foot can develop gangrene, which may then lead to amputation of the foot. Finally, in male patients, there are problems with reproductive function that generally result in impotence.

The mechanism responsible for the development of these long-term complications of diabetes is genetic in origin and dependent on the amount of time the tissues are exposed to the elevated plasma glucose concentrations. As an animal ages, most of its cells become less efficient in replacing damaged material, while its tissues lose their elasticity and gradually stiffen. For example, the lungs and heart muscle expand less successfully, blood vessels become increasingly rigid, and ligaments tighten. These apparently diverse age-related changes are accelerated in diabetes, and the causative agent is glucose. Glucose becomes chemically attached to proteins and deoxyribonucleic acid (DNA) in the body without the aid of enzymes to speed the reaction along. What is important is the duration of exposure to the elevated glucose concentrations. Once glucose is bound to tissue proteins, a series of chemical reactions is triggered that, over the passage of months and years, can result in the formation and eventual accumulation of cross-links between adjacent proteins. The higher glucose concentrations in diabetics accelerate this process, and the effects become evident in specific tissues throughout the body.

Understanding the chemical basis of protein cross-linking in diabetes has permitted the development and study of compounds that can intervene in this process. Certain compounds, when added to the diet, can limit the glucose-induced cross-linking of proteins by preventing their formation. One of the best-studied compounds, aminoguanidine, can help prevent the cross-linking of collagen; this fact is shown in a decrease in the accumulation of trapped lipoproteins on artery walls. Aminoguanidine also prevents thickening of the capillary basement membrane in the kidney. Aminoguanidine acts by blocking glucose's ability to react with neighboring proteins. Vitamins C and B_6 are also effective in reducing cross-linking.

Alternatively, transplantation of the entire pancreas is an effective means of achieving an insulin-independent state in persons with Type I diabetes mellitus. Both the technical problems of pancreas transplantation and the possible rejection of the foreign tissue, however, have limited this procedure as a treatment for diabetes. Diabetes is usually manageable; therefore, a pancreas transplant is not necessarily lifesaving. Some limited success in treating diabetes has been achieved by transplanting only the insulin–producing islet cells from the pancreas or grafts from fetal pancreas tissue. It may one day be possible to use genetic engineering to permit cells of the liver to self-regulate glucose concentrations by synthesizing and releasing their own insulin into the blood.

CONTROLLING TYPE II DIABETES

Some of the less severe forms of Type II diabetes mellitus can be controlled by the use of oral hypoglycemic agents that bring about a reduction in blood glucose. These drugs can be taken orally to drive the beta cells to release even more insulin than usual. These drugs also increase the ability of insulin to act on the target cells, which ultimately reduces the insulin requirement. The use of these agents remains controversial, because they overwork the already strained beta cells. If a diabetic person is reliant on these drugs for extended periods of time, the insulin cells could "burn out" and completely lose their ability to synthesize insulin. In this situation, the previously non-insulin-dependent person would have to be placed on insulin therapy for life.

If obesity is a factor in the expression of Type II diabetes, the best therapy is a combination of a reduction of calorie intake and an increase in activity. More than any other disease, Type II diabetes is related to lifestyle. It is often the case that people prefer having an injection or taking a pill to improving their quality of life by changing their diet and level of activity. Attention to diet and exercise results in a dramatic decrease in the need for drug therapy in nine out of ten diabetics. In some cases, the loss of only a small percentage of body weight results in an increased sensitivity to insulin. Exercise is particularly helpful in the management of both types of diabetes, because working muscle does not require insulin to metabolize glucose. Thus, exercising muscles take up and use some of the excess glucose in the blood, which reduces the overall need for insulin. Permanent weight reduction and exercise also help to prevent long-term complications and permit a healthier and more active lifestyle.

Research into a Cure

Although insulin, when combined with an appropriate diet and exercise, alleviates the symptoms of diabetes to such an extent that a diabetic can lead an essentially normal life, insulin therapy is not a cure. The complications that arise in diabetics are typical of those found in the general population except that they happen much earlier in the diabetic.

In the mid-1970's, Anthony Cerami introduced the concept of the nonenzymatic attachment of glucose to protein and recognized its potential role in diabetic complications. A decade later, this development led to the discovery of aminoguanidine, the first compound to limit the cross-linking of tissue proteins and thus delay the development of certain diabetic complications.

In 1974, Josiah Brown published the first report showing that diabetes could be reversed by transplanting fetal pancreatic tissue. By the mid-1980's, procedures had been devised for the isolation of massive numbers of human islets that could then be transplanted into diabetics. For persons with diabetes, both procedures represent more than a treatment; they may offer a cure for the disease.

—Hillar Klandorf

See also Childbirth complications; Exercise; Exercise and children; Exercise and the elderly; Genetic diseases; Obesity; Obesity and aging; Obesity and children; Prenatal care; Screening; Sexual dysfunction; Transplantation; Yeast infections.

FOR FURTHER INFORMATION:

Biermann, June, and Barbara Toohey. *The Diabetic's Book*. 4th ed. New York: G. P. Putnam's Sons, 1998. This extremely helpful book deals with both Type I and Type II diabetes. It is filled with useful information to help patients live a more healthful and satisfying life and contains answers to 130 frequently asked questions about the disease, including lifestyle, diet, and therapy.

Cerami, Anthony, Helen Vlassara, and Michael Browlee. "Glucose and Aging." *Scientific American* 256 (May, 1987): 90-96. A pioneering article written by experts in the field of diabetic complications. This important work clearly explains the development of cross-linking in the tissues and challenges the reader with new approaches to treating a very old problem. Contains excellent figures and diagrams of the processes involved.

Jovanovic-Peterson, Lois, Charles M. Peterson, and Morton B. Stori. *A Touch of Diabetes*. Minneapolis: Chronimed, 1995. A straightforward guide for people with Type II diabetes. Provides useful information on the disease and suggestions of how to change eating habits and monitor one's lifestyle.

Krall, Leo P., and Richard S. Beaser. *Joslin Diabetes Manual*. 12th ed. Philadelphia: Lea & Febiger, 1989. First published in 1918, this book serves as a guide for people with diabetes. Its intent is to help diabetics understand the disease and permit them to take control of their lives.

Powers, Margaret A., ed. *Handbook of Diabetes Medical Nutrition Therapy*. Rev. ed. Gaithersburg, Md.: Aspen, 1996. A comprehensive book written by dietitians for persons interested in the nutritional treatment of diabetes; blends new scientific knowledge and thought with recent advances in clinical practice.

✧ DISABILITIES

Type of issue: Economic issues, mental health, occupational health, social trends

Definition: Physical or mental impairments that substantially limit major life activities.

Persons with physical disabilities have the ability and the legal right to participate fully in family and community life, but this requires that everyone make special accommodations for their unique needs

In the United States, disability is legally defined as any physical or mental impairment that substantially limits one or more of a person's major life activities. Temporary impairment due to an illness or injury from which the person can completely recover are not considered to be disabilities. Employment, education, use of public facilities, parenting, and social contact are all major life activities that can be limited by physical disabilities unless disabled persons, families, and communities work together to remove barriers in the way of full participation. The challenges faced by persons with disabilities affect everyone not only by law, but also because of the large numbers of disabled persons. One in six Americans has a disability, and one in eight has a physical disability. Almost every nuclear or extended family in America has at least one member who is or will be affected by a disability at some point during the life span.

TYPES OF PHYSICAL DISABILITIES

There are four types of physical disabilities. The first is impairment in the sensory system (vision and hearing). The most common type of all physical disabilities is hearing impairment, which affected 22 million Americans by the late twentieth century. Hearing impairment ranges in severity from complete lack of sound perception to loss of only a portion of normal hearing. Vision impairment is less common than hearing impairment. The majority of vision-impaired persons are totally blind—that is, they have no functional sight. Legally blind persons have some sight but are limited in some life activities because of their limited acuity of vision (clarity and sharpness) or field of vision (the amount of area the eye can see at one time). Many people with sensory impairments can achieve nearly normal perception with the help of hearing aids, glasses, or surgery. Even though a disability can be completely compensated for, persons are still regarded as having a disability if they need continuing medical assistance to be able to fully engage in major life activities.

The second type of physical disability is impairment of a person's ability to move or control the body. This can include loss of control over involuntary functions such as bowel, bladder, breathing, or sexual activity. Persons with motor impairments may have difficulty eating or speaking. Most people with motor impairments use some type of equipment to help them move around, including wheelchairs, canes, walkers, and orthotic devices that keep paralyzed or spastic body parts in correct alignment. The most severe motor impairments include paraplegia, or paralysis in the legs and lower body, and quadriplegia, or paralysis in the upper and lower body. The majority of motor impairments affect only some body parts and functions, leaving others completely healthy. For example, a person with paraplegia due to spinal cord damage may have no sensation or movement in the legs, but may have bowel and bladder control and normal sexual functioning. Most people with motor impairments have the same cognitive ability as others, although individuals with severe mental retardation often have both sensory and motor impairments.

The third type of physical disability is disfigurement of one or more body parts. Even if disfigurements do not cause motor or sensory impairments, they can contribute to social isolation or loss of self-esteem, presenting a barrier to many major life activities.

The fourth type of physical disability includes chronic, incurable illnesses that interfere with major life activities. Such illnesses may include epilepsy, diabetes, human immunodeficiency virus (HIV) infection, autoimmune diseases such as multiple sclerosis (which affects the nervous system) or lupus erythematosus (which can affect all body tissues), and severe respiratory problems such as asthma or emphysema. These are only considered to be disabilities if they are severe enough to interfere with daily activities.

CAUSES OF PHYSICAL DISABILITIES

There are three causes of physical disabilities, each of which presents families with unique challenges. The first is congenital or developmental problems. Congenital problems are present at birth and have many sources. Some congenital problems are inherited, as is true of some types of cataracts that result in blindness and some forms of hearing impairments. Others may be the result of prenatal exposure to toxic substances, drugs, or a disease such as German measles. Congenital problems can also be the result of random genetic accidents that are not inherited and can affect anyone, such as Down syndrome. Problems during pregnancy and childbirth, including anoxia (lack of oxygen) and illnesses contracted by expectant mothers can also create problems that lead to disabilities. Some problems start before birth, but are not apparent at birth. These often result in disabilities later in life as children grow and are called developmental problems because they appear during childhood. Many conditions that affect motor control, speech, and eating are only discovered when children fail to develop these abilities at the same time as other children of the same age.

The second cause of physical disabilities is accidental injury. Such disabilities affect adolescents and young adults more than any other group. The leading cause of motor disabilities is head injuries, which most often occur in bicycle or automobile accidents. Automobile accidents are also responsible for most cases of spinal cord injuries that result in paralysis.

The third cause of physical disabilities is physical deterioration and illnesses that sometimes accompany aging. Persons who have been healthy and unimpaired all their lives can become disabled by strokes, arthritis, chronic illnesses, and chronic pain.

FAMILY ISSUES

No two individuals with a physical disability, even the same disability, are alike. No two families will face the same challenges and experiences in dealing with disabilities. How families cope and the types of support they need depend on the types of disabilities, the causes of the disabilities, and families' strengths and vulnerabilities.

Disabilities that require a great deal of physical assistance are the most time-consuming for family members, who may take time away from work and education to care for disabled persons. There are some sources of funding in the United States and Canada for in-home help, ranging from caregiving for an evening to live-in aides. Family members with the most severe motor disabilities still require a great deal of family time and planning, even with such assistance.

The causes of disabilities present different challenges to every family. Parents of children with congenital or developmental problems may blame themselves for their children's impairments. This natural tendency toward self-blame is aggravated by the difficulty, present in most cases, of identifying the problem and finding appropriate treatment and support, a process which can take many years. Parents also face the financial and emotional responsibility of providing for children who may need assistance well into adulthood. When adolescents or adults are suddenly disabled by illness or injury, the issues are different but no less difficult. Persons who have been disabled by head injuries or strokes or who take medication to control pain may undergo personality changes in addition to suffering from their physical disability. Many people who become disabled later in life feel depressed and angry for a time after being injured, which can put a strain on family relationships. Like developmental problems, it can take many years to diagnose and treat chronic illnesses, leaving families on a roller coaster of hope and disappointment.

The strongest factor contributing to family member satisfaction and the disabled person's sense of fulfillment is not the cause or type of disability, as challenging as this may be. Nor is it the family's financial status, education, or the number of family members, all of which can affect the amount of effort each member must devote to the care of the disabled. The strongest factor is the emotional climate before onset of the disability. Families in which communication has been good, the emotional climate has been positive, and family members' needs have been met before the onset of disability are best able to cope when a disability occurs. This does not mean that emotionally strong families do not experience the self-blame, depression, and anger that normally accompany adjusting to a disability. Nor does it mean that families who faced emotional problems before the onset of disability will be unable to cope. It does mean that all family members must learn to communicate and meet each others' emotional needs in order to cope with the disability when it arises.

How Families Cope with Disabilities

Many families who are faced with the challenges of disability have a strong desire to help the disabled person. Sometimes one or more family members devote all their energy and attention to the disabled person. This is a pattern of coping that does not work well either for the disabled person or for the family. Disabled children who receive too much help, attention, and pity may find it difficult to become as independent as they can be. Adults who suddenly become disabled often do not want help or extra attention; most such adults want life and family relationships to return to normal. Family members who devote all their energies to disabled relatives may feel either depleted of energy and feeling or neglected and angry.

There are ways of coping with disabilities that help disabled persons as well as their families. First, every member of the family should feel free to discuss their caregiving responsibilities, feelings, and needs openly. Second, responsibilities should be divided as equitably as possible, allowing all family members to pursue their own lives. Third, families should seek as much help as they can get—financial, practical, and emotional. Fourth, nondisabled family members can find ways to value and enjoy the company of their disabled relatives as they are, while encouraging them to pursue their own goals and achieve independence. Finally, and most important, disabled persons should be active parts of their families' coping processes; they should be included in any decisions that affect them or the family. By recognizing disabled persons' right to be contributing members of the family, families help the disabled to see themselves as fully capable, independent, and valuable persons.

Full Inclusion

For the first time in North American history, government programs and disability rights legislation have shown communities how to take responsibility for protecting and accommodating the needs of persons with disabilities. In the 1990's, 26 percent of disabled adults were fully employed. Every public school classroom included children with disabilities, and every college campus enrolled students with disabilities. Persons with disabilities, once segregated and kept out of sight, were involved in every aspect of community, social, and family life. As medical care has improved and people live longer, a result of the fact that once-fatal injuries have become only disabling, the number of families affected by disability may increase. The sharing of responsibility between families and communities may help families to cope with disability. Furthermore, research has shown that the inclusion of disabled persons in family and community life has persuaded more persons to believe that they can lead meaningful, productive lives—with or without a disability.

—*Kathleen M. Zanolli*

See also AIDS; AIDS and children; AIDS and women; Alzheimer's disease; Autism; Birth defects; Chronic fatigue syndrome; Cleft lip and palate; Down syndrome; Dyslexia; Fetal alcohol syndrome; Foot disorders; Genetic counseling; Genetic diseases; Learning disabilities; Macular degeneration; Mental retardation; Mobility problems in the elderly; Parkinson's disease; Physical rehabilitation; Safety issues for children; Safety issues for the elderly; Speech disorders; Spina bifida; Strokes.

FOR FURTHER INFORMATION:

Albrecht, Donna G. *Raising a Child Who Has a Physical Disability.* New York: John Wiley & Sons, 1995. Written by a parent of two children with physical disabilities, this book explains how to find funding, set up a support network, navigate the medical and educational system, and how to cope with guilt and stress.

Kissane, Sharon. *Career Success for People with Physical Disabilities.* Lincolnwood, Ill.: VGM Career Horizons, 1997. Provides many strategies for persons with disabilities in selecting, training for, finding, and keeping employment.

LaPlante, Mitchell P. *Families with Disabilities in the United States.* Washington, D.C.: U.S. Department of Education, 1996. Describes in detail the facts of disability and its effect on families, with national, regional, and state breakdowns as well as descriptions of model programs for persons with disabilities.

Sullivan, Tom. *Special Parent, Special Child.* New York: Putnam, 1995. Written by a visually impaired person from a unique and interesting perspective, this book relates the stories of families dealing with children's disabilities.

Tracey, William R. *Training Employees with Disabilities.* New York: Amacom, 1995. Detailed description of the legal, ethical, and training issues involved in hiring and managing persons with disabilities, pointing out that by the year 2000 the majority of the workforce, including persons with disabilities, will be protected by civil rights legislation.

✧ DOMESTIC VIOLENCE

Type of issue: Children's health, elder health, ethics, mental health, social trends, women's health

Definition: Assaultive behavior intended to punish, dominate, or control another in an intimate family relationship; physicians are often best able to identify situations of domestic violence and assist victims to implement preventive interventions.

Domestic or family violence is the intentional use of violence against an intimate partner. The purpose of the violence is to assert domination, to control the victim's actions, or to punish the victim for some actions. Family violence generally occurs as a pattern of behavior over time rather than as a single, isolated act.

Common Traits of All Domestic Abuse

Forms of family violence include child physical abuse, child sexual abuse, spousal or partner abuse, and elder abuse. These forms of violence are related, in that they occur within the context of the family unit. Therefore, the victims and perpetrators know one another, are related to one another, may live together, and may love one another. These various forms of violence also differ insofar as victims may be children, adults, or frail, elderly adults. The needs of victims differ with age and independence, but there are also many similarities between the different types of violence.

One such similarity is the relationship between the offender and the victim. Specifically, victims of abuse are always less powerful than abusers. Power includes the ability to exert physical and psychological control over situations. For example, a child abuser has the ability to lock a child in a bathroom or to abandon him or her in a remote area in order to control access to authorities. A spouse abuser has the ability to physically injure a spouse, disconnect the phone, and keep the victim from leaving for help. An elder abuser can exert similar control. Such differences in power between victims and offenders are seen as a primary cause of abuse; that is, people batter others because they can.

Families that are violent are often isolated. The members usually keep to themselves and have few or no friends or relatives with whom they are involved, even if they live in a city. This social isolation prevents victims from seeking help from others and allows the abuser to establish rules for the relationship without answering to anyone for these actions. Abuse continues and worsens because the violence occurs in private, with few consequences for the abuser.

Victims of all forms of family violence share common experiences. In addition to physical violence, victims are also attacked psychologically, being told they are worthless and responsible for the abuse that they receive. Because they are socially isolated, victims do not have an opportunity to take social roles where they can experience success, recognition, or love. As a result, victims often have low self-esteem and truly believe that they cause the violence. Without the experience of being worthwhile, victims often become severely depressed and anxious, and they experience more stress-related illnesses such as headaches, fatigue, or gastrointestinal problems.

Inherited Abuse

Child and partner abuse are linked in several ways. About half of the men who batter their wives also batter their children. Further, women who are battered are more likely to abuse their children than are nonbattered women. Even if a child of a spouse-abusing father is not battered, living in a violent home and observing the father's violence has negative effects. Such children often experience low self-esteem, aggression toward other children, and school problems. Moreover, abused children are more likely to commit violent offenses as adults. Children, especially males, who have observed violence between parents are at increased risk of assaulting their partners as adults. Adult sexual offenders have an increased likelihood of having been sexually abused as children.

Yet, while these and other problems are reported more frequently by adults who were abused as children than by adults who were not, many former victims do not become violent. The most common outcomes of childhood abuse in adults are emotional problems. Although much less is known about the relationship between child abuse and future elder abuse, many elder abusers did suffer abuse as children. While most people who have been abused do not themselves become abusers, this intergenerational effect remains a cause for concern.

PATTERNS OF ABUSE AND CYCLES OF VIOLENCE

Family violence typically consists of a pattern of behavior occurring over time and involving both hands-on and hands-off violence. Hands-on violence consists of direct attacks against the victim's body. Such acts range from pushing, shoving, and restraining to slapping, punching, kicking, clubbing, choking, burning, stabbing, or shooting. Hands-on violence also includes sexual assault, ranging from forced fondling of breasts, buttocks, and genitals; to forced touching of the abuser; to forced intercourse with the abuser or with other people.

Hands-off violence includes physical violence that is not directed at the victim's body but is intended to display destructive power and assert domination and control. Examples include breaking through windows or locked doors, punching holes through walls, smashing objects, destroying personal property, and harming or killing pet animals. The victim is often blamed for this destruction and forced to clean up the mess. Hands-off violence also includes psychological control, coercion, and terror. This includes name calling, threats of violence or abandonment, gestures suggesting the possibility of violence, monitoring of the victim's whereabouts, controlling of resources (such as money, transportation, and property), forced viewing of pornography, sexual exposure, or threatening to contest child custody. These psychological tactics may occur simultaneously with physical assaults or may occur separately. Whatever the pattern of psychological and physical tactics, abusers exert extreme control over their partners.

Neglect—the failure of one person to provide for the basic needs of another dependent person—is another form of hands-off abuse. Neglect may involve failure to provide food, clothing, health care, and shelter. Children, older adults, and developmentally delayed or physically handicapped people are particularly vulnerable to neglect.

Family violence differs in two respects from violence directed at strangers. First, the offender and victim are related and may love each other, live together, share property, have children, and share friends and relatives. Hence, unlike victims of stranger violence, victims of family violence cannot quickly or easily sever ties with or avoid seeing their assailants. Second, family violence often increases slowly in intensity, progressing until victims feel immobilized, unworthy, and responsible for the violence that is directed toward them. Victims may also feel substantial and well-grounded fear about leaving their abusers or seeking legal help, because they have been threatened or assaulted in the past and may encounter significant difficulty obtaining help to escape. In the case of children, the frail and elderly, or people with disabilities, dependency upon the caregiver and cognitive limitations make escape from an abuser difficult. Remaining in the relationship increases the risk of continued victimization. Understanding this unique context of the violent family can help physicians and other health care providers understand why battered victims often have difficulty admitting abuse or leaving the abuser.

Family violence follows a characteristic cycle that begins with escalating tension and anger in the abuser. Victims describe a feeling of "walking on eggs." Next comes an outburst of violence. Outbursts of violence sometimes coincide with episodes of alcohol and drug abuse. Following the outburst, the abuser may feel remorse and expect forgiveness. The abuser often demands reconciliation, including sexual interaction. After a period of calm, the abuser again becomes increasingly tense and angry. This cycle generally repeats, with violence becoming increasingly severe. In partner abuse, victims are at greatest risk when there is a transition in the relationship such as pregnancy, divorce, or separation. In the case of elder abuse, risk increases as the elder becomes increasingly dependent on the primary caregiver, who may be inexperienced or unwilling to provide needed assistance. Without active intervention, the abuser rarely stops spontaneously and often becomes more violent.

IDENTIFYING CHILD ABUSE

Because children do not usually tell a physician directly if they are being abused physically or sexually, physicians use several strategies to identify child and adolescent victims. Physicians screen for abuse during regular checkups by asking children if anyone has hurt them, touched them in private places, or scared them. To accomplish this screening with five-year-old patients having a routine checkup, physicians may teach their young patients about private areas of the body; let them know that they can tell a parent, teacher, or doctor if anyone ever touches them in private places; and ask the patients if anyone has ever touched them in a way that they did not like. For fifteen-year-old patients, physicians may screen potential victims by providing information on sexual abuse and date rape, then ask the patients if they have ever experienced either.

A second strategy that physicians use to identify children who are victims of family violence is to remain alert for general signs of distress that may indicate a child or youth lives in a violent situation. General signs of distress in children, which may be caused by family violence or by other stressors, include depression, anxiety, low self-esteem, hyperactivity, disruptive behaviors, aggressiveness toward other children, and lack of friends.

In addition to general signs of distress, certain specific signs and symptoms of physical and sexual abuse in children indicate that the child has probably been exposed to violence. For example, bruises that look like a handprint, belt mark, or rope burn would indicate abuse. X rays can show a history of broken bones that are suspicious. Intentional burns from hot water, fire, or cigarettes often have a characteristic pattern. Sexually transmitted diseases in the genital, anal, or oral cavity of a child who is aged fourteen or under would suggest sexual abuse.

A physician observing specific signs of abuse or violence in a child, or even suspecting physical or sexual abuse, has an ethical and legal obligation to provide this information to state child protective services. Every state has laws that require physicians to report suspected child abuse. Physicians do not need to find proof of abuse before filing a report. In fact, the physician should never attempt to prove abuse or interview the child in detail because this can interfere with interviews conducted by experts in law, psychology, and the medicine of child abuse. When children are in immediate danger, they may be hospitalized so that they may receive a thorough medical and psychological evaluation while also being removed from the dangerous situation. In addition to filing a report, the physician records all observations in the child's medical chart. This record includes anything that the child or parents said, drawings or photographs of the injury, the physician's professional opinion regarding exposure to violence, and a description of the child abuse report.

IDENTIFYING PARTNER ABUSE

Physicians also play a key role in helping victims of partner violence. Like children and adolescents, adult victims will usually not disclose violence. Therefore physicians should screen for partner violence and ask about partner violence whenever they notice specific signs of abuse or general signs of distress. Physicians screen for current and past violence during routine patient visits, such as during initial appointments; school, athletic, and work physicals; premarital exams; obstetrical visits; and regular checkups. General signs of distress include depression, anxiety disorders, low self-esteem, suicidal ideation, drug and alcohol abuse, stress illnesses (headache, stomach problems, chronic pain), or patient comments about a partner being jealous, angry, controlling, or irritable. Specific signs of violence include physical injury consistent with assault, including those requiring emergency treatment.

When a victim reports partner violence, there are five steps that a physician can take to help. Communicating belief and support is the first step. Sometimes abuse is extreme and patient reports may seem incredible. The physician validates the victim's experience by expressing belief in the story and exonerating the patient of blame. The physician can begin this process by making eye contact and telling the victim, "You have a right to be safe and respected" and "No one should be treated this way."

The second step is helping the patient assess danger. This is done by asking about types and severity of violent acts, duration and frequency of violence, and injuries received. Specific factors that seem to increase the risk of death in violent relationships include the abuser's use of drugs and alcohol, threats to kill the victim, and the victim's suicidal ideation or attempts. Finally, the physician should ask if the victim feels safe returning home. With this information, the physician can help the patient assess lethal potential and begin to make appropriate safety plans.

The third step is helping the patient identify resources and make a safety plan. The physician begins this process by simply expressing concern for the victim's safety and providing information about local resources such as mandatory arrest laws, legal advocacy services, and shelters. For patients planning to return to an abusive relationship, the physician should encourage a detailed safety plan by helping the patient identify safe havens with family members, friends, or a shelter; assess escape routes from the residence; make specific plans for dangerous situations or when violence recurs; and gather copies of important papers, money, and extra clothing in a safe place in or out of the home in the event of a quick exit. Before the patient leaves, the physician should give the patient a follow-up appointment within two weeks. This provides the victim with a specific, known resource. Follow-up visits should continue until the victim has developed other supportive resources.

The physician's final step is documentation in the patient's medical chart. This written note includes the victim's report of violence, the physician's own observations of injuries and behavior, assessment of danger, safety planning, and follow-up. This record can be helpful in the event of criminal or civil action taken by the victim against the offender. The medical chart and all communications with the patient are kept strictly confidential. Confronting the offender about the abuse can place the victim at risk of further, more severe violence. Improper disclosure can also result in loss of the patient's trust, precluding further opportunities for help.

The physician should not encourage a patient to leave a violent relationship as a first or primary choice. Leaving an abuser is the most dangerous time for victims and should be attempted only with adequate planning and resources. The physician should not recommend couples counseling. Couples counseling endangers victims by raising the victim's expectation that issues can be discussed safely. The abuser often batters the victim after disclosure of sensitive information. Finally, the physician should not overlook violence if the violence appears to be "minor." Seemingly minor acts of aggression can be highly injurious.

IDENTIFYING ABUSE OF THE ELDERLY AND DISABLED

Physicians also play an important role in helping adults who are older, developmentally delayed, or physically disabled. People in all three groups experience a high rate of family violence. Each group presents unique challenges for the physician. One common element among all three groups is that the victims may be somewhat dependent upon other adults to meet their basic needs. Because of this dependence, abuse may sometimes take the form of failing to provide basic needs such as adequate food or medical care. In many states, adults who are developmentally delayed are covered by mandatory child abuse reporting laws.

The signs and symptoms of the abuse of elders are similar to the other forms of family violence. These include physical injuries consistent with assault, signs of distress, and neglect, including self-neglect. Elder abuse victims are often reluctant to reveal abuse because of fear of retaliation, abandonment, or institutionalization. Therefore, a key to intervention is coordinating with appropriate social service and allied health agencies to support an elder adequately, either at home or in a care center. Such agencies include aging councils, visiting nurses, home health aids, and respite or adult day care centers. Counseling and assistance for caregivers is also an important part of intervention.

Many states require physicians to report suspected elder abuse. Because many elder abuse victims are mentally competent, however, it is important that they be made part of the decision-making and reporting process. Such collaboration puts needed control in the elder's hands and therefore facilitates healing. Many other aspects of intervention described for partner abuse apply to working with elders, including providing emotional support, assessing danger, safety planning, and documentation.

A PUBLIC HEALTH EPIDEMIC

In its various forms, family violence is a public health epidemic in the United States. Once thought to be rare, family violence occurs with high frequency in the general population. Although exact figures are lacking and domestic violence tends to be underreported, it is estimated that each year 1.9 million children are physically abused; 250,000 children are sexually molested; 1.6 million women are assaulted by their male partners; and between 500,000 and 2.5 million elders are abused. Rates of violence directed toward unmarried heterosexual women, married heterosexual women, and members of homosexual male and female couples tend to be similar. Victims come from all social classes, races, and religions. Partner violence directed toward heterosexual men, however, is rare and usually occurs in relationships in which the male hits first.

Because family violence is so pervasive, physicians encounter many victims. One out of every three to five women visiting emergency rooms is seeking medical care for injuries related to partner violence. In primary care clinics, including family medicine, internal medicine, and obstetrics and gynecology, one out of every four female patients reports violence in the past year, and two out of five report violence at some time in their lives. It is therefore reasonable to expect all physicians and other health care professionals working in primary care and emergency rooms to provide services for victims of family violence.

—L. Kevin Hamberger and Bruce Ambuel

See also Addiction; Alcoholism; Alcoholism among teenagers; Alcoholism among the elderly; Child abuse; Depression; Depression in children; Depression in the elderly; Drug abuse by teenagers; Elder abuse; Ethics; Recovery programs; Schizophrenia; Stress.

FOR FURTHER INFORMATION:

Barnett, Ola W., Cindy-Lou Miller-Perrin, and Robert D. Perrin. *Family Violence Across the Lifespan: An Introduction.* Thousand Oaks, Calif.: Sage Publications, 1997. Provides information about the different ways that domestic violence, and the warning signs associated with it, may be recognized at various stages in the life spans of individuals and families.

Dutton, Donald G. *The Abusive Personality: Violence and Control in Intimate Relationships.* New York: The Guilford Press, 1998. Dutton, a psychologist, began as a disciple of social learning theory and eventually came to understand that theory alone was inadequate to explain the multifaceted origins of spousal abuse. He takes the reader through a journey across the various explanations of the male batterer, eventually arriving at an in-depth discussion of the cyclical abuser.

Raphael, Jody. *Saving Bernice: Battered Women, Welfare, and Poverty.* Boston: Northeastern University Press, 2000. Raphael uses the case study of one welfare mother and survivor of domestic violence to exemplify the broader issues connecting domestic violence and poverty. In interviews taped during 1995-1999, Bernice, a mother of two and on welfare for eight years, recounts the trauma of abuse, harassment, and stalking by her former partner.

Wilson, K. J. *When Violence Begins at Home: A Comprehensive Guide to Understanding and Ending Domestic Violence.* Alameda, Calif.: Hunter House, 1997. Wilson seeks to share her wealth of knowledge stemming from experience as the current training director at the Austin Center for Battered Women, as an educator, and as a survivor of domestic abuse. She targets a range of audiences, from domestic violence opponents, victims, family, and friends of survivors to a myriad of helping professionals.

Wolfe, David A., Christine Wekerle, and Katreena Scott. *Alternatives to Violence: Empowering Youth to Develop Healthy Relationships.* Thousand Oaks, Calif.: Sage Publications, 1997. Offers information about how to recognize problems related to the development of violence in relationships, as well as strategies to help adolescents develop healthy relationship habits.

✧ DOWN SYNDROME

Type of issue: Children's health, mental health

Definition: A congenital abnormality characterized by moderate to severe mental retardation and a distinctive physical appearance caused by a chromosomal aberration, the result of either an error during embryonic cell division or the inheritance of defective chromosomal material.

Down syndrome results from an incorrect transfer of genetic material in the formation of cells. This disease is also termed trisomy 21 because it most commonly results from the presence of a third, extra copy of the smallest human chromosome, chromosome 21. Actually, it is not the entire extra chromosome 21 that is responsible, but rather a small segment of the long arm of this chromosome. Most incidences of Down syndrome are a consequence of a nondisjunction during meiosis. In about 75 percent of these cases, the extra chromosome is present in the egg. About 1 percent of Down syndrome cases occur after the fertilization of normal gametes from a mitosis nondisjunction, producing a mosaic in which some of the embryo's cells are normal and some exhibit trisomy. The degree of mosaicism and its location will determine the physiological consequences of the nondisjunction. Although mosaic individuals range from apparent normality to completely affected, typically the disorder is less severe.

In about 4 percent of all Down syndrome cases, the individual possesses not an entire third copy of chromosome 21 but rather extra chromosome 21 material, which has been incorporated via a translocation into a nonhomologous chromosome. In translocation, pieces of arms are swapped between two nonrelated chromosomes, forming hybrids. The most common translocation associated with Down syndrome is that between the long arm (Down gene area) of chromosome 21 and an end of chromosome 14. The individual in whom the translocation has occurred shows no evidence of the aberration, since the normal complement of genetic material is still present, only at different chromosomal locations. The difficulty arises when this individual forms gametes.

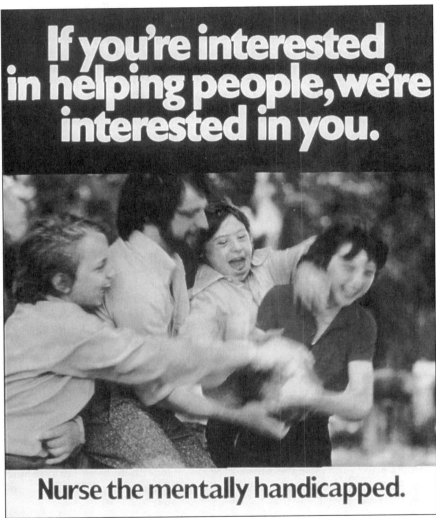

Many agencies offer social and emotional support for people with Down syndrome and their families. (National Library of Medicine)

A mother who possesses the 21/14 translocation, for example, has one normal 21, one normal 14, and the hybrid chromosomes. She is a genetic carrier for the disorder, because she can pass it on to her offspring even though she is clinically normal. This mother could produce three types of viable gametes: one containing the normal 14 and 21; one containing both translocations, which would result in clinical normality; and one containing the normal 21 and the translocated 14 having the long arm of 21. If each gamete were fertilized by normal sperm, two apparently normal embryos and one partial trisomy 21 Down syndrome embryo would result. Down syndrome that results from the passing on of translocations is termed familial Down syndrome and is an inherited disorder.

THE EFFECTS OF DOWN SYNDROME

The presence of an extra copy of the long arm of chromosome 21 causes defects in many tissues and organs. One major effect of Down syndrome is mental retardation. The intelligence quotients (IQs) of affected individuals are typically in the range of 40-50. The IQ varies with age, being higher in childhood than in adolescence or adult life. The disorder is often accompanied by physical traits such as short stature, stubby fingers and toes, protruding tongue, and an unusual pattern of hand creases. Perhaps the most recognized physical feature is the distinctive slanting of the eyes, caused by a vertical fold (epicanthal fold) of skin near the nasal bridge which pulls and tilts the eyes slightly toward the nostrils. For normal Caucasians, the eye runs parallel to the skin fold below the eyebrow; for Asians, this skin fold covers a major portion of the upper eyelid. In contrast, the epicanthal fold in trisomy 21 does not cover a major part of the upper eyelid.

It should be noted that not all defects associated with Down syndrome are found in every affected individual. About 40 percent of Down syndrome patients have congenital heart defects, while about 10 percent have intestinal blockages. Affected individuals are prone to respiratory infections and contract leukemia at a rate twenty times that of the general population. Although Down syndrome children develop the same types of leukemia in the same proportions as other children, the survival rate of the two groups is markedly different. While the survival rate for non-Down syndrome patients after ten years is about 30 percent, survival beyond five years is negligible in Down syndrome patients. It appears that the extra copy of chromosome 21 not only increases the risk of contracting the cancer but also exerts a decisive influence on the disease's outcome. Reproductively, males are sterile while some females are fertile. Although many Down syndrome infants die in the first year of life, the mean life expectancy is about thirty years. This reduced life expectancy results from defects in the immune system, causing a high susceptibility to infectious disease. Most older Down syndrome individuals develop an Alzheimer's-like condition, and less than 3 percent live beyond fifty years of age.

Risk Factors

Trisomy 21 is one of the most common human chromosomal aberrations, occurring in about 0.5 percent of all conceptions and in one out of every seven hundred to eight hundred live births. About 15 percent of the patients institutionalized for mental deficiency suffer from Down syndrome.

Even before the chromosomal basis for the disorder was determined, the frequency of Down syndrome births was correlated with increased maternal age. For mothers at age twenty, the incidence of Down syndrome is about 0.05 percent, which increases to 0.9 percent by age thirty-five and 3 percent for age forty-five. Studies comparing the chromosomes of the affected offspring with both parents have shown that the nondisjunction event is maternal about 75 percent of the time. This maternal age effect is thought to result from the different manner in which the male and female gametes are produced. Gamete production in the male is a continual, lifelong process, while it is a one-time event in females early in embryonic life, somewhere between the eighth and twentieth weeks. It appears that the frequency of nondisjunction events increases with the length of the storage period.

Studies have demonstrated that cells in a state of meiosis are particularly sensitive to environmental influences such as viruses, X rays, and cytotoxic chemicals. It is possible that environmental influences may play a role in nondisjunction events. Up to age thirty-two, males contribute an extra chromosome 21 as often as do females. Beyond this age, there is a rapid increase in nondisjunctional eggs, while the number of nondisjunctional sperm remains constant.

Testing for Down Syndrome

Techniques such as amniocentesis, chorionic villus sampling, and alpha-fetoprotein screening are available for prenatal diagnosis of Down syndrome in fetuses. Amniocentesis, the most widely used technique for prenatal diagnosis, is generally performed between the fourteenth and sixteenth weeks of pregnancy. In this technique, about one ounce of fluid is removed from the amniotic cavity surrounding the fetus by a needle inserted through the mother's abdomen. Although some testing can be done directly on the fluid (such as the assay for spina bifida), more information is obtained from the cells shed from the fetus that accompany the fluid. The mixture obtained in the amniocentesis is spun in a centrifuge to separate the fluid from the fetal cells. Unfortunately, the chromosome analysis for Down syndrome cannot be conducted directly on the amount of cellular material obtained. Although the majority of the cells collected are nonviable, some will grow in culture. These cells are allowed to grow and multiply in culture for two to four weeks, and then the chromosomes undergo karyotyping, which will detect both trisomy 21 and translocational aberration.

In karyotyping, the chromosomes are spread on a microscope slide, stained, and photographed. Each type of chromosome gives a unique, observable banding pattern when stained which allows it to be identified. The chromosomes are then cut out of the photograph and arranged in homologous pairs, in numerical order. Trisomy 21 is easily observed, since three copies of chromosome 21 are present, while the translocation shows up as an abnormal banding pattern. Termination of the pregnancy in the wake of an unfavorable amniocentesis diagnosis is complicated, because the fetus at this point is usually about eighteen to twenty weeks old, and elective abortions are normally performed between the sixth and twelfth weeks of pregnancy. Earlier sampling of the amniotic fluid is not possible because of the small amount of fluid present.

An alternate testing procedure called chorionic villus sampling became available in the mid-1980's. In this procedure, a chromosomal analysis is conducted on a piece of placental tissue that is obtained either vaginally or through the abdomen during the eighth to eleventh week of pregnancy. The advantages of this procedure are that it can be done much earlier in the pregnancy and that enough tissue can be collected to conduct the chromosome analysis immediately, without the cell culture step. Consequently, diagnosis can be completed during the first trimester of the pregnancy, making therapeutic abortion an option for the parents. Chorionic villus sampling does have some negative aspects. One disadvantage is the slightly higher incidence of test-induced miscarriage as compared to amniocentesis—around 1 percent (versus less than 0.5 percent). Also, because tissue of both the mother and the fetus are obtained in the sampling process, they must be carefully separated, complicating the analysis. Occasionally, chromosomal abnormalities are observed in the tested tissue that are not present in the fetus itself.

Prenatal maternal alpha-fetoprotein testing has also been used to diagnose Down syndrome. Abnormal levels of a substance called maternal alpha-fetoprotein are often associated with chromosomal disorders. Several research studies have described a high correlation between low levels of maternal alpha-fetoprotein and the occurrence of trisomy 21 in the fetus. By correlating alpha-fetoprotein levels, the age of the mother, and specific female hormone levels, between 60 percent and 80 percent of fetuses with Down syndrome can be detected. Although techniques allow Down syndrome to be detected readily in a fetus, there is no effective intrauterine therapy available to correct the abnormality.

CARING FOR CHILDREN WITH DOWN SYNDROME

The care of a Down syndrome child presents many challenges for the family unit. Until the 1970's, most of these children spent their lives in institutions. With the increased support services available, however, it is now common for such children to remain in the family environment. Although many Down syndrome children have happy dispositions, a significant number have behavioral problems that can consume the energies of the parents, to the detriment of the other children. Rearing a Down syndrome child often places a large financial burden on the family: Such children are, for example, susceptible to illness; they also have special educational needs. Since Down syndrome children are often conceived late in the parents' reproductive period, the parents may not be able to continue to care for these children throughout their offspring's adult years. This is problematic because many Down syndrome individuals do not possess sufficient mental skills to earn a living or to manage their affairs without supervision.

For parents who have produced a Down syndrome child, genetic counseling can be beneficial in determining their risk factor for future pregnancies. The genetic counselor determines the specific chromosomal aberration that occurred utilizing chromosome studies of the parents and affected child, along with additional information provided by the family history. If the cause was nondisjunction and the mother is young, the recurrence risk is much less than 1 percent; for mothers over the age of thirty-four, it is about 5 percent. If the cause was translocational, the Down syndrome is hereditary and risk is much greater—statistically, a one-in-three chance. In addition, there is a one-in-three chance that clinically normal offspring will be carriers of the syndrome, producing it in the next generation.

—*Arlene R. Courtney*

See also Amniocentesis; Birth defects; Children's health issues; Disabilities; Genetic counseling; Genetic diseases; Health problems and families; Learning disabilities; Mental retardation; Prenatal care; Screening.

FOR FURTHER INFORMATION:

Holtzman, Neil A. *Proceed with Caution: Predicting Genetic Risks in the Recombinant DNA Era.* Baltimore: The Johns Hopkins University Press, 1989. Discusses genetic counseling, how genetic disorders are diagnosed, and social implications.

Pueschel, Siegfried. *A Parent's Guide to Down Syndrome.* 2d ed. Baltimore: Paul H. Brookes, 2000. An informative guide highlighting the important developmental stages in the life of a child with Down syndrome.

Rondal, Jean A., et al., eds. *Down's Syndrome: Psychological, Psychobiological, and Socioeducational Perspectives.* San Diego: Singular, 1996. An academic text on issues surrounding Down syndrome. Includes references and an index.

Shaw, Michael, ed. *Everything You Need to Know About Diseases.* Springhouse, Pa.: Springhouse Press, 1996. This well-illustrated consumer reference, compiled by more than one hundred doctors and medical experts, describes five hundred illnesses and conditions, their causes, symptoms, diagnosis, treatment, and prevention. A valuable reference book for everyone interested in health and disease. Of particular interest is chapter 21, "Genetic Disorders."

Tingey, Carol, ed. *Down Syndrome: A Resource Handbook*. Boston: Little, Brown, 1988. A practical resource for rearing a Down syndrome child, including guidelines on daily life, developmental expectations, and health and medical needs.

✧ DROWNING

Type of issue: Children's health, public health
Definition: Submersion in water or other fluid, resulting in death.

When a person is submerged in water, the first step toward drowning is spasm of the larynx, followed by decreased oxygen and often the aspiration of water or other fluid. This is followed by decreased blood circulation to the brain. Damage to brain cells begins after about six minutes of submersion and is considered irreversible after about nine minutes. Up to one-fifth of drowning victims have no water in their lungs. These incidents are termed dry drownings.

The temperature of the water is an important factor in drowning or near-drowning. Being suddenly submerged in cold water may cause an involuntary gasp that draws water into the lungs. Cold water also causes loss of consciousness. As the body temperature cools, abnormal heart rhythms may occur. On the other hand, hypothermia does reduce the oxygen requirements of the brain and may be protective. In some cases of submersion, especially in icy water, the so-called mammalian diving reflex is triggered, causing the circulation to slow dramatically and the brain to require less oxygen to survive undamaged. For this reason, victims who appear to have drowned should receive resuscitation until they are thoroughly warm, even if this takes a prolonged period of time.

Victims of near-drowning have the best chance of a good outcome if they do not require cardiopulmonary resuscitation (CPR), if they have no lung-related symptoms following the near-drowning, and if they were submerged in cold, clean water. Serious neurological problems occur in about 10 percent of victims who are victims of near-drowning.

RESUSCITATION

Initial treatment of someone who has apparently drowned is mouth-to-mouth resuscitation beginning in the water, if necessary. Once the victim is on dry land, full CPR measures may be started if a pulse is absent. If there is any evidence of neck injury, the rescuers must take appropriate precautions against further damage. Also, it is important to take precautions against the victim vomiting and choking on the vomited material. Rewarming should begin at the scene: Rescuers should remove the victim's wet clothing and cover the body with dry blankets.

In the hospital setting, emergency care is governed by the ABC's: management of the airway, breathing, and circulation. The victim should be rewarmed by means appropriate to the core body temperature. Sometimes, victims can be reheated with radiant warmers; other times, they require warmed intravenous solutions. Abnormal heart rhythms may also be a problem. The length of the emergency room stay and the need for hospital admission depends on the patient's condition. Some victims do well initially but show significant respiratory problems after twelve or more hours.

The victim of near-drowning may recover without any brain damage or may suffer from significant problems. Factors that are associated with a poorer outcome include submersion for more than ten minutes, the need for CPR, a delay in beginning CPR, arrival at the emergency room in a coma, and a core body temperature of less than 30 degrees Celsius (86 degrees Fahrenheit).

THE RISK TO CHILDREN

Among children between the ages of one and fourteen, drowning is the third most common cause of death, and among all children and adolescents, it is the second most common cause of accidental death. Drownings take place not only in lakes and streams but also in toilets and washing machines. Although all children are at risk for drowning, toddlers and adolescents (particularly males) are the groups most at risk.

About 40 percent of childhood drownings occur with children less than four years old, most of whom drown in swimming pools. More than half of all adolescent drowning deaths are associated with alcohol use. Drowning deaths among teenagers are largely the result of boating accidents or diving and swimming in unsafe areas. Not surprisingly, most drowning deaths occur in the summer and are more common in warm-weather areas, such as California and Florida. In the case of drowning in a child who is not able to walk or crawl, child abuse or neglect should be considered.

Childhood drownings are nearly all preventable. Babies and toddlers should never be left alone in a bathtub; indeed, most drownings in children under the age of one are bathtub drownings. Toddlers have been known to drown in as little as one inch of water and in buckets of paint, so constant supervision is essential. Children with epilepsy are at particular risk of drowning and should be monitored even when they get older.

Laws regarding the fencing of swimming pools must be rigorously enforced. Alcohol consumption near water recreation areas should be strictly limited. Other public health measures include the easy availability of rescue equipment and widespread training in CPR. All children should be taught to swim, but such a measure does not decrease the need for careful supervision.

—Rebecca Lovell Scott

See also Children's health issues; Choking; First aid; Safety issues for children.

FOR FURTHER INFORMATION:
Berkow, Robert, ed. *The Merck Manual of Medical Information, Home Edition.* Whitehouse Station, N.J.: Merck Research Laboratories, 1997.
Fein, Joel A., Dennis R. Durbin, and Steven M. Selbst. "Injuries and Emergencies." In *Rudolph's Fundamentals of Pediatrics,* edited by Abraham M. Rudolph and Robert K. Kamei. 2d ed. Stamford, Conn.: Appleton and Lange, 1998.
Fulcher, William. "Thermal and Environmental Injuries." In *Textbook of Family Practice,* edited by Robert E. Rakel. 5th ed. Philadelphia: W. B. Saunders, 1995.
Hay, William W., et al., eds. "Emergencies, Injuries, and Poisoning." In *Current Pediatric Diagnosis and Treatment.* 15th ed. New York: McGraw-Hill, 2000.
Schmitt, Barton D. *Your Child's Health: The Parents' Guide to Symptoms, Emergencies, Common Illnesses, Behavior, and School Problems.* Rev. ed. New York: Bantam Books, 1991.

✧ DRUG ABUSE BY TEENAGERS

Type of issue: Children's health, mental health, social trends
Definition: A behavioral disorder characterized by dependence on and/or abuse of psychoactive substances.

Drug abuse is a broad term subsuming a range of abused substances, including nicotine, alcohol, marijuana, cocaine, opiates, hallucinogens, amphetamine, and many others, including many prescription medications. The term also includes several disorders, including physical addiction and psychological dependence as well as experimental and recreational drug abuse. The latter two are disproportionately found among juvenile drug abusers. The causes of each form of abuse vary, as do the medical, behavioral, and social consequences.

THE BIGGER PICTURE

Most experimental and recreational abuse declines with maturity (unlike addiction or dependence). Nevertheless, in the short term, the associated behaviors are highly dangerous, including binge drinking, multiple substance abuse, and risk taking associated with intoxication. Thus, drug abuse is strongly linked to other juvenile behavioral disorders and problems, including automobile and other accidents, pregnancy, sexually transmitted diseases, and delinquent behavior. Academic problems also may result from, as well as be causally linked to, substance abuse.

Addiction and dependence in juveniles are commonly associated with dysfunctionality in the home life. A combination of home stress, lack of parental supervision, modeling of abusive behavior, and genetic predisposition are likely involved. In addition, low socioeconomic status is commonly associated with addiction, probably owing to high stress and the accessibility of the criminal and drug subculture in many low-income neighborhoods. Not all addicts, however, come from such backgrounds. One of the risks that concerns counselors is that many addicts began the process of dependence while engaged in recreational drug abuse.

Recreational and experimental drug abuse are also linked to home life and socioeconomic factors, although in a more complex fashion. High socioeconomic status is linked to certain forms of abuse, such as cocaine, while in general low socioeconomic status is associated with a higher general rate of substance abuse. Home stress can contribute to drug abuse, but adolescents from stable homes may be influenced by parental attitudes condoning recreational abuse. Additional causes include cultural factors such as the mass media (which may be seen as condoning recreational abuse), role models among celebrities and athletes, peer culture and conformity, and the general developmental processes associated with adolescent identity formation and autonomy seeking. The latter concerns cause problems in interpreting whether a particular instance of drug abuse indicates a more general psychological disorder or whether it is a part of "normal" development. Parents may become concerned that recreational drug abuse indicates addiction or dependence; a danger of overdiagnosis of these disorders exists.

CONSEQUENCES OF DRUG USE

The physical consequences of drug abuse depend on the drug and on the nature of the abusive behavior. In addition to the noted link with risk-taking behavior, most of the abused substances are intrinsically dangerous. Overuse can lead to death through overdose, especially in cases of multiple drug abuse. Binge drinking is commonly the source of overdoses in cases involving alcohol alone. Combining prescription medications (especially tranquilizers) with alcohol is especially dangerous, leading to accidental overdoses.

Some overdoses may be deliberate, or in other cases involve deliberate recklessness. Long-term addiction is associated in many cases with damage to internal systems, particularly the liver, although these effects are cumulative over a lifetime and are not typically seen in adolescents.

Psychological problems can occur even with limited use. In addition to the poor judgment associated with intoxication, counselors worry about the impact on general motivation, especially with marijuana. Involvement with a drug subculture can interfere with peer relationships and foster anti-authority attitudes.

JUVENILE DRUG TREATMENT

Treatment programs need to separate addicts from other substance abusers. This separation is in the interests of both addicts, who need intensive treatment, and nonaddicts, who can be harmed by extended contact with those with more serious abuse problems.

Juvenile addicts may require home removal because of poor home environments and the need for supervised treatment. Because of expense and other practical considerations, treatment is frequently conducted on an outpatient basis, although this is generally considered less effective. Inpatient addiction programs for juveniles must ensure that education is not disrupted as a consequence of treatment. Eclectic approaches, combining insight-oriented therapies (both individually and in groups) along with behavior modification and training in social skills, are essential in treating this multifaceted problem. Family therapy is also frequently recommended. The long-term concern is with the high relapse rate, common to adult as well as juvenile addicts but further complicated by the lack of control that teenage clients have in constructing their own social environments upon leaving the treatment program. Follow-up outpatient care is recommended but is not always available or heeded.

Treatment for nonaddicted abusers may be either as an outpatient or as an inpatient. The biggest risk is association with addicts and the labeling of one's behavior by the patient and others. Family therapy can be particularly important in this context. Some therapists emphasize abstinence from all drugs; others emphasize learning responsible use, especially in the case of alcohol. Disruptions in academic and social development occurring as a result of abuse also need attention, with particular concern for the incident that led to referral (possibly an arrest or an accident).

PREVENTION OF DRUG USE

Most experts agree that prevention is more effective than treatment. One approach to prevention is through the legal system, either regulating or prohibiting use of psychoactive substances. Substance abuse experts are often concerned about the unintended consequences of many such approaches, such as the lack of regulation of illegal drugs, the fear of abusers to seek treatment (including during pregnancy), and the creation of contact with the criminal world in order to obtain illegal drugs. In addition, variations in the legal status of abused substances may send unintended messages. For example, alcohol use is often associated with proof of maturity.

In the United States, legal efforts aimed at stopping the illegal drug trade have led to mandatory sentencing of many drug offenders. An increasing proportion of the prison population consists of such people, who ironically often end up with longer sentences than violent offenders who are not covered by such policies and who may receive early release in order to relieve prison overcrowding. Many legal experts have expressed concern with the lack of judicial discretion, especially for the convicted who might benefit from rehabilitation efforts. Juvenile drug abusers are not typically directly affected by these laws, unless charged with a crime as an adult (in some states, automatically so as young as age seventeen). Critics are also concerned about the ultimate diversion of public resources toward punishment and away from rehabilitation programs and education and prevention efforts.

Thus, most experts advocate an emphasis on drug education. Efforts have included "scare tactics," including graphic visual images of withdrawal or accident victims; straightforward information about risks; and broader programs aimed at developing the social skills and attitudes associated with resisting pressures to abuse drugs. The consensus is that the broader programs (combining information and skills training) are more successful, and especially so when begun before the ages at which children have been found abusing drugs—that is, earlier than age nine. Important social skills include resisting peer pressure, developing appropriate stress management, finding alternative social outlets, and handling anger. These skills need to be practiced through role play and other exercises. Thus, these programs require more than a single presentation by an outside speaker, as has been characteristic of less successful drug education programs. Information must be presented honestly; loss of credibility is a serious concern with many of the scare tactic approaches, although scaring teenagers with accurate information can be highly successful.

Most experts also agree that the temptations to abuse drugs are intrinsic to human life, with its stresses and the escape or relief that drugs provide. It is for this reason that many programs emphasize responsible use, rather than abstinence, at least with alcohol. These programs emphasize the issue of responsibility, the avoidance of intoxication, and such practical safety methods as the use of designated drivers. Nevertheless, despite treatment and prevention efforts, drug abuse is likely to remain as a social problem.

SOCIAL ISSUES

Several trends in juvenile drug use raise legitimate concerns. Drug abuse is occurring at ever-younger ages. The impact of these behaviors on puberty is not fully understood; moreover, interference with academic and social development from ages as young as nine is extremely serious. Such considerations drive the younger ages at which drug education is occurring in the United States.

Political and social considerations lead to multiple difficulties in interpreting the dangers associated with specific drugs. The legal status of nicotine and alcohol may lead to an underestimation of their dangers. Political debates are not resolved concerning the relative dangers of marijuana. Social considerations can lead either to an argument for more leniency to avoid criminalizing relatively harmless behavior or, conversely, to more efforts at prohibition by those who consider marijuana a "gateway drug" that leads to the abuse of more dangerous drugs. Cocaine abuse is associated with high socioeconomic status, whereas crack abuse is associated with lower status. The harsher legal penalties for crack use have led to accusations of both social class and racial bias. Finally, keeping track of fads with regard to LSD, PCP, inhalants, and other substances is a constant worry to counselors, law enforcement officers, health professionals, and parents. All these issues end up as concerns in the counseling and education processes.

Moreover, legal policies, as noted with regard to mandatory sentencing, influence the consequences of drug abuse, as well as the location of many drug rehabilitation programs. Increasingly, these programs are directly associated with prisons and juvenile detention centers. Most patients in drug treatment programs are not there entirely of their own choice but are required to be in such programs by schools or parents. Voluntary compliance with rehabilitation is highly associated with successful outcomes; the involvement of legally mandated treatment can complicate this issue further. In some cases, a legal requirement may be the only way to begin treatment that ultimately may be successful. In other cases, it can produce resentment that may interfere with the trust essential in any counselor/client relationship.

Preventing drug abuse among juveniles must occur with each new generation. Cigarette use declined sharply among teenagers during the 1980's but increased again in the 1990's. Many experts attribute this increase in part to complacency over the success of education about nicotine. This example contains important lessons for all drug education programs.

—Nancy E. Macdonald

See also Addiction; Alcoholism among teenagers; Children's health issues; Depression in children; Recovery programs; Smoking; Suicide among children and teenagers; Tobacco use by teenagers.

For Further Information:

Boyd, Gayle M., Jan Howard, and Robert A. Zucker, eds. *Alcohol Problems Among Adolescents: Current Directions in Prevention Research.* Hillsdale, N.J.: Lawrence Erlbaum Associates, 1995. This volume contains eleven articles addressing a variety of issues in alcohol abuse prevention, including family influence, decision making, high-risk adolescents, and alcohol price policies.

Gonet, Marlene Miziker. *Counseling the Adolescent Substance Abuser: School-Based Intervention and Prevention.* Thousand Oaks, Calif.: Sage Publications, 1994. The author provides detailed information on the needs of school-based counseling programs, including individual, group, and family counseling. Case examples are provided.

Males, Mike A. *The Scapegoat Generation: America's War on Adolescents.* Monroe, Maine: Common Courage Press, 1996. The author argues that political interests lead to an exaggeration of a number of social problems involving adolescents, including delinquency and drug abuse. This book provides a useful perspective to consider in responding to real and potential behavioral problems, including drug abuse.

Miller, William R., and Nick Heather, eds. *Treating Addictive Behaviors: Processes of Change.* 2d ed. New York: Plenum Press, 1998. This book, written by medical and psychological scientists, is an overview of treatment strategies for problems ranging from nicotine to opiate addiction. Psychological, behavioral, interpersonal, familial, and medical approaches are outlined and discussed.

Yoslow, Mark. *Drugs in the Body: Effects of Abuse.* New York: Franklin Watts, 1992. This book provides highly readable, straightforward information on the effects of cocaine and crack, the opiates, cannabis drugs, hallucinogens, and amphetamines.

✧ Dyslexia

Type of issue: Children's health, mental health
Definition: Severe reading disability in children with average to above-average intelligence.

Nearly 25 percent of the individuals in the United States and of many other industrialized societies who otherwise possess at least average intelligence cannot read well. Many such people are viewed as suffering from a neurological disorder called dyslexia. This term was first introduced by the German ophthalmologist Rudolf Berlin in the nineteenth century. He defined it as designating all those individuals who possessed average or above-average intelligence quotients (IQs) but who could not read adequately because of their inability to process language symbols.

The modern definition of the disorder is based on long-term, extensive studies of dyslexic children that have identified dyslexia as a complex syndrome composed of a large number of associated behavioral dysfunctions that are related to visual-motor brain immaturity and/or brain dysfunction. These problems include a poor memory for details, easy distractibility, poor motor skills, visual letter and word reversal, and the inability to distinguish between important elements of the spoken language.

EXPLAINING DYSLEXIA

Understanding dyslexia in order to correct this reading disability is crucial and difficult. To learn to read well, an individual must acquire many basic cognitive and linguistic skills. First, it is necessary to pay close attention, to concentrate, to follow directions, and to understand the language spoken in daily life. Next, one must develop an auditory and visual memory, strong sequencing ability, solid word decoding skills, the ability to carry out structural-contextual language analysis, the capability to interpret the written language, a solid vocabulary which expands as quickly as is needed, and speed in scanning and interpreting written language. These skills are taught in good developmental reading programs, but some or all are found to be deficient in dyslexic individuals.

Two basic explanations have evolved for dyslexia. Many physicians propose that it is caused by brain damage or brain dysfunction. Evolution of the problem is attributed to accident, disease, and/or hereditary faults in body biochemistry. Here, the diagnosis of dyslexia is made by the use of electroencephalograms (EEGs), computed tomography (CT) scans, and related neurological technology. After such evaluation is complete, medication is often used to diminish hyperactivity and nervousness, and a group of physical training procedures called patterning is used to counter the neurological defects in the dyslexic individual.

In contrast, many special educators and other researchers believe that the problem of dyslexia is one of dormant, immature, or undeveloped learning centers in the brain. Many proponents of this concept strongly encourage the correction of dyslexic problems by the teaching of specific reading skills. While such experts agree that the use of medication can be of great value, they attempt to cure dyslexia mostly through a process called imprinting. This technique essentially trains dyslexic individuals and corrects their problems via the use of exaggerated, repeated language drills.

TYPES OF DYSLEXIA

A number of experts propose three types of dyslexia. The most common type and the one most often identified as dyslexia is called visual dyslexia, the lack of ability to translate the observed written or printed language into meaningful terms. The major difficulty is that afflicted people see certain words or letters backward or upside down. The resultant problem is that—to the visual dyslexic—any written sentence is a jumble of many letters whose accurate translation may require five or more times as much effort as is needed by an unafflicted person.

The other two problems viewed as dyslexia are auditory dyslexia and dysgraphia. Auditory dyslexia is the inability to perceive individual sounds of spoken language. Despite having normal hearing, auditory dyslexics are deaf to the differences between certain vowel and/or consonant sounds, and what they cannot hear they cannot write. Dysgraphia is the inability to write legibly. The basis for this problem is a lack of the hand-eye coordination that is required to write clearly.

Many children who suffer from visual dyslexia also exhibit elements of auditory dyslexia. This complicates the issue of teaching many dyslexic students because only one type of dyslexic symptom can be treated at a time. Also, dyslexia appears to be a sex-linked disorder, being much more common in boys than in girls. Estimates vary between three and seven times as many boys having dyslexia as girls.

Diagnosing Dyslexia

The early diagnosis and treatment of dyslexia is essential to its eventual correction. Many experts agree that if a treatment begins before the third grade, there is an 80 percent probability that the dyslexia can be corrected. If the disorder remains undetected until the fifth grade, however, success at treating dyslexia is cut in half. If treatment does not begin until the seventh grade, the probability of successful treatment drops below 5 percent.

The preliminary identification of a dyslexic child can be made from symptoms that include poor written schoolwork, easy distractibility, clumsiness, poor coordination, poor spatial orientation, confused writing and/or spelling, and poor left-right orientation. Because numerous nondyslexic children also show many of these symptoms, a second step is required for such identification: the use of written tests designed to identify dyslexics. These tests include the Peabody Individual Achievement Test, the Halstead-Reitan Neuropsychological Test Battery, and the SOYBAR Criterion Tests.

Correcting the Disorder

Once conclusive identification of a dyslexic child has been made, it becomes possible to begin corrective treatment. Such treatment is usually the preserve of special education programs. These programs are carried out by the special education teacher in school resource rooms. They also involve special classes limited to children with reading disabilities and schools that specialize in treating learning disabilities.

An often-cited method used is that of Grace Fernald, which utilizes kinesthetic imprinting, based on combined language experience and tactile stimulation. In this popular method or adaptations of it, a dyslexic child learns to read in the following way. First, the child tells a spontaneous story to the teacher, who transcribes it. Next, each word that is unknown to the child is written down by the teacher, and the child traces its letters repeatedly until he or she can write the word without using the model. Each word learned becomes part of the child's word file. A large number of stories are handled this way. Though the method is quite slow, many reports praise its results. Nevertheless, no formal studies of its effectiveness have been made.

A second common teaching technique that is utilized by special educators is the Orton-Gillingham-Stillman method, which was developed in a collaboration between two teachers and a pediatric neurologist, Samuel T. Orton. The method evolved from Orton's conceptualization of language as developing from a sequence of processes in the nervous system that ends in its unilateral control by the left cerebral hemisphere. He proposed that dyslexia arises from conflicts between this cerebral hemisphere and the right cerebral hemisphere, which is usually involved in the handling of nonverbal, pictorial, and spatial stimuli.

Consequently, the corrective method that is used is a multisensory and kinesthetic approach, like that of Fernald. It begins, however, with the teaching of individual letters and phonemes. Then, it progresses to dealing with syllables, words, and sentences. Children taught by this method are drilled systematically, to imprint them with a mastery of phonics and the sounding out of unknown written words. They are encouraged to learn how the elements of written language look, how they sound, how it feels to pronounce them, and how it feels to write them down. Although the Orton-Gillingham-Stillman method is as laborious as that of Fernald, it is widely used and appears to be successful.

Another treatment aspect is the use of therapeutic drugs in the handling of dyslexia. Most physicians and educators propose the use of these drugs as a useful adjunct to the special education training of those dyslexic children who are restless and easily distracted and who have low morale because of continued embarrassment in school in front of their peers. The drugs that are utilized most often are amphetamine, Dexedrine, and methylphenidate (Ritalin).

These stimulants, given at appropriate dose levels, will lengthen the time period during which certain dyslexic children function well in the classroom and can also produce feelings of self-confidence. Side effects of their overuse, however, include loss of appetite, nausea, nervousness, and sleeplessness. Furthermore, there is also the potential problem of drug abuse. When they are administered carefully and under close medical supervision, however, the benefits of these drugs far outweigh any possible risks.

A proponent of an entirely medical treatment of dyslexia is psychiatrist

Harold N. Levinson. He proposes that the root of dyslexia is in inner ear dysfunction and that it can be treated with the judicious application of proper medications. Levinson's treatment includes amphetamines, antihistamines, drugs used against motion sickness, vitamins, health food components, and nutrients mixed in the proper combination for each patient. He asserts that he has cured more than ten thousand dyslexics and documents many cases. Critics of Levinson's work pose several questions, including whether the studies reported were well controlled and whether the patients treated were actually dyslexics. A major basis for the latter criticism is Levinson's statement that many of his cured patients were described to him as outstanding students. The contention is that dyslexic students are never outstanding students and cannot work at expected age levels.

An important aspect of dyslexia treatment is parental support of these children. Such emotional support helps dyslexics to cope with their problems and with the judgment of their peers. Useful aspects of this support include a positive attitude toward an afflicted child, appropriate home help that complements efforts at school, encouragement and praise for achievements, lack of recrimination when repeated mistakes are made, and positive interaction with special education teachers.

—Sanford S. Singer

See also Attention deficit disorder (ADD); Children's health issues; Learning disabilities; Speech disorders.

For Further Information:
Huston, Anne Marshall. *Understanding Dyslexia: A Practical Approach for Parents and Teachers.* Rev. ed. Lanham, Md.: Madison Books, 1992. Explains dyslexia, describes its three main types, identifies causes and treatments, and covers useful teaching techniques. A bibliography, a useful glossary, appendices, and teaching materials are valuable additions.

Levinson, Harold N. *Smart but Feeling Dumb.* Rev. ed. New York: Warner Books, 1994. Based on "thousands of cases cured," this book explains the basis and treatment of dyslexia as inner ear dysfunction that can be cured with judicious application of the correct medications. Included are an overview, case studies, a summary, useful appendices, and a bibliography.

Routh, Donald K. "Disorders of Learning." In *The Practical Assessment and Management of Children with Disorders of Development and Learning,* edited by Mark L. Wolraich. Chicago: Year Book Medical Publishers, 1987. This succinct article summarizes salient facts about learning disorders, including etiology, assessment, management, and outcome. Interested readers will also find many useful references.

Snowling, Margaret. *Dyslexia: A Cognitive Developmental Perspective.* 2d ed. New York: Basil Blackwell, 2000. Covers aspects of dyslexia, including its identification, associated cognitive defects, the basis for language skill development, and the importance of phonetics. Also contains many references.

Valett, Robert E. *Dyslexia: A Neuropsychological Approach to Educating Children with Severe Reading Disorders.* Belmont, Calif.: David S. Lake, 1980. This text, containing hundreds of references, is of interest to readers wishing detailed information on dyslexia and on educating dyslexics. Its two main sections are the neuropsychological foundations of reading (including neuropsychological factors, language acquisition, and diagnosis) and a wide variety of special education topics.

✦ EATING DISORDERS

Type of issue: Children's health, mental health, social trends, women's health

Definition: A set of emotional disorders centering on body image that lead to misuse of food in a variety of ways—through overeating, overeating and purging, or undereating—that severely threaten the physical and mental well-being of the individual.

The presence of an eating disorder in a patient is defined by an abnormal mental and physical relationship between body image and eating. While obesity is considered an eating disorder, the most prominent conditions are anorexia nervosa and bulimia nervosa. Anorexia nervosa (the word "anorexia" comes from the Greek for "loss of appetite") is an illness characterized by the relentless pursuit of thinness and fear of gaining weight. Bulimia nervosa (the word "bulimia" comes from the Greek for "ox appetite") refers to binge eating followed by self-induced vomiting. These conditions are related in intimate, yet ill-defined ways.

ANOREXIA NERVOSA

Anorexia nervosa affects more women than men by the overwhelming ratio of nineteen to one. It most often begins in adolescence and is more common among the upper and middle classes of the Western world. According to most studies, its incidence increased severalfold from the 1970's to the 1990's. Prevalence figures vary from 0.5 to 0.8 cases per one hundred adolescent girls. A familiar pattern of anorexia nervosa is often present, and studies indicate that 16 percent of the mothers and 23 percent of the fathers of anorectic patients had a history of significantly low adolescent weight or weight phobia.

The criteria for anorexia nervosa include intense fear of becoming obese, which does not diminish with the progression of weight loss; disturbance of body image, or feeling "fat" even when emaciated; refusal to maintain body weight over a minimal weight for age and height; the loss of 25 percent of original body weight or being 25 percent below expected weight based on standard growth charts; and no known physical illness that would account for the weight loss. Anorexia nervosa is also classified into primary and secondary forms. The primary condition is the distinct constellation of behaviors described above. In secondary anorexia nervosa, the weight loss results from another emotional or organic disorder.

The most prominent symptom of anorexia nervosa is a phobic avoidance of eating that goes beyond any reasonable level of dieting in the presence of striking thinness. Attending this symptom is the characteristic distorted body image and faulty perceptions of hunger and satiety, as well as a pervasive sense of inadequacy.

The distortion of body image renders patients unable to evaluate their body weight accurately, so that they react to weight loss by intensifying their desire for thinness. Patients characteristically describe themselves as "fat" and "gross" even when totally emaciated. The degree of disturbance in body image is a useful prognostic index. Faulty perception of inner, visceral sensations, such as hunger and satiety, extends also to emotional states. The problem of nonrecognition of feelings is usually intensified with starvation.

Other cognitive distortions are also common in anorectic patients. Dichotomous reasoning—the assessment of self or others—is either idealized or degraded. Personalization of situations and a tendency to overgeneralize are common. Anorectics display an extraordinary amount of energy, directed to exercise and schoolwork in the face of starvation, but may curtail or avoid social relationships. Crying spells and complaints of depression are common findings and may persist in some anorectic patients even after weight is gained.

Sleep disturbances have also been reported in anorectics. Obsessive and/or compulsive behaviors, usually developing after the onset of the eating symptoms, abound with anorexia. Obsession with cleanliness and house cleaning, frequent handwashing, compulsive studying habits, and ritualistic behaviors are common.

As expected, the most striking compulsions involve food and eating. Anorectics' intense involvement with food belies their apparent lack of interest in it. The term "anorexia" is, in fact, a misnomer because lack of appetite is rare until late in the illness. Anorectics often carry large quantities of sweets in their purses and hide candies or cookies in various places. They frequently collect recipes and engage in elaborate meal preparation for others. Anorectics' behavior also includes refusal to eat with their families and in public places. When unable to reduce food intake openly, they may resort to such subterfuge as hiding food or disposing of it in toilets. If the restriction of food intake does not suffice for losing weight, the patient may resort to vomiting, usually at night and in secret. Self-induced vomiting then becomes associated with bulimia. Some patients also abuse laxatives and diuretics.

Commonly reported physical symptoms include constipation, abdominal pain, and cold intolerance. With severe weight loss, feelings of weakness and lethargy replace the drive to exercise. Amenorrhea (cessation of menstruation) occurs in virtually all cases, although it is not essential for a diagnosis of anorexia. Weight loss generally precedes the loss of the menstrual cycle. Other physical symptoms reveal the effects of starvation. Potassium depletion is the most frequent serious problem occurring with both anorexia and bulimia. Gastrointestinal disturbances are common, and death may occur from either infection or electrolyte imbalance.

TREATING ANOREXIA

The management of anorectic patients, in either hospital or outpatient settings, may include individual psychotherapy, family therapy, behavior modification, and pharmacotherapy. Many anorectic patients are quite physically ill when they first consult a physician, and medical evaluation and management in a hospital may be necessary at this stage. A gastroenterologist or other medical specialist familiar with this condition may be required to evaluate electrolyte disturbance, emaciation, hypothermia, skin problems, hair loss, sensitivity to cold, fatigue, and cardiac arrhythmias. Starvation may cause cognitive and psychological disturbances that limit the patient's cooperation with treatment.

Indications for hospitalization are weight loss exceeding 30 percent of ideal body weight or the presence of serious medical complications. Most clinicians continue the hospitalization until 80 percent to 85 percent of the ideal body weight is reached. The hospitalization makes possible hyperalimentation (intravenous infusion of nutrients) when medically necessary. Furthermore, individual and family psychiatric evaluations can be performed and a therapeutic alliance established more rapidly with the patient hospitalized.

Most programs utilize behavior modification during the course of hospitalization, making increased privileges such as physical and social activities and visiting contingent on weight gain. A medically safe rate of weight gain is approximately one-quarter of a pound a day. Patients are weighed daily, after the bladder is emptied, and daily fluid intake and output are recorded. Patients with bulimic characteristics may be required to stay in the room two hours after each meal without access to the bathroom to prevent vomiting. Some behavior modification programs emphasize formal contracting, negative contingencies, the practice of avoidance behavior, relaxation techniques, role-playing, and systematic desensitization.

The goal of dynamic psychotherapy is to achieve patient autonomy and independence. The female anorectic patient often uses her body as a battleground for the separation or individuation struggle with her mother.

The cognitive therapeutic approach begins with helping the patient to articulate beliefs, change her view of herself as the center of the universe, and render her expectations of the consequences of food intake less catastrophic. The therapist acknowledges the patient's beliefs as genuine, particularly the belief that her self-worth is dependent on achieving and maintaining a low weight. Through a gradual modification of self-assessment, the deficits in the patient's self-esteem are remedied. The therapist also challenges the cultural values surrounding body shape and addresses behavioral and family issues such as setting weight goals and living conditions.

Bulimia

Bulimia usually occurs between the ages of twelve and forty, with greatest frequency between the ages of fifteen and thirty. Unlike anorectics, bulimics usually are of normal weight, although some have a history of anorexia or obesity. Like anorectics, however, they are not satisfied by normal food intake. The characteristic symptom of bulimia is episodic, uncontrollable binge eating followed by vomiting or purging. The binge eating, usually preceded by a period of dieting lasting a few months or more, occurs when patients are alone at home and lasts about one hour. In the early stages of the illness, patients may need to stimulate their throat with a finger or spoon to induce vomiting, but later they can vomit at will. At times, abrasions and bruises on the back of the hand are produced during vomiting. The binge-purge cycle is usually followed by sadness, self-deprecation, and regret. Bulimic patients have troubled interpersonal relationships, poor self-concept, a high level of anxiety and depression, and poor impulse control. Alcohol and drug abuse are not uncommon with bulimia, in contrast to their infrequency with anorexia.

From the medical perspective, bulimia is nearly as damaging to its practitioners as anorexia. Dental problems, including discoloration and erosion of tooth enamel and irritation of gums by highly acidic gastric juice, are frequent. Electrolyte imbalance, such as metabolic alkalosis or hypokalemia (low potassium levels) caused by the self-induced vomiting, is a constant threat. Parotid gland enlargement, esophageal lacerations, and acute gastric dilatation may occur. Cardiac irregularities may also result. The chronic use of emetics such as ipecac to induce vomiting after eating may result in cardiomyopathy (disease of the middle layer of the walls of the heart, the myocardium), occasionally with a fatal outcome. While their menstrual periods are irregular, these patients are seldom amenorrheic.

Treating Bulimia

The behavioral management of bulimia includes an examination of the patient's thinking and behavior toward eating and life challenges in general.

The patient is made fully aware of the extent of her binging by being asked to keep a daily record of her eating and vomiting practices. A contract is then established with the patient to help her restrict her eating to three or four planned meals per day. The second stage of treatment emphasizes self-control in eating as well as in other areas of the patient's life. In the final stage of treatment, the patient is assisted in maintaining her new, more constructive eating behaviors.

Almost all clinicians work intensively with the family of anorectic patients, particularly in the initial stage of treatment. Family treatment begins with the current family structure and later addresses the early family functioning that can influence family dynamics dramatically. Multigenerational sources of conflict are also examined.

Family therapy with bulimics explores the sources of family conflicts and helps the family to resolve them. Particular attention is directed toward gender roles in the family, as well as the anxiety of the parents in allowing their children autonomy and self-sufficiency. The roots of impulsive and depressive behaviors and the role of parental satisfaction with the patients' lives and circumstances are often explored and addressed.

OBESITY

Another eating disorder, obesity, is the most prevalent nutritional disorder of the Western world. Using the most commonly accepted definition of obesity—a body weight greater than 20 percent above an individual's normal or desirable weight—approximately 35 percent of adults in the United States were considered obese in the early 1990's. This figure represents twice the proportion of the population that was obese in 1900. Evidently, more sedentary lifestyles strongly contributed to this increase, since the average caloric intake of the population decreased by 5 percent since 1910. Although the problem affects both sexes, obesity is found in a larger portion of women than men. In the forty- to forty-nine-year-old age group, 40 percent of women, while only 30 percent of men, were found to meet the criterion for obesity. Prevalence of obesity increases with both age and lower socioeconomic status.

While results of both animal and human studies suggest that obesity is genetically influenced to some degree, most human obesity is reflective of numerous influences and conditions. Evidence indicates that the relationship between caloric intake and adipose tissue is not as straightforward as had been assumed. In the light of this evidence, the failure to lose unwanted pounds and the failure to maintain hard-won weight loss experienced by many dieters seem much more understandable. In the past, obese individuals often were viewed pejoratively by others and by themselves. They were seen as having insufficient willpower and self-discipline. It was incorrectly assumed that it is no more difficult for most obese individuals to lose fat by decreasing caloric intake than it is for individuals in a normal weight range and that it would be just as easy for the obese to maintain normal weight as it is for those who have never been obese.

Treating Obesity

In the treatment of obesity, the use of a reduced-calorie diet regimen alone does not appear to be an effective approach for many patients, and it is believed that clinicians may do more harm than good by prescribing it. In addition to the high number of therapeutic failures and possible exacerbation of the problem, negative emotional responses are common side effects. Depression, anxiety, irritability, and preoccupation with food appear to be associated with dieting. Such responses have been found to occur in as many as half of the general obese population while on weight-loss diets and are seen with even greater frequency in the severely obese.

Some researchers conclude that some cases are better off with no treatment. Their reasoning is based not only on the ineffectiveness of past treatments and the evidence of biological bases for differences in body size but also on the fact that mild to moderate obesity does not appear to put women (or men) at significant health risk. Moreover, an increase in the incidence of serious eating disorders in women has accompanied the increasingly stringent cultural standards of thinness for women. Given the present level of knowledge, it may be that some individuals would benefit most by adjusting to a weight that is higher than the culturally determined ideal.

When an individual of twenty-five to thirty-four years of age is more than 100 percent above normal weight level, however, there is a twelvefold increase in mortality, and the need for treatment is clear. Although much of the increased risk is related to the effects of extreme overweight on other diseases (such as diabetes, hypertension, and arthritis), these risks can decrease with weight loss. Conservative treatments have had very poor success rates with this group, both in achieving weight reduction and in maintaining any reductions accomplished. Inpatient starvation therapy has had some success in reducing weight in the severely obese but is a disruptive, expensive, and risky procedure requiring very careful medical monitoring to avoid fatality. Furthermore, for those patients who successfully reduce their weight by this method, only about half will maintain the reduction.

Severe obesity seems to be treated most effectively by surgical measures, which include wiring the jaws to make oral intake nearly impossible, reducing the size of the stomach by suturing methods, or short-circuiting a portion of the intestine so as to reduce the area available for uptake of nutrients. None of these methods, however, is without risk.

—Genevieve Slomski

See also Addiction; Anorexia nervosa; Children's health issues; Depression; Depression in children; Infertility in women; Malnutrition among children; Menstruation; Nutrition and aging; Nutrition and children; Nutrition and women; Obesity; Obesity and aging; Obesity and children; Recovery programs; Stress; Weight changes with aging; Weight loss medications; Women's health issues.

For Further Information:

Brownell, Kelly D., and Christopher G. Fairburn, eds. *Eating Disorders and Obesity: A Comprehensive Handbook*. New York: Guilford Press, 1995. This text addresses all eating disorders, particularly obesity. Includes references and an index.

Garner, David M., and Paul E. Garfinkel, eds. *Handbook of Treatment for Eating Disorders*. 2d ed. New York: Guilford Press, 1997. This is an updated source on the diagnosis, assessment, and treatment of eating disorders, as well as key issues associated with developing eating disorders.

Hsu, L. K. George. *Eating Disorders*. New York: Guilford Press, 1990. The work provides a summary of the knowledge about the eating disorders of anorexia and bulimia, a historical development of the concepts, their clinical features, methods of diagnostic evaluation, and various treatment options.

Moe, Barbara. *Understanding the Causes of a Negative Body Image*. New York: Rosen, 1999. Designed for students in grades seven and above, who are bombarded by misinformation and media images of the perfect young adult, this book looks at the causes behind a negative body image and stresses that self-esteem is more important than personal size.

Monroe, Judy. *Understanding Weight-Loss Programs*. New York: Rosen, 1999. Designed for students in grades seven and above, who are bombarded by misinformation and media images of the perfect young adult, this book makes it clear that most weight-loss programs are shams and should be viewed with a critical eye.

✧ Elder abuse

Type of issue: Elder health, ethics, mental health, social trends

Definition: A form of domestic violence against the elderly, including neglect and verbal, psychological, physical, economic, and sexual abuse, often committed by their primary caregivers.

Social gerontologists and other professionals who study and work with older persons report that the prevalence of elder abuse is much greater than was previously realized and that it takes multiple forms. Neglect and verbal, psychological, physical, economic, and sexual abuse do not typically occur at the hands of strangers or in unfamiliar surroundings. More often, the perpetrators of elder abuse are the primary caretakers or neighbors of the victims, and the setting is the victims' own homes, neighborhoods, or institutions charged with their care. Researchers, social workers, medical professionals, and law-enforcement officials have agreed that documented cases of elder abuse represent a small proportion of all such incidents, which are increasing in frequency.

ABUSE BY FAMILY CARETAKERS

The phrase "graying of America" alludes to the fact that the fastest-growing American age group is the sixty-five-and-over population and that the category of Americans older than eighty-five has the fastest growth rate of all. As Americans become ever older, the probability of their experiencing a degree of physiological or cognitive dysfunction that makes them dependent on others for their care increases. Members of any age group who depend on others for survival are the most likely targets of domestic abuse. The infirm elderly are the most often abused; they typically become more submissive to protect themselves from abandonment by their family caretakers.

Although the prevalence of elder abuse, as with other forms of domestic violence, is impossible to assess accurately, of greatest concern are cases involving perpetrators closely related to the victims. Not only is the specter of abuse by a family member, as opposed to a stranger, especially disturbing, but a majority of incidents occur in domestic settings. The number of documented cases of domestic elder abuse, a mere fraction of real existing instances of the problem, is increasing geometrically. Between 1986 and 1994, officially reported cases steadily increased from 117,000 to 241,000. Most cases go unreported, and 70 percent or more of documented cases are reported by someone other than the victim. Estimates of the actual number of such cases range between one and two million annually.

Data from the 1990's show that substantiated cases of reported domestic elder abuse took every form imaginable. Neglect accounted for 58.5 percent of these cases, physical abuse 15.7 percent, financial exploitation 12.3 percent, psychological and emotional abuse 8.1 percent, and sexual abuse 0.5 percent. These same data indicate that close relatives of the victims are responsible for two-thirds of the cases. Perpetrators were victims' adult children in about 38 percent of the reports, spouses in about 14 percent, and other family members in about 15 percent.

Sociologists assert that, given the strong cultural normative prescriptions for intergenerational support and affection, domestic elder abuse constitutes a violation of a social taboo—the most serious category of social infractions. This form of deviant behavior is difficult to analyze because of the complexity of its causes. Researchers who attempt to understand such dysfunctional behavior in family settings contend that like all forms of domestic violence, the causes involve a combination of psychological, social, economic, and health-related characteristics of the perpetrators and the victims.

In some cases, the stress associated with caring for an infirm elderly family member may lead to abuse, especially if the caregiver perceives the demands on time, energy, and financial resources as excessive or if the caregiver is not well prepared for the task. Some studies have found that the incidence of abuse increases when the continued physical or mental decline of the older person heightens the caretaker's responsibilities. Some domestic elder abuse is related to the perpetrator's personal problems, such as chronic financial difficulties, pathological emotional or mental conditions, or addiction to alcohol or other drugs. In these cases, the abuser is often dependent on the victim for financial support and housing, and the frustration of failing to function as an independent adult manifests itself in abusive episodes. Furthermore, some researchers report that abusers who have experienced or witnessed domestic violence in their households as children may have learned to abuse in response to conflicts or stress, resulting in an intergenerational transfer of violence. Complex combinations of these and other possible factors underlie each individual case of domestic elder abuse.

ABUSE IN INSTITUTIONAL SETTINGS

Although only about 5 percent of older Americans reside in nursing and convalescent homes, they represent half of the long-term-care patients. As the eighty-five-and-over population continues to increase, the population of institutionalized older Americans is projected to grow from 1.5 million in 1990 to 2.6 million by the year 2020. The risk of abuse is especially high for this group of elderly Americans. Physicians have often recommended institutionalization as a way to prevent or stop abuse, but a potential for serious abuse in these settings has been demonstrated.

Assessing the prevalence of elder abuse in health care settings is difficult. Studies in which nursing home staff were assured of confidentiality and anonymity, however, have shown that a problem does exist. In one such study involving almost six hundred nursing home workers, 45 percent said that they had yelled at, cursed, or threatened residents; 10 percent admitted physically abusing patients by hitting, pinching, or violently grabbing them; another 3 percent stated that they had hit patients with objects or thrown objects at them; and 4 percent had denied patients food or privileges. Such research efforts have probably underestimated levels of abuse by paid caregivers, and none are likely to produce reliable results regarding sexual abuse and theft.

ADULT PROTECTIVE SERVICES

A number of public agencies include elder abuse among their concerns: police and sheriffs' departments, district attorneys' offices, acute-care licensing and certification agencies, and State Long-Term Care Ombudsman's offices, which were created by the federal Older Americans Act of 1965 and organized under State Agencies on Aging to investigate elder abuse in nursing homes. However, the agencies most responsible for investigating, intervening in, and resolving cases of domestic elder abuse in most states are Adult Protective Services (APS), which are usually part of the county departments of social services. Although APS offices deal with abuse of anyone older than eighteen, 70 percent of their cases involve elder abuse.

APS responses to elder abuse have varied according to the severity and nature of the abuse. The problem is often addressed by APS caseworkers with a plan to provide assistance to family caregivers by linking them to public service, volunteer, and church-related agencies that assist in caregiving functions and even counsel abusive family caretakers. Caseworkers monitor caregiving plans to determine their effectiveness and the need for adjustments. In the most severe cases, the APS offices take more drastic measures, such as institutionalizing elderly persons or calling in law enforcement agencies. In cases requiring institutionalization, the State Long-Term Care Ombudsman program is often called upon to monitor the safety of abuse victims.

APS faces great challenges in its attempts to prevent future abuse and improve the quality of life of abuse victims. Investigators' interactions with family members are usually tense at best, because elder abuse, like spousal and child abuse, is often a well-kept family secret. Furthermore, caseworkers are prohibited from revealing the identities of the persons who report abuse, which often frustrates the families, and the interventions sometimes confuse the victims because they seldom report the abuse themselves.

Not all APS elder abuse cases are successfully resolved. Agency intervention in cases involving chronic domestic violence, regardless of the victims' ages, is especially difficult. Moreover, elder abuse intervention is often thwarted because older persons, unlike children, are beyond the age of majority and can thus refuse assistance if they fear institutionalization, abandonment, or retribution. APS caseworkers must be able to investigate cases, assess victims' physical and psychological health, know about available elder services, work within the criminal justice system, deal with crisis situations, and protect themselves from violence at the hands of abusers. There are only a few thousand APS investigators in the United States, and their large caseloads are growing constantly.

CRIME

Although most forms of elder abuse, including willful neglect in many states, are illegal, crimes against elderly victims committed by noncaretakers are of growing concern to law enforcement officials and older persons. Conventional analyses of crime statistics have indicated that the elderly have been far less victimized than the general adult population. There is a growing consensus, however, that these statistics have grossly underestimated the magnitude of elderly victimization. Older Americans appear to be the targets of certain types of crime, and the incidents most often occur in the victims' homes or neighborhoods. Most victims of con artists, for example, are older persons. Con games take many forms, including phony insurance schemes, hearing aid scams, medical quackery of all types, real estate swindles, and investment fraud. Moreover, elderly persons are the main victims of purse snatchers, pickpockets, and petty thieves, whereby the victims are often assaulted. The perpetrators of these attacks are most often young males who live in their victims' neighborhoods.

Another form of crime-related elder abuse stems from older persons' fear of crime, which research has indicated is the greatest single concern among older Americans. Although crime statistics indicate that the elderly are less likely than younger adults to be victims of most violent crimes, the consequences of physical abuse can be especially devastating to the aged. Young or middle-aged persons might sustain minimal injuries during an assault that would cripple older victims. Even a purse snatching can result in an older person requiring hip replacement surgery or long-term medical care for internal injuries. In addition, larceny can significantly affect the economic independence of older persons with limited and fixed incomes. Fear of crime itself compromises the quality of life of many older Americans, causing them to live reclusively, afraid to leave their homes. Furthermore, some studies have concluded that few crimes against the elderly are reported, because the victims fear retribution by neighborhood criminals and pressure from family and friends to give up living independently because of their limited ability to protect themselves.

—Jack Carter

See also Aging; Alcoholism among the elderly; Alzheimer's disease; Child abuse; Dementia; Depression in the elderly; Domestic violence; Nursing and convalescent homes.

For Further Information:

Baumhover, Lorin A., and S. Coleen Beall, eds. *Abuse, Neglect, and Exploitation of Older Persons: Strategies for Assessment and Intervention.* Baltimore: Health Professions Press, 1996. Essays focusing on the causes and nature of elder abuse, with an emphasis on responses to the problem by health-care professionals.

Byers, Bryan, and James E. Hendricks, eds. *Adult Protective Services: Research and Practice.* Springfield, Ill.: Charles C Thomas, 1993. Papers by social scientists from several disciplines examining elder abuse, highlighting the challenges facing government agencies.

Filinson, Rachel, and Stanley R. Ingman, eds. *Elder Abuse: Practice and Policy.* New York: Human Sciences Press, 1989. Contributors discuss the problem, focusing on federal and state policy responses to it.

Lustbader, Wendy, and Nancy R. Hooyman. *Taking Care of Aging Family Members.* New York: Free Press, 1994. Discusses neglect and abuse and the caregiving stress that can lead to it.

O'Connell, James J., Jean Summerfield, and F. Russell Kellogg. "The Homeless Elderly." In *Under the Safety Net: The Health and Social Welfare of the Homeless in the United States,* edited by Philip W. Brickner et al. New York: W. W. Norton, 1990. Essay examining the demographics of elderly homelessness, the problems that plague these people, and the programs designed to help them in several large American cities.

✧ ELECTRICAL SHOCK

Type of issue: Children's health, public health
Definition: The physical effect of an electrical current entering the body and the resulting damage.

Electrical shock ranges from a harmless jolt of static electricity to a power line's lethal discharge. The severity of the shock depends on the current flowing through the body, and the current is determined by the skin's electrical resistance. Dry skin has a very high resistance; thus 110 volts produces a small, harmless current. The resistance for perspiring hands, however, is lower by a factor of 100, resulting in potentially fatal currents. Because of their proximity to the heart, currents traveling between bodily extremities are particularly dangerous.

Electrical shock causes injury or death in one of three ways: paralysis of the breathing center in the brain, paralysis of the heart, or ventricular fibrillation (extremely rapid and uncontrolled twitching of the heart muscle).

The threshold of feeling (the minimum current detectable) ranges from 0.5 to 1.0 milliamperes. Currents up to 5.0 milliamperes, the maximum harmless current, are not hazardous, unless they trigger an accident by involuntary reaction. Currents in this range create a tingling sensation. The minimum current that causes muscular paralysis occurs between 10 and 15 milliamperes. Currents of this magnitude cause a painful jolt. Above 18 milliamperes, the current contracts chest muscles and breathing ceases. Unconsciousness and death follow within minutes unless the current is interrupted and respiration resumed. A short exposure to currents of 50 milliamperes causes severe pain, possible fainting, and complete exhaustion, while currents in the 100 to 300 milliampere range produce ventricular fibrillation, which is fatal unless quickly corrected. During ventricular fibrillation, the heart stops its rhythmic pumping and flutters uselessly. Since blood stops flowing, the victim dies from oxygen deprivation to the brain in a matter of minutes. This is the most common cause of death for victims of electrical shock.

Relatively high currents (above 300 milliamperes) may produce ventricular paralysis, deep burns in the body's tissue, or irreversible damage to the central nervous system. Victims are more likely to survive a large but brief current, even through smaller, sustained currents are usually lethal. Burning or charring of the skin at the point of contact may be a contributing factor to the delayed death that often follows severe electrical shock. Very high voltage discharges of short duration, such as a lightning strike, tend to disrupt the body's nervous impulses, but victims may survive. On the other hand, any electric current large enough to raise body temperature significantly produces immediate death.

TREATING ELECTRICAL SHOCK

Before medical treatment can be applied, the current must be stopped or the shock victim must be separated from the current source without being touched. Nonconducting materials such as dry, heavy blankets or pieces of wood can be used for this purpose. If the victim is not breathing, artificial respiration immediately applied provides adequate short-term life support, though the victim may become stiff or rigid in reaction to the shock. Victims of electrical shock may suffer from severe burns and permanent aftereffects, including eye cataracts, angina, or disorders of the nervous system.

Electrical shock can usually be prevented, particularly in children, by strictly adhering to safety guidelines and using commonsense precautions. Careful inspection of appliances and tools, compliance with manufacturers' safety standards, and the avoidance of unnecessary risks greatly reduce the chance of an electrical shock. Electrical appliances or tools should never be used when standing in water or on damp ground, and dry gloves, shoes, and floors provide considerable protection against dangerous shocks from 110-volt circuits.

Electrical safety is also provided by isolation, guarding, insulation, grounding, and ground fault interrupters. Isolation means that high-voltage wires strung overhead are not within reach, while guarding provides a barrier around high voltage devices, such as are found in television sets.

Old wire insulation may become brittle with age and develop small cracks. Defective wires are hazardous and should be replaced immediately. Most modern power tools are double-insulated; the motor is insulated from the plastic insulating frame. These devices do not require grounding, as no exposed metal parts become electrically live if the wire insulation fails.

In a home, grounding is accomplished by a third wire in outlets, connected through a grounding circuit to a water pipe. If an appliance plug has a third prong, it will ground the frame to the grounding circuit. In the event of a short circuit, the grounding circuit provides a low resistance path, resulting in a current surge which trips the circuit breaker.

In some instances, however, the current may be inadequate to trip a circuit breaker (which usually requires 15 or 20 amperes), but current in excess of 10 milliamperes could still be lethal to humans. A ground-fault interrupter ensures nearly complete protection by detecting leakage currents as small as 5 milliamperes and breaking the circuit. This relatively inexpensive device operates very rapidly and provides an extremely high degree of safety against electrocution in the household. Many localities now have codes which require the installation of ground-fault interrupters in bathrooms, kitchens, and other areas where water is used.

—*George R. Plitnik*

See also Burns and scalds; Children's health issues; First aid; Resuscitation; Safety issues for children.

For Further Information:

Atkinson, William. "Electric Injuries Can Be Worse than They Seem." *Electric World* 214, no. 1 (January/February, 2000): 33-36. Whether an electrical shock initially seems serious or mild, it is always a cause for concern. Aspects of electrical shock injuries are explored.

Bridges, J. E., et al., eds. *International Symposium on Electrical Shock Safety Criteria.* New York: Pergamon Press, 1985. The summary of a symposium covering the physiological effects of shock, bioelectrical conditions, and safety measures.

Hewitt, Paul G. *Conceptual Physics.* 8th ed. Reading, Mass.: Addison-Wesley, 1998. Comprehensive coverage of physics for the layperson that includes detailed discussions of the laws of electricity and electrical devices.

Liu, Lynda. "Pullout Emergency Guide: Electric Shock." *Parents* 75, no. 1 (January, 2000): 65-66. A pull-out emergency guide for the prevention and treatment of electrical shock in children. Household hazards and electricity dos and don'ts are among the tips offered.

U.S. Department of Labor. Occupational Safety and Health Administration. *Controlling Electrical Hazards.* Washington, D.C.: Government Printing Office, 1991. A report which identifies common electrical hazards and discusses their prevention.

✧ Emphysema

Type of issue: Elder health, environmental health, occupational health, public health

Definition: A lung disease characterized by increased shortness of breath on exertion, often a natural accompaniment of aging but also initiated or aggravated by cigarette smoking or a heritable specific protein deficiency.

Emphysema is one of the two major clinical conditions encompassed in the terms "chronic obstructive pulmonary disease" (COPD) and "chronic airflow obstruction" (CAO). Fourteen million individuals in the United States suffer from emphysema or the other, more frequent condition, chronic bronchitis.

Emphysema involves the lung tissue associated with the exchange of oxygen and carbon dioxide between the blood and the air. There is destruction of the walls of the alveoli, the small sacs where blood and air are in closest contact, so that permanent enlargement of the alveolar volume occurs. Clinically, patients with chronic bronchitis tend to an extreme characterized by marked decrease of oxygen in the blood, a bluish discoloration of the skin (cyanosis), and swelling of the legs (peripheral edema) as a result of heart failure. Such patients are sometimes referred to as "blue bloaters." In contrast, patients with emphysema tend to an extreme characterized by marked shortness of breath on exertion, a pinkish complexion, and little, if any, peripheral edema. Such patients are sometimes referred to as "pink puffers." Chronic bronchitis and emphysema may coexist in a given individual to a greater or lesser degree.

With the increases in life expectancy and actual longevity in the United States, the number of individuals significantly affected by emphysema can be expected to increase with time. Most older individuals show some evidence of emphysema at death. Even without emphysema, however, aging is associated with a decrease in lung or pulmonary functions such that physical activities become more limited. These normal declines in pulmonary function cannot yet be reversed or even arrested and are the result of tissue changes occurring over time. They can be markedly aggravated if emphysema, such as that caused by cigarette smoking, is superimposed on the normal processes. The life span of affected individuals may be shortened significantly.

RISK FACTORS, EPIDEMIOLOGY, AND NATURAL HISTORY

The incidence of emphysema increases with age and is much more common in men than in women. The dominant cause is cigarette smoking. The one other major identified cause is a deficiency of alpha-1 antitrypsin, a protein that inhibits the destruction of alveolar walls by enzymes. Other factors that may play significant but less certain roles are environmental pollution (including oxidants), hazardous occupations, socioeconomic status, diet, low birth weight, and severe childhood respiratory illnesses.

Although the diagnosis of emphysema is made in slightly less than 1 percent of the population, the incidence is much higher in cigarette smokers. Thus, in one study, 2.9 percent of nonsmoking males showed moderate changes associated with emphysema at autopsy, 25 percent of individuals smoking less than twenty cigarettes per day showed moderate changes, and 32.7 percent of those smoking twenty or more cigarettes per day showed such changes. Of the latter group, nearly 20 percent showed marked changes.

COPD was the fourth leading cause of death in the United States at the end of the twentieth century. Between 80 and 90 percent of the cases of COPD could be attributed to cigarette smoking. Cigarette smoking clearly limits longevity; cessation of smoking increases life expectancy and decreases the rate of decline of pulmonary functions. One measure of pulmonary function is the volume of air that can be expelled forcibly from the lungs in one second after a maximal inspiratory effort. This measure normally peaks at age twenty-five and decreases to 75 percent of the value at age twenty-five when age seventy-five is reached. In those individuals whose pulmonary functions are affected by cigarette smoking, the measure drops to about 75 percent at age forty-five. If smoking continues, the life expectancy falls to well below seventy-five years. If smokers stop at about age fifty, however, the deterioration is slowed and their life expectancy is increased, although they may show significant disability by age seventy-five or eighty. Cessation of smoking beyond the age of fifty, for example at sixty-five, is associated with lesser benefits because much damage

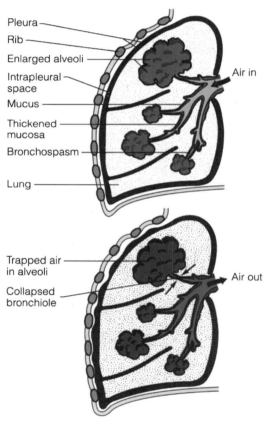

In emphysema, the body releases enzymes in response to inhaling irritants in the air, such as cigarette smoke; these enzymes reduce the lung's elasticity, compromising the bronchioles' ability to expand and contract normally. Air becomes trapped in the alveoli upon inhalation (top) and cannot escape upon exhalation (bottom). Over time, breathing becomes extremely difficult. (Hans & Cassidy, Inc.)

has already been done and there is superposition of the damage caused by cigarette smoking on the changes occurring with age.

Of major importance to the cigarette smoker is the number of cigarettes smoked, calculated as pack years (number of packs of cigarettes smoked per day times the number of years the individual has smoked). For smokers with twenty-one to forty pack years, pulmonary function declines to about 90 percent of the predicted value for that age. For smokers with sixty-one or more pack years, it declines to less than 80 percent of the predicted value.

Not all smokers are so affected. Indeed, 10 to 15 percent of smokers escape the effects mentioned, for reasons unknown. That some smokers are affected so much more than others might stem from intrinsic sensitivity of the airways, effects in childhood of environmental pollution or passive smoking, genetic factors, or manner of smoking (for example, whether they inhale deeply).

FUNCTIONAL AND TISSUE CHANGES

The patient with emphysema is generally thin, may purse the lips during expiration, is older (fifty to seventy-five years of age), and experiences increased limitation of exercise tolerance because of shortness of breath (dyspnea on exertion). This portrait is in contrast with the patient with chronic bronchitis, who has a chronic cough, excessive sputum production, and cyanosis at forty to fifty-five years of age. Chest radiographs (X rays) and computed tomography (CT) and magnetic resonance imaging (MRI) scans typically show that the patient with emphysema has a small heart, an increased lung and chest volume, lowering and flattening of the diaphragm, and areas of radiolucency (indicating decreased lung tissue density) and large bubbles or bullae (indicating the absence of any lung tissue in those areas). The patient with chronic bronchitis, in contrast, may show increased markings indicating changes in the walls of the bronchial airways and of vascular engorgement.

Pulmonary function tests (PFTs) in patients with emphysema typically show marked increases in lung volumes, particularly the total lung capacity (essentially the maximal air content) and the residual air volume (RV), the volume remaining after full expiration. The RV is an indicator of air trapped because of airway closure. The rate of flow in expiration is decreased. The elastic recoil, the driving pressure of the lungs during expiration, is decreased because of tissue changes. The action of the diaphragm is also decreased because these muscles are flattened instead of being domed and cannot move as freely as in normal individuals. In addition, because of the destruction of lung tissue there is a reduction in the pulmonary diffusing capacity, which indicates that the rate of exchanges of oxygen between the air and the blood in the pulmonary vessels is reduced. The lungs must work at a mechanical disadvantage so that with the decrease of alveolar ventilation, the work of breathing and oxygen consumption are increased. With the destruction of lung tissue, the surface of the lungs available for gas exchanges is decreased. So while the demand for oxygen is increased, the delivery is decreased, particularly during exertion.

The tissue changes in cigarette smokers differ somewhat from those observed in patients with alpha-1 antitrypsin deficiency. In the former, the respiratory bronchioles are mainly affected, with relatively normal alveolar ducts and alveoli. The bronchioles widen and may fuse. In the latter, the alveolar walls are destroyed more uniformly throughout the lungs, so that mainly vascular, bronchial, and supporting structures are left. In both types of emphysema, proteases, enzymes that degrade structural proteins such as collagen and particularly elastin, overwhelm their inhibitors such as the antitrypsins. In cigarette smokers, the inflammatory response to the irritants in smoke is associated with macrophages (scavenger cells) and neutrophils, cells that respond to inflammation and produce proteases which not only attack tissues but also destroy antiproteases. Individuals with antiprotease deficiency have impaired defense mechanisms and are at greater risk of serious damage. Emphysema can be considered to occur as the result of imbalance between proteases and antiproteases. The resultant irreversible tissue changes in the peripheral parts of the lungs lead to overinflation of the alveolar air sacs and in turn may lead to compression of some of the remaining unaffected lung tissue.

PREVENTION AND TREATMENT

In cigarette smokers, the single most effective treatment is cessation of smoking. In most cases, cessation will slow the decline in respiratory functions and in exercise tolerance. The best prevention is discouraging young individuals from ever starting to smoke. Only 10 to 15 percent of cigarette smokers develop emphysema, and relatively few of them have alpha-1 antitrypsin deficiency. Nevertheless, abolition of cigarette smoking could have not only major health benefits but also major economic benefits in reducing the costs of care for an aging population already faced with declining respiratory function and exercise tolerance.

Other recognized measures for the treatment of emphysema include long-term supplemental oxygen administration as needed, bronchodilators, corticosteroids when airway inflammatory changes are present, antibiotics for infections, and diuretics and vasodilators for heart failure. Physical training programs and mechanically assisted ventilation can be extremely helpful. In patients with homozygous alpha-1 antitrypsin deficiency, replacement therapy with the purified protein should be considered.

Controlled clinical trials employing the surgical reduction of lung volume began in 1997 under the joint auspices of the National Institutes of Health (NIH) and the Health Care Financing Administration. This approach is based on the fact that the overinflation of the lungs is not uniform throughout the organs. It had been suggested in the 1950's that surgical removal of the overinflated areas could improve pulmonary functions by permitting more normal positioning of the diaphragm and increasing elastic recoil. Early attempts in this direction were associated with marked subjective improvement in some patients, but the overall postoperative morbidity and mortality were very high. More recently, improved surgical techniques and intensive care procedures have resulted in better clinical results. However, the criteria for application of the procedure, the short-term benefits, and the long-term outcomes, together with cost-benefit considerations, have not yet been evaluated fully. The prospects for the controlled program, undertaken at nineteen centers in the United States, are encouraging.

Emphysema will remain a major issue in an aging population for many years. Probably the most effective means of limiting the problem will be cessation of smoking for those who do smoke and efforts to discourage younger generations from ever smoking at all.

—*Francis P. Chinard*

See also Cancer; Illnesses among the elderly; Lung cancer; Smoking.

FOR FURTHER INFORMATION:
Cherniack, N. S. *Chronic Obstructive Pulmonary Disease.* Philadelphia: W. B. Saunders, 1991.
Fishman, Alfred P., ed. *Fishman's Pulmonary Diseases and Disorders.* 3d ed. 2 vols. New York: McGraw-Hill, 1998.
Haas, François, and Sheila Sperber Haas. *The Chronic Bronchitis and Emphysema Handbook.* Rev. and expanded ed. New York: John Wiley & Sons, 2000.
Jenkins, Mark. *Chronic Obstructive Pulmonary Disease: Practical, Medical, and Spiritual Guidelines for Daily Living with Emphysema, Chronic Bronchitis, and Combination Diagnosis.* Center City, Minn.: Hazelden Information Education, 1999.
Staton, G. W., and R. H. Ingram. "Chronic Obstructive Diseases of the Lungs." In *Scientific American Medicine,* edited by D. C. Dale and D. D. Federman. New York: Scientific American, 1998.

✧ ENDOMETRIOSIS

Type of issue: Women's health
Definition: A condition in which the endometrial tissue that lines the uterus grows in other parts of the body; it affects many women during their reproductive years, seriously impairing all aspects of their quality of life and sometimes resulting in infertility.

Endometriosis is a condition in which the endometrial tissue of the uterus grows into other parts of the body, usually into the ovaries, pelvic cavity, intestines, or bladder but occasionally in more distant locations such as the lungs. Like the uterine lining, this endometrial tissue also responds to the hormonal changes of the menstrual cycle. The blood and cells that are sloughed off by this tissue cannot leave the body during menstruation, and the results can be internal bleeding, the formation of cysts, and the creation of scar tissue. The primary symptom of endometriosis is intense pain connected with the menstrual cycle, particularly during ovulation and menstruation, but other symptoms include intestinal problems and infertility.

The cause of endometriosis is not fully known. One theory associates it with a backward reflux of the menstrual flow, which permits endometrial tissue to attach and grow on other organs in the abdomen. Other theories connect endometriosis with hormonal problems or with an abnormal response by the immune system. Another suggestion is the dispersal of endometrial cells through the blood or lymph systems. Most likely, a combination of these and other elements causes this condition.

Endometriosis is difficult to diagnose because only exploratory abdominal surgery can offer a definitive diagnosis. Such surgery is usually done by laparoscopy, in which a fiber-optic tube inserted into the abdomen allows the physician to view the pelvic organs directly. The successful treatment of endometriosis is even more difficult since the underlying causes of this condition are poorly understood. The two primary approaches are hormonal therapy and surgery. Because the growth of endometrial tissue responds to sex hormones, various kinds of hormonal treatment may improve the condition. Surgery can also be used to remove the tissue. New techniques such as laser laparoscopy are less invasive. In extreme cases, however, a hysterectomy (the removal of the uterus), often with the removal of the Fallopian tubes and the ovaries as well, may be indicated.

Statistical information about endometriosis is hard to obtain because of the difficulty of diagnosis and the fairly recent acceptance within the medical community of the seriousness of this condition. It is estimated that at least five million women suffer from endometriosis during their reproductive years. The condition has been associated in the medical literature and the popular mind with white, educated, career-oriented women in their twenties and thirties. In fact, endometriosis occurs in women of all races, economic levels, and ages from puberty to the menopause. Many women are severely disabled because of endometriosis. The disease often restricts their ability to bear children, and it may substantially limit their productive capacity in a working environment. Increasingly, especially through the educational and lobbying efforts of the Endometriosis Association in the United States and similar organizations in other countries, the myths about endometriosis are being dispelled. Ongoing research into the causes and treatment of endometriosis will improve the outlook and relieve the physical pain and psychological stigma associated with this major problem in women's health.

—Karen Gould

See also Cervical, ovarian, and uterine cancers; Hysterectomy; Menstruation; Women's health issues.

FOR FURTHER INFORMATION:
Ballweg, Mary Lou, with Endometriosis Association. *The Endometriosis Sourcebook.* NTC/Contemporary, 1995. Provides information about research; surgical and medical treatments; alternative treatments; common myths about the disease; pregnancy, labor, and postpartum experiences of women with endometriosis; and advice for coping physically and emotionally.
Phillips, Robert H., and Glenda J. Motta. *Coping with Endometriosis: A Practical Guide to Understanding, Treating, and Living with Chronic Endometriosis.* Los Angeles: Jeremy P. Tarcher, 2000. In addition to the latest research on treatment of endometriosis, this book addresses the psychological and emotional concerns brought on by its diagnosis.
Venturini, Pier Luigi, and Johannes L. H. Evers, eds. *Endometriosis: Basic Research and Clinical Practice.* New York: Parthenon, 1999. Contains important information for clinicians treating endometriosis patients with pain or infertility problems. Covers the basic aspects of epidemiology, pathogenesis, and immunology, then clinical appearance, infertility and pelvic pain, medical treatment by endocrine modulation, and new methods of surgical treatment.
Weinstein, Kate. *Living with Endometriosis.* Reading, Mass.: Addison-Wesley, 1987. The main divisions of this handy book are medical aspects, treatments and outcomes, emotional problems, and pain and psychiatric problems.

✧ ENVIRONMENTAL DISEASES

Type of issue: Environmental health, public health
Definition: A wide variety of conditions and diseases resulting from largely human-mediated hazards in both the natural and humanmade (for example, home and workplace) environments; an area of special concern given rapid environmental degradation during the twentieth century.

Almost any condition except those of purely genetic origin could be considered as environmentally caused or having an environmental component, but the term "environmental disease" is usually applied to the effects of human alterations in the physical environment and excludes transmissible disease caused by pathogenic organisms, except in cases where human alteration of the environment is an important factor in epidemiology. Health hazards generally classed as environmental include air and water (including groundwater) pollution, toxic wastes, lead, asbestos, pesticides and herbicides, ionizing and nonionizing radiation, noise, and light.

AIR AND WATER POLLUTION

In the United States, the Clean Air Act of 1970 established maximum levels for sulfur and nitrogen dioxide, particulates, hydrocarbons, ozone, and carbon monoxide—the most common air pollutants of concern in urban environments. Even with increasingly stringent controls on emissions from automobiles and industry, air quality in urban areas frequently does not meet minimum standards. Carbon monoxide lowers the oxygen-carrying capacity of the blood, nitrogen and sulfur dioxide react with water to form acids which damage lung tissue, ozone damages tissue directly, and particulates may accumulate in the lungs. The result is decreased lung capacity and function.

Indoor air quality poses additional concerns. Emphasis on energy efficiency in building design decreases air exchange. Carpets and furniture release organic compounds, and cleaning solvents leave a volatile residue. Formaldehyde from foam stuffing and insulation inhibits liver function and is a suspected carcinogen. Breathing in an enclosed space decreases atmospheric oxygen and increases carbon dioxide. In some areas, radioactive radon gas released by the soil becomes concentrated in buildings. A ventilation system which draws its air from a polluted outdoor environment, such as a loading dock, will fail to perform its function. Secondhand cigarette smoke poses the same hazards of emphysema and lung cancer to people chronically exposed to it in an enclosed environment as to the smokers themselves. The phenomenon known as sick building syndrome, in which large numbers of people in one building complain of respiratory illness, headaches, and impaired concentration, results from a combination of these factors.

Inhalation of asbestos fibers carries a high risk of developing lung cancer after an interval of twenty or thirty years, a connection first established among shipyard workers. Between 1940 and 1970, asbestos was used extensively in public buildings as insulation. It is estimated that three to five million workers in the United States were exposed to unacceptably high levels of airborne fibers during this period, and millions of people continue to be exposed when building materials deteriorate. Asbestos abatement adds considerably to the cost of renovating old public buildings.

A category of severe lung disease affects workers in environments with a high concentration of particulate matter in the air: black lung disease, from coal dust in coal mines; silicosis, from fine rock powder in mines; and byssinosis, from textile fibers in spinning and weaving mills. The result of long-term breathing of particulates is obstruction and emphysema, which may be fatal.

Lead additives in gasoline were once a significant source of atmospheric lead, but they are being phased out; unfortunately, they leave a permanent residue in soils of high-traffic areas. Levels of 20 micrograms per deciliter of lead in the blood inhibit hemoglobin production, slow the transmission of nerve impulses, and are suspected of causing cognitive impairment in children; higher levels cause anemia, weakness, stomach pains, and nervous system impairment. Even levels below 5 micrograms may be hazardous to children. Because of lead in the paint and plumbing in old houses and soil contamination, blood lead levels high enough to cause developmental impairment in children occur frequently in older parts of cities; low-income residents are most likely to be at risk.

Mercury, another metallic neurotoxin, is introduced into water in small amounts through industrial effluent but becomes concentrated in the food chain, where it poses a hazard to people who eat large quantities of fish. Any waterborne pollutant that is not rapidly degraded has the potential for being concentrated in the food chain. Shellfish, which filter nutrients from seawater, can concentrate toxins. The most notorious cause of shellfish poisoning is a naturally occurring neurotoxic alga, but polychlorinated biphenyls (PCBs) and pesticides have also been implicated. Some metals, including lead, arsenic, and mercury, remain toxic indefinitely and are exceedingly difficult to remove from an environment into which they have been introduced.

Urban drinking water in industrialized countries is monitored for hazardous contaminants; there is some question as to whether chlorine and fluoride, added for legitimate health reasons, are completely without negative effects. Well water in irrigated agricultural areas may have high levels of nitrates, which decrease blood oxygen and have been implicated in miscarriages and birth defects.

TOXIC WASTES, RADIATION, AND OTHER HAZARDS

Organic chemical compounds make up 60 percent of the hazardous wastes generated by industry. This category includes PCBs (including dioxin), chlorofluorocarbons (CFCs), phthalate esters, chlorinated benzenes, chloromethanes, solvents (such as benzene and carbon tetrachloride), plasticizers, fire retardants, pesticides, and herbicides. Many are acutely toxic—dioxin is one of the most potent toxins known—and require elaborate precautions to prevent worker exposure or accidental contamination of foodstuffs. PCBs, which are used in a wide variety of manufacturing processes, have been shown to cause cancer and reproductive disorders in laboratory animals and have been linked to these conditions in humans. The herbicide 2,4,5-T, the defoliant Agent Orange used during the Vietnam War, is the subject of continuing claims against the manufacturer and the Veterans Administration by soldiers who later developed neurological symptoms, immune disorders, or cancer or who had children with birth defects.

The burial of toxic by-products of manufacturing processes in landfills has created an ongoing environmental health crisis as containers rupture and chemicals leach into the surrounding soil. Underground fuel storage tanks pose a similar problem. Toxins leached from a waste dump eventually enter streams and become disseminated or, if volatile, enter the atmosphere. Residents of the infamous Love Canal site in New York State were made ill by fumes from contaminated soil and groundwater.

Exposure to industrial solvents has been a significant source of workplace illness. Among the most dangerous solvents are benzene, used in a variety of processes and produced as a by-product in the coking industry; vinyl chloride, used in plastics manufacture; and formaldehyde. All these chemicals are carcinogenic.

High energy from X-ray sources and radioactive materials is termed "ionizing" because such radiation can cause chemical changes in molecules, including genetic material. Chronic exposure to ionizing radiation poses a high risk of cancer, inheritable mutations, and fetal malformation. Exposure may be occupational, as with workers in the nuclear power industry or hospital radiology laboratories. Some radioactive by-products of nuclear weapons testing and reactor accidents (such as strontium 90 or carbon 14) are exceptionally hazardous because they are structurally incorporated into living tissue and become concentrated in the food chain. The by-products of the nuclear reactor accident in Chernobyl, Ukraine, in 1987 were disseminated across international boundaries and will continue to endanger the health of millions of people in Belarus, Ukraine, and Eastern Europe. Whether widespread atmospheric testing of nuclear weapons in the 1950's caused radiation damage in the population at large is unknown; military personnel involved in the testing and inhabitants of the regions near test sites report increased rates of suspected radiation-induced illness.

Hazards of nonionizing radiation (visible, ultraviolet, infrared, or microwave) are less well established. Intense visible light can damage vision. Artificial lighting is known to disrupt reproductive cycles in plants and invertebrates and could have subtle effects on human biology. That the level of microwave radiation to which the public at large is inadvertently exposed is well below levels known to produce adverse effects is not completely reassuring. Ultraviolet light, principally from sunlight, is a factor in skin cancer, which is increasing both because of the popularity of sunbathing and because ozone depletion increases ultraviolet exposure.

Electromagnetic fields produced by power lines and electrical devices are an area of increasing controversy as electricity becomes more ubiquitous.

One study found a higher-than-average rate of childhood leukemia near high-tension power lines; other studies have failed to confirm this finding. Women who work constantly at video display terminals have somewhat higher miscarriage rates than other office workers.

SOCIETAL INTERVENTION

It is notoriously difficult to prove that an illness has an environmental cause. Suspicion arises when epidemiological statistics on reportable illnesses show that some condition known to be influenced by environmental factors—such as cancer, endocrine disorders, reproductive disorders, or immunodeficiency—occurs at an unusually high frequency in some subset of the population, occurs in a restricted geographical area, or is increasing throughout the general population.

The time interval between exposure and illness can be as long as twenty or thirty years, during which the exposed population may have dispersed and may no longer be readily identifiable. Subtle effects such as mild immunosuppression or cognitive impairment may escape detection or be dismissed as psychosomatic. Multiple environmental, behavioral, and even genetic factors are often involved, confounding efforts to pinpoint a cause. In the United States and Western Europe, high rates of exposure to pollutants are correlated with poverty and thus with higher-than-normal rates of malnutrition, alcohol and drug abuse, and inadequate access to health care. Tobacco smoking is a common confounding behavioral factor in environmental diagnosis. Where liability is involved, there are powerful financial incentives on the side of disproving the environmental or occupational linkage.

When a new technology or chemical is introduced, regulations in most countries require an assessment of health impact, which includes experimentation with animal models and risk assessment to determine the probable impact on the human population. Animal experimentation is most effective at demonstrating short-term and acute effects of toxic materials, but it is poor at demonstrating effects of long-term, low-level exposure. Risk assessment must take into consideration unusually susceptible individuals (pregnant women, for example), deliberate or accidental overexposure, and synergistic effects. In the realm of environmental legislation, risk assessment is also influenced by psychology; people are more willing to accept familiar risks over which they have personal control.

The increase in the proportion of morbidity and mortality attributable to environmental factors in the late twentieth century was the result not only of the exponential increase in energy use and the output of complex synthetic chemicals but also of changing demographics. Effects of low-level exposure to toxins may take decades to produce disease and may never become apparent in populations with a low life expectancy. In developing countries, where environmental protection is rudimentary and life expectancies are increasing rapidly, the adverse health effects of environmental degradation are particularly visible.

In the United States, specific legislation addresses compensation for miners, asbestos workers, and other specific victims of exposure to hazardous materials. On a worldwide basis, monitoring of hazardous substances is a prime concern of the World Health Organization.

—*Martha Sherwood-Pike*

See also Allergies; Asbestos; Asthma; Birth defects; Cancer; Chlorination; Chronic fatigue syndrome; Fluoridation of water sources; Food irradiation; Food poisoning; Frostbite; Genetically engineered foods; Hazardous waste; Heat exhaustion and heat stroke; Holistic medicine; Lead poisoning; Lice, mites, and ticks; Lung cancer; Lyme disease; Mad cow disease; Mercury poisoning; Multiple chemical sensitivity syndrome; Noise pollution; Occupational health; Parasites; Pesticides; Plague; Poisoning; Poisonous plants; Radiation; Radon; Seasonal affective disorder (SAD); Secondhand smoke; Sick building syndrome; Skin cancer; Skin disorders with aging; Smog; Smoking; Snakebites; Sunburns; Water quality; Worms; Zoonoses.

For Further Information:

Cooper, M. G., ed. *Risk: Man-Made Hazards to Man*. Oxford, England: Clarendon Press, 1985. A book about how people perceive and assess risks, factors that affect environmental legislation. In addition to a discussion of statistics and the effects of publicity, this British publication adopts a conservative view that hazards are often overstated.

Greenberg, Michael R., ed. *Public Health and the Environment: The United States Experience*. New York: Guilford Press, 1987. This text explores modern environmental problems from the point of view of public health. Part 1, a survey of the contribution of the environment to disease, includes sections on worker health and lifestyle as a factor in chronic disease.

National Research Council. Committee on Environmental Epidemiology. *Public Health and Hazardous Wastes*. Vol. 1 in *Environmental Epidemiology*. Washington, D.C.: National Academy Press, 1991. The report of a committee assigned to investigate the question of whether the federal hazardous waste programs in the United States actually protect human health. Reviews agencies and the methodologies of exposure assessment, the extent of the problem in the United States, and specific examples of hazardous wastes in air, groundwater, soil, and food. Includes charts and maps summarizing data and extensive bibliographies. A lengthy glossary is provided. A good factual reference on many aspects of environmental health.

Rom, William N., ed. *Environmental and Occupational Medicine*. 2d ed. Boston: Little, Brown, 1992. The emphasis in this textbook is on industrial occupational safety, with approximately a third of the work devoted to the diagnosis and pathology of occupational lung diseases, including byssinosis and black lung disease. The effects of acute and chronic exposure to heavy metals, solvents, and other toxic substances are organized by agent. Intended as a guide for medical practitioners treating patients with environmental illnesses and as a guide to the prevention of exposure for professionals concerned with workplace safety.

Steenland, Kyle, and David A. Savits. *Topics in Environmental Epidemiology.* New York: Oxford University Press, 1997. A comprehensive survey of the epidemiology of common environmental exposures, this volume covers diet, water, particulates in outdoor air, nitrogen dioxide, ozone, environmental tobacco smoke, radon in homes, electromagnetic fields, and lead.

✧ Epidemics

Type of issue: Environmental health, epidemics
Definition: Incidences of contagious, often widespread disease in human populations.

An epidemic is characterized by a large increase in the frequency of a disease within a population. Until relatively recently, the term was used primarily for outbreaks of contagious diseases caused by infectious agents, but current epidemiology also concerns itself with environmentally caused diseases, such as radiation-induced cancers, and with mental and behavioral problems, such as drug use. Outbreaks of diseases in plants and animals are also loosely termed epidemics but are more properly termed epiphytotics and epizootics, respectively.

The defining characteristic of an epidemic is not the absolute frequency of the disease or its severity, but the abrupt increase in its frequency. In contrast, an endemic disease is one whose frequency within a population does not vary markedly with time. An epidemic may be local in scope and limited in its effects; an endemic disease may be widespread and an important source of mortality within a population.

The extreme case is a pandemic, an epidemic which transcends national boundaries and affects huge numbers of individuals on a worldwide basis. The most notorious pandemics in recorded history were the bubonic plague that swept Eurasia in the fourteenth century, killing an estimated one-third of the population of Europe, and the influenza epidemic of 1918-1919, which killed approximately 20 million people worldwide. The acquired immunodeficiency syndrome (AIDS) epidemic, not recognized in the United States and Europe as a major public health threat until the early 1980's, has reached pandemic status; because of its predominantly sexual mode of transmission and relatively low infectivity, however, the number of infected individuals is far lower than would be the case for a disease transmitted by casual contact.

Pathogens and Populations

The nature and severity of an epidemic of infectious disease are influenced by the nature of the pathogen and by the physical and social makeup of the affected population. Characteristics of the pathogen include transmissibility (the ease with which a pathogen is passed from one host to another), infectivity (its ability to grow and multiply in that host), pathogenicity (its ability to produce clinical disease), and virulence (the severity of the disease produced). The worst epidemic diseases, such as smallpox, are highly transmissible, infective, pathogenic, and virulent. Chickenpox is highly transmissible and infective but not very virulent. Diseases that are not highly transmissible, such as leprosy, or are selectively pathogenic, such as tuberculosis, are more likely to be endemic than epidemic.

Each infectious disease has characteristic modes of transmission that must be understood for the purpose of disease prevention. Respiratory diseases transmitted as airborne particles—smallpox, influenza, measles, pneumonic plague—spread rapidly and are difficult to control through sanitation and quarantine. Diseases spread through fecal contamination of water and food—cholera, hepatitis, typhoid, poliomyelitis—are more easily avoided and, in industrialized countries, tend to occur in localized outbreaks with identifiable sources. Blood-borne diseases transmitted by biting arthropods—malaria, yellow fever, typhus, bubonic plague—can erupt in devastating epidemics when both host and vector populations are high. Localized outbreaks of arthropod-transmitted diseases that have natural animal reservoirs (including yellow fever, St. Louis encephalitis, bubonic plague, murine typhus, and Lyme disease) occur throughout the world, but human-to-human chains of transmission are most likely to occur in Third World countries beset by social upheaval. The spread of sexually transmitted diseases is also aided by war and social dislocation. The transmission of blood-borne viral diseases through contaminated hypodermic needles became significant in the latter part of the twentieth century.

Human resistance to disease is a function of genetic makeup, age, and general health. The impact of a measles epidemic illustrates these relationships. Europeans, through many generations of epidemics that killed the most susceptible individuals, inherit an immune system which is effective at fighting this virus. Disease resistance decreases with increasing age. Although no specific treatment for measles existed until a vaccine was developed in the 1960's, mortality rates in the United States declined dramatically between 1850 and 1950 as a result of improved nutrition and housing and better nursing care. The mortality rate of untreated measles among American children in the 1950's was one in two hundred or three hundred, among poor European slum dwellers in the nineteenth century was one in twenty or thirty, and among Amerindians and Polynesians, who were both impoverished and lacking genetic resistance, was one in two or three.

BEHAVIOR, ENVIRONMENT, AND DISEASE

Diseases caused by behavioral and environmental factors can also be viewed as occurring in epidemics. A major explanation for the increased prominence of noninfectious diseases as causes of mortality and morbidity has been an increasing life span; the cumulative effects of environmental toxins and unhealthy behavior exhibit themselves only as an individual ages. The age-specific frequency of Alzheimer's disease in the United States remained relatively constant in the twentieth century, but because of increasing longevity, the frequency increased dramatically.

Both longevity and changes in behavior contributed to the increase in mortality from lung cancer in industrialized countries in the twentieth century. The various lines of investigation linking this epidemic to tobacco smoking are a good example of epidemiological research. Recent increases in the incidence of skin cancer seem to be linked partly to the popularity of sunbathing and partly to increases in ultraviolet radiation caused by pollution.

Localized clusters of disease and mortality often point to a single environmental hazard. The long-term adverse effects of lead, asbestos, and herbicides have been identified and characterized based on observations of groups of peoples with high levels of exposure to these substances.

PREVENTION, DIAGNOSIS, AND TREATMENT

The discoveries by Robert Koch, Louis Pasteur, and others linking specific microorganisms to human disease ushered in an era when the most effective method for improving human health was the prevention of infection, principally through epidemiological public health measures. Sewage treatment, water purification, and the inspection of food preparation facilities reduced the incidence of cholera, typhoid, and hepatitis; draining and channeling stagnant water to control mosquitoes made malaria and yellow fever rare diseases in the United States and southern Europe. The pesticide DDT (although subsequently condemned because of the serious environmental problems that it caused) performed a laudable service to human health in the aftermath of World War II, killing the vectors of louse-borne typhus and other diseases.

Statistics are the raw material of epidemiological investigation. Death certificates record both the primary and contributing causes of death, the age and sex of the deceased, and the place of death. Census figures give a picture of the community in which epidemiological events occur, such as its racial and socioeconomic composition, age structure, and population density. Physicians and hospitals are required to notify the public health authorities of the occurrence of certain "reportable" diseases, such as AIDS, syphilis, and tuberculosis. Hospital admission records will reflect increases in conditions requiring hospitalization, while school and workplace attendance figures reflect outbreaks of milder communicable diseases.

Some outbreaks are routine and predictable, and the measures for controlling them are well established. When influenza cases increase, public health authorities identify the strain responsible and take steps to immunize those individuals who are most at risk for severe disease. Identifying the source of contaminated food or water is critical to controlling outbreaks of hepatitis A and typhoid in industrialized countries. When war or natural disaster disrupts the normal infrastructure of modern life, it is considered prudent to inoculate the affected population against a variety of infectious diseases.

The history of the discovery of Lyme disease illustrates how epidemiology works. Physician and hospital records indicated a clustering of cases diagnosed as juvenile arthritis near Lyme, Connecticut. By comparing the cases and observing their common characteristics, epidemiologists deduced that an arthropod-transmitted organism normally found on wild animals was probably responsible. Armed with this information, they surveyed microorganisms found in biting arthropods and were able to establish that the same spirochete was found in wild deer, deer ticks, and patients exhibiting symptoms of juvenile arthritis. This organism, and the chronic disease that it causes, proved to be widespread, although not particularly common among humans. Knowing the etiology of the disease enabled physicians to diagnose the condition correctly and to treat it.

Environmentally and behaviorally caused diseases are less amenable to control by health professionals alone, and consequently can prove much more intractable. This is particularly true when there are powerful economic factors working at cross purposes to disease control measures. The epidemiologist can demonstrate that the increase in lung cancer in the twentieth century paralleled an increase in tobacco consumption and that smokers account for most cases of lung cancer. The biomedical investigator studying etiology can show that tobacco derivatives cause cancer in laboratory animals and may ultimately be able to explain how this is brought about at the molecular level. Physicians can advise patients not to smoke, and psychologists can devise therapies to help people quit smoking. None of these efforts, however, will achieve definitive success as long as there are powerful forces encouraging people to smoke and undermining the efforts of the health professionals. The difficulty is compounded, as with any addictive drug, by the active participation of the very people who are the victims of the epidemic in perpetuating the conditions that favor it.

PROGRESS IN CONTROLLING EPIDEMICS

Tremendous progress was made in controlling epidemic disease over the course of the twentieth century, so much so that there was a period when epidemics of life-threatening contagious diseases were viewed as past history in industrialized countries and there was optimism that the same result could be achieved in the Third World as well. The gradual elimination of smallpox was viewed as a model. Yet the worldwide epidemic of AIDS and the resurgence of malaria, tuberculosis, and cholera as epidemic diseases in the late twentieth century are ample evidence that the epidemiological battle against disease is far from won, and that medical science's current arsenal of weapons against infectious disease has serious inadequacies. The factors favoring an increase in epidemics of transmissible disease in the last decades of the twentieth century included an increase in the speed and frequency of international travel, the emergence of drug-resistant strains of a wide variety of pathogens, and a high level of political and social instability in developing nations.

AIDS is only one notable example of dozens of tropical diseases that have the potential for causing lethal worldwide epidemics. Another is Ebola virus, a virulent pathogen responsible for a 1976 epidemic in Zaire in which 90 percent of the victims died. A related virus, lethal to monkeys and infective but nonvirulent in humans, swept a primate quarantine facility in Maryland, and another member of this virus group caused a localized lethal epidemic among monkeys and laboratory workers in Marburg, Germany. Many other lethal transmissible viruses have been identified.

AIDS, the widespread use of immunosuppressant drugs, and the aging of the population have created significant numbers of individuals who have weakened immune systems and are susceptible to infection by animal pathogens. It is worth noting that the worst pandemic in recorded human history, the fourteenth century bubonic plague epidemic, occurred when an animal pathogen became established in a human population and then mutated from a moderately transmissible, arthropod-borne disease to a highly transmissible, airborne infection. The likelihood that animal pathogens will spread to humans and that they will be disseminated internationally is increasing, and the chances of a mutation toward increased transmissibility or virulence increases with the number of infected individuals. The potential for a worldwide pandemic capable of overwhelming the efforts of modern medical science certainly exists, although its probability cannot be estimated.

—*Martha Sherwood-Pike*

See also AIDS; AIDS and children; AIDS and women; Childhood infectious diseases; Food poisoning; Herpes; Illnesses among the elderly; Influenza; Lice, mites, and ticks; Lyme disease; Mad cow disease; Meningitis; Necrotizing fasciitis; Occupational health; Parasites; Plague; Poisoning; Sexually transmitted diseases (STDs); Tuberculosis; Water quality; Worms; Zoonoses.

For Further Information:
Clegg, E. J., and J. P. Garlick, eds. *Disease and Urbanization*. London: Taylor & Francis, 1980. A series of papers discussing the impact of the growth of cities on the frequency of disease. One paper compares the relative impacts of improved living standards and urban services versus specific medical intervention in reducing disease mortality, concluding that the former is far more important.

Goldsmid, John. *The Deadly Legacy: Australian History and Transmissible Disease*. Kensington, New South Wales, Australia: New South Wales University Press, 1988. Because of its isolation before the eighteenth century, the epidemiological history of Australia is more completely documented than that of any other continent. This book discusses the disease history of Aborigines and settlers, as well as the history of government efforts to control epidemics from the early nineteenth century to the late twentieth century, with good coverage of the control measures in effect in 1988.

Preston, Richard. "A Reporter at Large: Crisis in the Hot Zone." *The New Yorker* 68 (October 26, 1992): 58. Focusing on how U.S. government epidemiologists controlled an outbreak of deadly Ebola virus in a primate quarantine facility in Maryland, this article gives a good overview of the various "new" human diseases that have surfaced, including AIDS, and the worldwide threat that they pose.

Ranger, Terence, and Paul Slack, eds. *Epidemics and Ideas: Essays on the Historical Perception of Pestilence*. Cambridge, England: Cambridge University Press, 1992. A collection of papers describing the interplay among perceptions of the etiology of disease, social and religious attitudes, and politics in epidemics from classical antiquity to the present. For example, in sixteenth century Italy, the transmission of plague from the poor to the upper classes was viewed as punishment from God visited on the rich for their lack of charity, whereas in nineteenth century England, the high incidence of disease among the lower classes was viewed as resulting from poor constitution and moral character.

Timmreck, Thomas C. *An Introduction to Epidemiology*. 2d ed. Boston: Jones and Bartlett, 1998. A book in the Jones and Bartlett series in health sciences. Discusses epidemiological methods. Includes a bibliography and an index.

✧ Ethics

Type of issue: Ethics
Definition: A philosophical discipline that attempts to analyze systematically the way in which moral decisions are made; in medicine, this involves defining appropriate patient care, humane biological research, an equi-

table distribution of scarce medical resources, and a just health care delivery system.

In the course of their work, health care professionals are faced with many situations that have moral significance. These situations are characterized by such questions as whether or when to proceed with treatment, which therapy to administer, which patient to see first, how to conduct research using human subjects, where to assign resources that are in short supply, or how to set up an equitable health care system. The discipline of medical ethics seeks to engage in a systematic examination of these questions which is as objective as possible.

Ethical questions in general fall into two categories. A quandary is a moral question about which detailed ethical analysis yields a single, undisputed answer. A dilemma, on the other hand, is a moral question to which there are at least two ethically defensible responses, with neither one taking clear precedence over the other. Ethical analysis consists of the application of primary principles to concrete, clinical situations. It also employs comparative reasoning, in which a particular problem is compared to other situations about which a moral consensus exists. Principled reasoning rests on four fundamental principles of biomedical ethics: respect for autonomy, nonmaleficence, beneficence, and justice.

PRINCIPLES OF REASONING

The principle of respect for autonomy requires that every person be free to take whatever autonomous action or make whatever autonomous decision he or she wishes without constraint by other individuals. An example of respect for autonomy is the doctrine of informed consent, which requires that patients or research subjects be provided with adequate information that they clearly understand before voluntarily submitting to therapy or participating in a research trial.

The principle of nonmaleficence states that one should not inflict evil or harm upon a patient. Although straightforward in its enunciation, it is clear that this principle may come into conflict with the principle of respect for autonomy in cases where a request for withdrawal of therapy is made. Similarly, this principle may come into conflict with obligations to promote the good of the patient, as many medical decisions involve the use of therapies or diagnostic procedures that have undesirable side effects. The principle of double effect in the Roman Catholic moral tradition has attempted to resolve this latter conflict by stating that if the intent of an action is to effect an overriding good, the action is defensible even if unintended but foreseen harmful consequences ensue. Some commentators suggest, however, that intent is an artificial distinction because all the consequences, both good and bad, are foreseen. As a result, the potential for harm should be weighed against the potential for benefit in deciding the best course of action. A formal evaluation of this kind is commonly referred to as a risk-benefit analysis. Individual interpretation of the principle of nonmaleficence lies at the heart of debates over abortion, euthanasia, and treatment withdrawal.

The principle of beneficence expresses an obligation to promote the patient's good. This can be construed as any action that prevents harm, supplants harm, or does active good to a person. As such, this principle provides the basis for all medical practice, be it preventive, epidemiologic, acute, or chronic care. Not all actions can be considered uniformly beneficial. Certain kinds of therapy that may prove to be lifesaving can leave a patient with what he or she finds to be an unacceptable quality of life. An examination of the positive and negative consequences of successful medical treatment is commonly called a benefit-burden analysis. In this context, the principle of beneficence most frequently comes into conflict with the principle of respect for autonomy. In situations such as these, the physician's appeal to beneficence is often considered paternalistic.

The principle of justice applies primarily to the distribution of health care resources in what can be considered to be a just and fair fashion. As there are many competing theories of justice, there is no one clear statement of this principle that can be succinctly applied to all situations. Nevertheless, the principle does require careful consideration of the means by which health care is allocated under conditions of scarcity. In the United States, scarce resources may comprise such entities as transplantable organs, intensive care beds, expensive medical technologies in general, and, in some circumstances, basic medical care itself. Under conditions of scarcity, one's understanding of justice can easily come into conflict with obligations to each of the three preceding principles. In general, the more scarce the resource, the more concerns about distributive justice will influence the deployment of that resource.

ETHICAL DISPUTES IN MEDICAL PRACTICE

Ethical issues in medicine can be divided into macrocosmic (large-scale) and microcosmic (small-scale) concerns. Macrocosmic issues are those which apply to a broad social constituency and therefore often intersect with both statutory and common law. Microcosmic concerns, on the other hand, are those which arise in the day-to-day practice of medicine, the discussion and resolution of which generally have less of a far-reaching impact on the society as a whole.

Primary among the macrocosmic ethical debates is the question of health care allocation. This centers largely on the development of health care delivery systems in particular and health care financing in general. Other issues being argued at the macrocosmic level are broad social policies regarding such concerns as euthanasia, physician-assisted suicide, voluntary abortion, and regulations governing the withholding and withdrawal of life-sustaining therapy. Biomedical research using fetal tissue from induced abortions and research aimed at precisely mapping the human genetic code have raised serious ethical questions regarding both the morality of these endeavors and the nature of life itself. The question of whether—and if so, how—to screen patients for the human immunodeficiency virus (HIV) that causes acquired immunodeficiency syndrome (AIDS) has been argued in both state and federal courts.

Mechanisms for Resolving Ethical Quandries

U.S. research involving human subjects is subjected to ethical review at both macrocosmic and microcosmic levels. Nationally, it is regulated by agencies such as the Food and Drug Administration (FDA). At the microcosmic level, the FDA mandates and supervises the administration of institutional review boards (IRBs), which are charged with the responsibility of assuring that human subjects are involved in creditable research, are treated in a humane manner, are not subjected to undue risks, and are fully cognizant both of the nature of the project in which they are participating and of any potential risks and benefits associated with it.

Resource allocation is a problem at the microcosmic as well as the macrocosmic level; however, the issues in small-scale settings revolve around who constitutes an appropriate candidate for a limited number of intensive care beds or what are the appropriate eligibility criteria for organ transplantation at a particular institution. Perhaps the most common microcosmic problems for hospitals and nursing homes are individual decisions regarding when to terminate life-sustaining therapy. Other common microcosmic dilemmas involve maternal-fetal conflict where the autonomous requests or medical best interests of the mother do not coincide with the presumed best interests of her unborn child.

Institutional Ethics Committees

In situations such as these, both acute and chronic health care facilities often solicit the assistance of institutional ethics committees. Such committees are characteristically composed of individuals representing a broad spectrum of professional disciplines as well as community members not directly employed by the facility. A typical committee might consist of representatives from physician and nursing staffs, social service, psychiatry, pastoral care, special care services (such as intensive care, AIDS management, and neonatal intensive care) that often have a greater number of patients with ethical concerns than others, and hospital administration. Many committees also employ the services of philosophers, attorneys, designated community representatives, or representatives of special interest groups.

In situations that require an institutional response, these committees will often assist in policy development. Examples include institutional policies specifying admission and discharge criteria for intensive care, or policies governing the procedures for withholding or withdrawing therapy. Ethics committees also serve as primary educational resources for both institutional staff and members of the surrounding community.

When the care of individual patients raises ethical questions, many committees have established mechanisms for case consultation or case review. Consultations of this type involve an in-depth review of the patient's clinical condition, as well as of various other social, religious, psychological, or family matters that may be pertinent. After a complete assessment of the facts of the case, consultants then investigate the various ethical arguments that support alternative courses of action before issuing a final recommendation. Case consultation is usually performed by a subcommittee of the institutional ethics committee and is sometimes offered by individual consultants who are not members of the committee. In most cases, the recommendations of the consultants are not binding. Certain models, however, require that some limited kinds of consultative recommendations determine the outcome in specific settings.

Although intervention by an ethics committee often allows for the resolution of ethical disputes within the walls of an institution, sometimes irreconcilable differences require judicial review by a court of law. Under these circumstances, the court's decision regarding a particular case becomes a matter of public record, providing precedent for future similar cases. In this way, certain ethical dilemmas that arise as microcosmic problems end up generating a body of common law which can have profound effects at the macrocosmic level.

—*John Arthur McClung, M.D.*

See also Abortion; Abortion among teenagers; Aging; Child abuse; Circumcision of boys; Circumcision of girls; Death and dying; Domestic violence; Elder abuse; Euthanasia; Fetal tissue transplantation; Genetic engineering; Genetically engineered foods; Health equity for women; Hippocratic oath; Hospice; Hysterectomy; In vitro fertilization; Law and medicine; Living wills; Malpractice; Mastectomy; Morning-after pill; Münchausen syndrome by proxy; Reproductive technologies; Resuscitation; Screening; Sterilization; Terminal illnesses; Transplantation.

FOR FURTHER INFORMATION:

Beauchamp, Tom L., and James F. Childress. *Principles of Biomedical Ethics.* 5th ed. New York: Oxford University Press, 2001. A lucidly written, basic textbook of bioethics. Although some commentators are critical of a primarily principle-based approach to bioethics, this book remains the most widely recognized introductory resource in the field.

Beauchamp, Tom L., and LeRoy Walters, eds. *Contemporary Issues in Bioethics.* 5th ed. Belmont, Calif.: Wadsworth, 1999. A composite of readings culled from legal decisions, seminal legislation, ethical codes of conduct, and the writings of well-known ethicists. The readings are organized by topic and are preceded by a short summary of ethical theory. This work serves as a good companion volume to a basic text.

Jonsen, Albert R., Mark Siegler, and William J. Winslade. *Clinical Ethics.* 4th ed. New York: McGraw-Hill, 1998. A handbook of medical ethics aimed primarily at the physician in training. The authors present a method for evaluating the ethical dimensions of clinical cases, after which the book is organized lexically so that commonly encountered problems can be located easily. A very concise reference which concentrates on practical rather than theoretical priorities.

Jonsen, Albert R., and Stephen Toulmin. *The Abuse of Casuistry: A History of Moral Reasoning.* Berkeley: University of California Press, 1988. A well-constructed history of the technique of case-based analysis which concludes with a practical description of how this approach can be used as an alternative to principle-based analysis in clinical situations.

Reich, Warren T., ed. *Encyclopedia of Bioethics.* 2d ed. New York: Free Press, 1992. A broad look at the entire field of bioethics. Probably the most comprehensive collection of readings currently available under one title.

✧ EUTHANASIA

Type of issue: Ethics

Definition: The intentional termination of a life, which may be active (resulting from specific actions causing death) or passive (resulting from the refusal or withdrawal of life-sustaining treatment), voluntary (with the patient's consent) or involuntary (on behalf of infants or others who are incapable of making this decision, such as comatose patients).

Euthanasia, sometimes called mercy killing, comes from a Greek word that can be translated as "good death." Most patients who express a wish to die more quickly are terminally ill; however, euthanasia is sometimes considered as a solution for nonterminal patients as well. An example of the latter would be seriously deformed or retarded infants whose futures are judged to have a poor "quality of life" and who would be a serious burden on their families and society.

TYPES OF EUTHANASIA

When discussing the ethical implications of euthanasia, the types of cases have been divided into various classes. A distinction is made between voluntary and nonvoluntary euthanasia. In voluntary euthanasia, the patient consents to a specific course of medical action in which death is hastened. Nonvoluntary euthanasia would occur in cases in which the patient is not able to make decisions about his or her death because of an inability to communicate or a lack of mental facility. Each of these classes has advocates and antagonists. Some believe that voluntary euthanasia should always be allowed, but others would limit voluntary euthanasia to only those patients who have a terminal illness. Some, although agreeing in principle that voluntary euthanasia in terminal situations is ethically permissible, nevertheless oppose euthanasia of any type because of the possibility of abuses.

With nonvoluntary euthanasia, the main ethical issues deal with when such an action should be performed and who should make the decision. If a person is in an irreversible coma, most agree that that person's physical life could be ended; however, arguments based on "quality of life" can easily become widened to include persons with physical or mental disabilities. Infants with severe deformities can sometimes be saved but not fully cured with medical technology, and some individuals would advocate nonvoluntary euthanasia in these cases because of the suffering of the infants' caregivers. Some believe that family members or those who stand to gain from the decision should not be allowed to make the decision. Others point out that the family is the most likely to know what the wishes of the patient would have been. Most believe that the medical care personnel, although knowledgeable, should not have the power to decide, and many are reluctant to institute rigid laws. The possibility of misappropriated self-interest from each of these parties magnifies the difficulty of arriving at well-defined criteria.

The second type of classification is between passive and active euthanasia. Passive euthanasia occurs when sustaining medical treatment is refused or withdrawn and death is allowed to take its course. Active euthanasia involves the administration of a drug or some other means that directly causes death. Once again, there are many opinions surrounding these two types. One position is that there is no difference between active and passive euthanasia because in each the end is premeditated death with the motive of prevention of suffering. In fact, some argue that active euthanasia is more compassionate than letting death occur naturally, which may involve suffering. In opposition, others believe that there is a fundamental difference between active and passive euthanasia. A person may have the right to die, but not the right to be killed. Passive euthanasia, they argue, is merely allowing a death which is inevitable to occur. Active euthanasia, if voluntary, is equated with suicide because a human being seizes control of death; if nonvoluntary, it is considered murder.

Passive euthanasia, although generally more publicly acceptable than active euthanasia, has become a topic of controversy as the types of medical treatment that can be withdrawn are debated. A distinction is sometimes made between ordinary and extraordinary means. Defining these terms is difficult, since what may be extraordinary for one patient is not for another, depending on other medical conditions that the patient may have. In addition, what is considered an extraordinary technique today may be judged ordinary in the future. Another way to assess whether passive euthanasia should be allowed in a particular situation is to weigh the benefits against the burdens for the patient. Although most agree that there are cases in which high-tech equipment such as respirators can be withdrawn, there is a question about whether administration of food and water should ever be discontinued. Here the line between passive and active euthanasia is blurred.

THE PHYSICIAN'S DILEMMA

C. Everett Koop, former surgeon general of the United States, differentiated between the positive role of a physician in providing a patient "all the life to which he or she is entitled" and the negative role of "prolonging the act of dying." Koop, opposed to euthanasia in any form, cautioned against the possibility of sliding down a slippery slope toward making choices about death that reflect the caregivers' "quality of life" more than the patient's.

Dr. Jack Kevorkian, a Michigan physician, became the most well known advocate of assisted suicide in the United States. From 1990 to 1997, Kevorkian assisted at least sixty-six people in terminating their lives. According to his lawyer, many other assisted suicides were not publicized. Kevorkian stated that physician-assisted suicide is a matter of individual choice and that it should be seen as a rational way to end tremendous pain and suffering. Most of the patients assisted by him spent many years suffering from extremely painful and debilitating diseases, such as multiple sclerosis, bone cancer, and brain cancer.

The American Medical Association (AMA) criticized this view, calling it a violation of professional ethics. When faced with pain and suffering, the AMA asserts that it is a doctor's responsibility to provide adequate "comfort" care, not death. In the AMA's view, Kevorkian is "a reckless instrument of death." Three trials in Michigan for assisting in suicide resulted in acquittals for Kevorkian before another trial delivered a guilty verdict on the charge of second-degree murder in March, 1999.

LEGAL RIGHTS AND RAMIFICATIONS

During the course of reevaluating the issues involved in terminating a life, the law has been in a state of flux. The decisions that are made by the courts act on the legal precedents of an individual's right to determine what is done to his or her own body and society's position against suicide. The balancing of these two premises has been handled legally by allowing refusal of treatment (passive euthanasia) but disallowing the use of poison or some other method that would cause death (active euthanasia). The latter is labeled suicide, and anyone who assists in such an act can be found guilty of assisting a suicide, or of murder. Following the Karen Ann Quinlan case in 1976, in which the family of a comatose woman secured permission to withdraw life-sustaining treatment, the courts routinely allowed family members to make decisions regarding life-sustaining treatment if the patient could not do so.

The area of greatest legal controversy involves the withdrawal of food and water. Some courts have charged doctors with murder for the withdrawal of basic life support measures such as food and water. Others have ruled that invasive procedures to provide food and water (intravenously, for example) are similar to other medical procedures and may be discontinued if the benefit to the patient's quality of life is negligible.

In 1994, 51 percent of the voters in Oregon passed the world's first "death with dignity" law. It allowed physician-assisted suicide. Doctors could begin prescribing fatal overdoses of drugs to terminally ill patients. The vote was reaffirmed in 1997 by 60 percent of the state's voters, despite opposition from the Roman Catholic Church, the AMA, and various anti-abortion and right-to-life groups. The 9th United States Circuit Court of Appeals in San Francisco then lifted a lower court order blocking implementation of the law.

Doctors in Oregon became free to prescribe fatal doses of barbiturates to patients with less than six months to live. Physicians were required to file forms with the Oregon Health Division before prescribing the overdose. Then, there would be a fifteen-day waiting period between the request for suicide assistance and the approval of the prescription. Opponents of the Oregon law charged that it perverted the practice of medicine and forced many suffering people to "choose" an early death to save themselves from expensive medical care or pain that could be manageable if physicians were aware of new methods of pain control. The National Right to Life Committee indicated that it would continue to fight implementation of the law in federal courts.

Although the laws vary from state to state, most states allow residents to make their wishes known regarding terminal health care either by writing a living will or by choosing a durable power of attorney. A living will is a document in which one can state that some medical treatments should not be used in the event that one becomes incapacitated to the point where one cannot choose. Living wills allow the patient to decide in advance and protect health care providers from lawsuits. Which treatment options can be terminated and when this action can be put into effect may be limited in some states. Most states have a specific format that should be followed when drawing up a living will and require that the document be signed in the presence of two witnesses. Often, qualifying additions can be made by the individual that specify whether food and water may be withdrawn and whether the living will should go into effect only when death is imminent or also when a person has an incurable illness but death is not imminent. A copy of the living will should be given to the patient's physician and become a part of the patient's medical records. The preparation or execution of a living will cannot affect a person's life insurance coverage or the payment of benefits. Since the medical circumstances of one's life may change and a person's ethical stance may also change, a patient may change the living will at any time by signing a written statement.

A second way in which a person can control what kind of decisions will be made regarding his or her death is to choose a decision maker in advance. This person assumes a durable power of attorney and is legally allowed to act on the patient's behalf, making medical treatment decisions. One advantage of a durable power of attorney over a living will is that the patient can choose someone who shares similar ethical and religious values. Since it is difficult to foresee every medical situation that could arise, there is more security with a durable power of attorney in knowing that the person will have similar values and will therefore probably make the same judgments as the patient. Usually a primary agent and a secondary agent are designated in the event that the primary agent is unavailable. This is especially important if the primary agent is a spouse or a close relative who could, for example, be involved in an accident at the same time as the patient.

An Age-Old Quandary

The famous Hippocratic oath for physicians acted in opposition to the prevailing cultural bias in favor of euthanasia. Contained in this oath is the statement, "I will never give a deadly drug to anybody if asked for it . . . or make a suggestion to this effect." The AMA reaffirmed this position in a policy statement: "the intentional termination of the life of one human being by another—'mercy killing'—is contrary to that for which the medical profession stands and is contrary to the policy of the American Medical Association."

Although these issues have been debated by physicians and philosophers for centuries, there is a heightened need for thoughtful discussion and resolution today. Clearly, the decisions surrounding the issue of euthanasia are very complicated. The choice is not simply between commitments to "sanctity of life" or "quality of life" viewpoints. No consensus has yet been reached across the spectrum of society, and instead a variety of alternatives are supported by groups of individuals. A clear understanding of all positions in the debate is the best preparation for making personal decisions at the time of death.

—Katherine B. Frederich; updated by Leslie V. Tischauser

See also Aging; Death and dying; Depression; Depression in the elderly; Ethics; Health insurance; Hippocratic oath; HMOs; Hospice; Hospitalization of the elderly; Law and medicine; Living wills; Pain management; Suicide; Suicide among the elderly; Terminal illnesses.

FOR FURTHER INFORMATION:
Gorovitz, Samuel. *Drawing the Line*. Reprint. New York: Oxford University Press, 1993. This book reflects on the author's seven-week sabbatical in residence at Beth Israel Hospital. Gorovitz presents numerous insights drawn from conversations with patients and medical personnel.
Leone, Daniel A. *The Ethics of Euthanasia*. San Diego, Calif.: Greenhaven Press, 1999. Part of a new anthology series that focuses a wide range of viewpoints onto a single controversial issue. This volume includes ten essays on the ethics and morality of euthanasia, potential abuse, distinctions between active and passive euthanasia, and whether euthanasia is consistent with Christian belief.
Spring, Beth, and Ed Larson. *Euthanasia*. Portland: Multnomah Press, 1988. This book considers the spiritual, medical, and legal issues in terminal health care, citing numerous perspectives from the religious community. Contains two chapters detailing practical guidelines for writing living wills and durable powers of attorney.
Torr, James D. *Euthanasia*. San Diego, Calif.: Greenhaven Press, 1999. Designed for high school students, this volume brings together essays by authorities in diverse vocations. The four chapters explore whether euthanasia is ethical, if it should be legalized, if legalization would lead to involuntary killing, and under what circumstances, if any, doctors should assist in suicide.
Wennberg, Robert N. *Terminal Choices*. Grand Rapids, Mich.: Wm. B. Eerdmans, 1989. The author presents a helpful history of the euthanasia debate and also discusses possible moral distinctions between treatment refusal and treatment withdrawal.

✧ Exercise

Type of issue: Prevention, public health, social trends
Definition: Various intensities and types of physical activity.

Low or moderate exercise intensity relies on oxygen to release energy for work. This process is often referred to as aerobic exercise. In the muscles, carbohydrates and fats are broken down to produce adenosine triphosphate (ATP), the basic molecule used for energy. Aerobic exercise can be sustained for several minutes to several hours.

Higher-intensity exercise is predominantly fueled anaerobically (in the absence of oxygen) and can be sustained for up to two minutes only. Muscle glycogen is broken down without oxygen to produce ATP. Anaerobic metabolism is much less efficient at producing ATP than is aerobic metabolism. During anaerobic metabolism, a by-product called lactic acid begins to accumulate in the blood as blood lactate. The point at which this accumulation begins is called the anaerobic threshold, or the onset of blood lactate accumulation. Blood lactate can cause muscle soreness and stiffness, but it also can be used as fuel during aerobic metabolism.

A third and less often used energy system is the creatine phosphate (ATP-CP) system. Utilizing the very limited supply of ATP that is stored in the muscles, phosphate molecules are exchanged between ATP and CP to provide energy. This system provides only enough fuel for a few seconds of maximum effort.

The type of muscle fiber recruited to perform a specific type of exercise is also dependent on exercise intensity. Skeletal muscle is composed of "slow-twitch" and two types of "fast-twitch" muscle fibers. Slow-twitch fibers are more suited to using oxygen than are fast-twitch fibers, and they are recruited primarily for aerobic exercise. One type of fast-twitch fiber also functions during aerobic activity. The second type of fast-twitch fiber serves to facilitate anaerobic, or high-intensity, exercise.

Exercise mode is also a factor in the physiological responses to exercise. Dynamic exercise (alternating muscular contraction and relaxation through a range of motion) using many large muscles requires more oxygen than does activity utilizing smaller and fewer muscles. The greater the oxygen requirement of the physical activity, the greater the cardiorespiratory benefits.

MEASURES OF INCREASING FITNESS

Many bodily adaptations occur over a training period of six to eight weeks, and other benefits are gradually manifested over several months. The positive adaptations include reduced resting and working heart rates. As the heart becomes stronger, there is a subsequent increase in stroke volume (the volume of blood the heart pumps with each beat), which allows the heart to beat less frequently while maintaining the same cardiac output (the volume of the blood pumped from the heart each minute). Another beneficial adaptation is increased metabolic efficiency. This is partially facilitated by an increase in the number of mitochondria (the organelles responsible for ATP production) in the muscle cells.

One of the most recognized representations of aerobic fitness is the maximum volume of oxygen (VO_{2max}) an individual can use during exercise. VO_{2max} is improved through habitual, relatively high-intensity aerobic activity. After three to six months of regular training, levels of high-density lipoproteins (HDLs) in the blood increase. HDL molecules remove cholesterol (a fatty substance) from the tissues to aid in protecting the heart from atherosclerosis.

Two major types of flexibility have been identified. One type consists of the flexibility through the range of motion of a muscle group or joint. This is called static flexibility. It can be measured using a metric stick or a protractor-type instrument called a goniometer. Dynamic flexibility is the other major identified type of flexibility. It is the torque of or resistance to movement. Methods to measure dynamic flexibility have not been developed.

Various internal and external factors influence the metabolic processes that take place during and after exercise. Internally, nutrition, degree of hydration, body composition, flexibility, sex, and age are some of the variables that play a role in the physiological responses. Other internal variables include medical conditions such as heart disease, diabetes, and hypertension (high blood pressure). Externally, environmental conditions such as temperature, humidity, and altitude alter how the exercising body functions.

Various modes of exercise testing and data collection are used to study the physiological responses of the body to exercise. Treadmills and cycle ergometers (instruments used to measure work and power output) are among the most common methods of evaluating maximum oxygen consumption. During these tests, special equipment and computers analyze expired air, heart rate is monitored with an electrocardiograph (ECG), and blood pressure is taken using a sphygmomanometer. Blood samples and muscle fiber samples can also be extracted to aid in identifying the fuel system and type of muscle fibers being used. Other data sometimes collected, such as skin temperatures and body core temperatures, can provide pertinent information.

Exercise and Body Composition

Another factor greatly affecting the physical response to exercise is body composition. The three major structural components of the body are muscle, bone, and fat. Body composition can be evaluated using a combination of anthropometric measurements. These measurements include body weight, standard height, measurements of circumferences at various locations using a tape measure, measurements of skeletal diameters using a sliding metric stick, and measurements of skinfold thicknesses using calipers.

Body fat can be estimated using several methods, the most accurate of which is based on a calculation of body density. This method is called hydrostatic weighing, which involves weighing the subject under water while taking into account the residual volume of air in the lungs. The principle underlying this measurement of body density is based on the fact that fat is less dense than water and will float, whereas bone and muscle, which are denser than water, will sink. One biochemical technique often used to determine levels of body fat is based on the relatively constant level of potassium 40 naturally existing in lean body mass. Another method utilizes ultrasound waves to measure the thickness of fat layers. X rays and computed tomography (CT) scanning can be used to provide images from which fat and bone can be measured. Bioelectrical impedance (BIA) is a method of estimating body composition based on the resistance imposed on a low voltage electrical current sent through the body. The most widely used and easily assessable method, however, involves measurement of skinfolds at various sites on the body using calipers. In all cases, mathematical formulas have been devised to interpret the collected data and provide the best estimate of an individual's body composition.

Other tests have been developed to determine muscular strength, muscular endurance, and flexibility. Muscular strength is often measured by performance of one maximal effort produced by a selected muscle group. Muscular endurance of a muscle or muscle group is often demonstrated by the length of time or number of repetitions a particular, submaximal workload or skill can be performed.

The Goals of Exercise

For the healthy adult participant, the American College of Sports Medicine, a widely recognized authoritative body on exercise prescription, recommends three to five sessions of aerobic exercise weekly. Each session should include a five- to ten-minute warm-up period, twenty to sixty minutes of aerobic exercise at a predetermined exercise intensity, and a five- to ten-minute cooldown period.

Determining an individual's maximum heart rate is important in choosing an appropriate aerobic exercise intensity. The best way to obtain this maximum heart rate is to take a maximal exercise test. Such a test can be supervised by an exercise physiologist or an exercise test technician; it is advisable, especially for the older participant, that a cardiologist also be in attendance. An ECG is monitored for irregularities as the subject walks, runs, cycles, or performs some dynamic exercise to exhaustion or until the onset of irregular symptoms or discomfort.

Adequate physical fitness can be defined as the ability to perform daily tasks with enough reserve for emergency situations. All aspects of health-related fitness direct attention toward this goal. Aerobic exercise often provides some conditioning for muscular endurance, but muscular strength and flexibility need to be addressed separately.

The ACSM recommends resistance training using the "overload principle," which involves placing habitual stress on a system, causing it to adapt and respond. For this training, it is suggested that eight to twelve repetitions of eight to ten strengthening exercises of the major muscle groups be performed a minimum of two days per week.

Flexibility of connective tissue and muscle tissue is essential to maximize physical performance and to limit musculoskeletal injuries. At least one stretching exercise for each major muscle group should be executed three to four times per week while the muscles are warm.

Exercise in Cardiac Rehabilitation

Cardiac rehabilitation takes exercise prescription a step further. Participation of the heart patient is more individualized than in wellness programs. The condition of the circulatory system, pulmonary system, and joints are only a few of the special concerns. Secondary conditions such as obesity, diabetes, and hypertension must also be considered. The responsibilities of cardiac rehabilitation specialists include monitoring blood sugar in diabetic patients and blood pressure in all patients, especially those with hypertension. Many drugs affect heart rate or blood pressure, and most of these participants are taking more than one type of medication. Patients with heart damage caused by a heart attack may display atypical heart rhythms, which can be seen on an ECG monitor. Furthermore, the stage of recovery of the postsurgical patient is a major factor in recommending the type, frequency, intensity, and duration of exercise.

Patient education is also important. Lifestyle is usually the main factor in the development of heart disease. Cardiac patients often have never participated in a regular exercise program. Frequently, they are smokers, are overweight, and have poor eating habits. Helping them to identify and correct destructive health-related behaviors is the focus of education for the heart patient.

Sports Medicine

Another application of the study of exercise physiology involves dealing with the competitive athlete. In this case, findings from the most recent research are constantly applied to yield the best athletic performance possible. A delicate balance of aerobic training, anaerobic training, strength training, endurance training, and flexibility exercises are combined with the optimum percentage of body fat, proper nutrition, and adequate sleep. The program that is designed must enhance the athletic qualities that are most beneficial to the sport in which the athlete participates.

The competitive athlete usually pushes beyond the boundaries of general exercise prescription in terms of intensity, duration, and frequency of exercise performance. As a result, the athlete risks suffering more injuries than the individual who exercises for health benefits. If the athlete sustains an injury, the exercise physiologist may work in conjunction with an athletic trainer or sports physician to return the athlete to competition as soon as possible.

—Kathleen O'Boyle

See also Biofeedback; Canes and walkers; Cardiac rehabilitation; Exercise and children; Exercise and the elderly; Hypertension; Mobility problems in the elderly; Muscle loss with aging; Obesity; Obesity and aging; Obesity and children; Physical fitness tests for children; Physical rehabilitation; Preventive medicine; Steroid abuse; Wheelchair use among the elderly; Yoga.

FOR FURTHER INFORMATION:

American College of Sports Medicine. *Guidelines for Exercise Testing and Prescription.* 6th ed. Philadelphia: Lippincott Williams & Wilkins, 2000. This manual provides guidelines for the professional working in preventive exercise programs or in cardiac rehabilitation. The recommendations are based on the most-up-to-date research available at the time of publication. Requirements for certification through the ACSM are also explained in detail.

_____. *Resource Manual for Guidelines for Exercise Testing and Prescription.* 3d ed. Baltimore: Williams & Wilkins, 1998. Based on the objective of providing safe and effective exercise programs for all individuals, this publication provides an excellent overview of many of the topics of concern to the exercise physiologist. Specific recommendations regarding stress testing and exercise prescription are included in the text.

McArdle, William D., Frank I. Katch, and Victor L. Katch. *Exercise Physiology: Energy, Nutrition, and Human Performance.* 4th ed. Baltimore: Williams & Wilkins, 1996. This textbook is designed for the serious student of exercise physiology. Provides relatively detailed explanations of various energy systems in the body.

Powers, Scott K., and Edward T. Howley. *Exercise Physiology: Theory and Application to Fitness and Performance.* Dubuque, Iowa: Wm. C. Brown, 1990. The upper-level undergraduate or beginning graduate student will find detailed information concerning exercise physiology in this useful textbook. Designed for students who are serious about the study of exercise science.

Sharkey, Brian J. *Physiology of Fitness.* 3d ed. Champaign, Ill.: Human Kinetics Books, 1990. Provides an excellent learning opportunity for the junior college student. Offers a guide to the prescription of exercise for health, fitness, and performance, but takes things a step further by explaining the scientific basis for these guidelines.

✧ EXERCISE AND CHILDREN

Type of issue: Children's health, prevention, public health
Definition: Exertion of the body to develop or maintain physical fitness.

In 1996 the U.S. surgeon general issued a report on physical activity and health. The report documented the benefits of regular physical activity to the health and well-being of both adults and children. The Centers for Disease Control and Prevention followed in 1997 with guidelines for promoting lifelong physical activity. This document identifies the benefits of physical activity for children and adolescents as improving strength and endurance, building healthy bones and muscles, controlling weight, reducing anxiety and stress, increasing self-esteem, and potentially improving blood pressure and cholesterol levels.

TYPES OF EXERCISE

Healthy individuals of all ages can benefit from regular exercise. General exercise regimens can be developed and may include training to improve flexibility, endurance, and strength. Specific exercise programs can also be prescribed to meet an individual's special needs.

Flexibility training primarily includes stretching to increase the range of motion in joints and to enhance freedom of movement. Healthy children can safely participate in stretching activities. To avoid injury and obtain the benefits of stretching, one must use good body mechanics and slow, controlled stretches. Fast, bouncing movements should be avoided. Moderation in stretching exercises is also recommended. Stretching for ballet, gymnastics, or other sports is necessary for competition purposes but goes beyond the level needed for normal healthy development. Regular stretching can contribute to an improved quality of life, as in the control of back pain, and has long-term health benefits.

Cardiovascular exercise, one component of endurance exercise, is believed to offer the greatest long-term health benefits. This form of exercise is commonly called aerobic. Aerobic exercise relies on oxygen. It demands sufficient oxygen from the cardiovascular system to maintain the activity for fifteen minutes or longer. Aerobic activity is vigorous, continuous, and rhythmical and uses the major muscle groups. The purest forms of aerobic exercise include repetitive activities such as walking, running, bicycling, cross-country skiing, and rowing. Many exercise machines are also good aerobic options, such as climbers and ski machines. Young children do not need to participate in these types of activities on a regular basis. They benefit most from games that have a high aerobic component and strengthen the cardiovascular system like soccer, basketball, and other games involving a lot of running. Games are beneficial because they develop the muscles, heart, and lungs and also help children learn motor skills. Older children and adolescents can participate in most aerobic activities because their bodies are developed enough to obtain the cardiovascular benefits.

Another component of endurance exercise is muscular endurance. This involves activities that focus on the muscles rather than the heart. While cardiovascular endurance activities generally improve muscular endurance, not all muscular endurance activities improve cardiovascular endurance. Muscular endurance activities involve contracting the same muscle group repeatedly. Examples include sit-ups, pull-ups, or push-ups. Although they are not aerobic, these exercises should be a component of any good exercise program. Adolescents can benefit from these activities as well and after reaching puberty can begin to include strength-training activities in their exercise routine. Strength training (or resistance training) is activity designed to increase the force of muscle contraction. Muscular endurance activities will increase strength as well, but not to the same extent as strength training. It is generally recommended that strength training be avoided until a child reaches adolescence and the hormone levels required to elicit increases in strength and muscle size are present. Prior to maturity, children will not obtain major increases in strength and size, and the risks to the growing body are much greater. If children do participate in strength-training programs, close, qualified adult supervision is absolutely required.

GOALS AND GUIDELINES

The goal of exercise programs for young people should be to promote lifelong physical activity. Children who mature into adults who exercise regularly are likely to have fewer cardiovascular risk factors. The major controllable risk factors include smoking, high blood pressure, high blood cholesterol, physical inactivity, and obesity. Physical activity may decrease blood pressure, improve blood cholesterol levels, and decrease obesity.

From one to six years of age, the focus of exercise should be on gross motor skill development. This includes activities such as walking, running, jumping, and skipping. These fundamental motor skills are necessary for the development of the more advanced skills that will be part of adult physical activity.

From seven years of age to maturity, the focus of physical activity should be on sport skill development. The type of sport is not important as long as the child continues to learn. Ball control, balance, eye-hand coordination, and body control are some of the useful skills. By developing these types of skills, children will be able to perform at a higher level in sports and, more important, to develop a good appreciation for lifelong exercise.

After children reach maturity, they can safely begin training programs that include strength training and serious cardiovascular endurance training. Prior to maturity, the bones are still growing and have not fused. Increased risk of growth plate fractures (which can severely damage the growth of the injured bone) and ruptured intervertebral disks is involved in lifting heavy weights. Furthermore, hormone levels, especially testosterone levels, are much lower prior to maturity and this affects the tissue-building capabilities of the body. The body is also better prepared to handle cardiovascular endurance exercise after reaching maturity. Although the risks of beginning cardiovascular training before maturity are less than those associated with strength training, it is best to keep the focus on skill development in young children.

The generally accepted guidelines for exercise in children recommend aerobic types of activities. However, these activities do not need to be continuous, as recommended for adults. Aerobic exercise can include various endurance games and activities. They should be done for thirty to sixty minutes duration at a time on a daily basis. The intensity of aerobic exercise is determined by a complicated set of equations and is based on the exercise heart rate for adults. The general recommendation for children is simply moderate intensity. The child's physician should be consulted about concerns regarding exercise. It is recommended that adolescents get similar amounts of exercise as young children with the addition of twenty minutes of continuous, vigorous activity three times per week as part of their regular routine.

Creating a Lasting Exercise Plan

Additional considerations for exercise among children must be noted. First, competitive running and other competitive activities are not necessary for attaining health benefits. Second, children have a greater chance of fatigue than do adults in high intensity activities. Third, children have a lower tolerance for high heat. Children should be monitored closely, drink plenty of fluids, and decrease the intensity of exercise under these conditions.

Organized youth sports are a popular type of physical activity for many children. However, with the goal of lifelong physical activity, poorly organized youth sports can have a negative effect. Children who do not get to play or who fail to develop new skills can quickly become discouraged with exercise in general. In a 1990 study called *American Youth and Sports Participation*, ten thousand students in grades seven to twelve were asked why they play their best sport. The top three reasons were to have fun, to improve skills, and to stay in shape. When asked what needed to change in order to get them involved again in a sport after quitting, the top answers were to make practices more fun, to play more, and for coaches to understand players more. These reasons provide valuable insight into the development of programs that have the goal of promoting long-term interest in exercise.

Safe exercise for children and adults begins with a good warm-up and ends with a good cooldown. The warm-up prepares the body for intense exercise by performing light activity for several minutes, such as a slow run. It slowly raises the heart rate and increases body temperature. This helps the body function more efficiently and loosens the muscles. The cooldown prepares the body for rest. Light activity for several minutes helps the heart slow down gradually and maintains good circulation. The cooldown helps the body readjust gradually to the decrease in many body functions that follows exercise.

Complications from exercise are a concern; however, healthy children are at much less risk than are adults. The aforementioned exercise guidelines have been developed to minimize problems during periods of physical activity. While the opportunity for injury increases during exercise, especially during competitive or contact sports, practicing these guidelines can ensure safe and effective exercise for children.

Physical activity is characteristic of all animals, including humans. Young animals begin with play; older animals use their physical skills to survive. Animals that are the most fit have the best chance for survival. Historically, this was true for humans. As technology has advanced and there has been less reliance on physical activity to survive, humans have become more sedentary. Children have become less active with the advent of television, videotapes, computers, and electronic games. These technological advances have led to an increasing concern about the fitness levels of children. Researchers have been studying the effects of lack of exercise and in the process have established important guidelines to help people better understand the relationship between inactivity and health. In addition, new exercise regimens and equipment, books, and magazines have created a better awareness of the role of exercise in a healthy lifestyle. The future challenge is to develop more strategies to get people moving. These strategies must include children. Good exercise habits, developed at an early age, will promote continuing interest in physical activity throughout life.

—*Bradley R. A. Wilson*

See also Children's health issues; Exercise; Exercise and the elderly; Obesity; Obesity and children; Physical fitness tests for children; Preventive medicine; Sports injuries among children; Steroid abuse.

FOR FURTHER INFORMATION:

Foster, Emily R., Karyn Hartinger, and Katherine A. Smith. *Fitness Fun.* Champaign, Ill.: Human Kinetics, 1992. This book is full of activities that can be used to promote physical fitness in children. Eighty-five games and activities develop at least one of the components of fitness.

Greene, Leon, and Matthew Adeyanju. "Exercise and Fitness Guidelines for Elementary and Middle School Children." *The Elementary School Journal* 91, no. 5 (May, 1991): 437-444. This paper clearly lists the factors important for exercise and fitness in young people.

Kalish, Susan. *Your Child's Fitness.* Champaign, Ill.: Human Kinetics, 1996. This easy-to-read book covers most of the major areas of children's physical fitness and exercise. Clear activities and assessments are presented.

Pangrazi, Robert P., Charles B. Corbin, and Gregory J. Welk. "Physical

Activity for Children and Youth." *Journal of Physical Education, Recreation, and Dance* 67, no. 4 (April, 1996): 38-43. This brief review of children and physical activity gets straight to the point. The most commonly asked questions are addressed in very understandable terms.

Rowland, Thomas W. *Exercise and Children's Health*. Champaign, Ill.: Human Kinetics, 1990. This book contains a thorough review of the relationship between exercise and the health of children. It is slightly technical but easy to read.

Waitz, Grete, with Gloria Averbuch. *On the Run: Exercise and Fitness for Busy People*. Emmaus, Pa.: Rodale Press, 1997. Geared to the family, this book has an excellent section on children's fitness and a section on children and running. It also includes information on how to begin a training program.

✧ EXERCISE AND THE ELDERLY

Type of issue: Elder health, prevention, public health, social trends
Definition: Regular physical activity undertaken for the purpose of maintaining or increasing physical and mental health.

The physiological deterioration commonly associated with aging is not entirely caused by the aging process; it is also caused by the physical inactivity that often accompanies aging. In the United States, it has been reported that adults over age fifty are the most sedentary members of the population. By the year 2030, it has been predicted that 22 percent of the population will be over age sixty-five. Increased physical activity is a frequently suggested mechanism for reducing the rising health care costs that accompany cardiovascular disease and deterioration of the musculoskeletal system. Even so, 50 percent of men and 70 percent of women over age sixty-five are not participating in enough regular exercise to have a sufficient impact on their health.

Four general components collectively represent physical fitness: cardiorespiratory endurance (aerobic capacity), anaerobic power, muscular strength and endurance, and body composition. All these components are susceptible to decline with aging; however, the magnitude of this decline is dependent upon the extent of physical inactivity and other health factors.

AEROBIC CAPACITY

Aerobic capacity refers to the body's ability to maximally transport and utilize oxygen to the cells (maximal volume of oxygen consumed, or VO$_2$max). The body requires a higher volume of oxygen (O$_2$) to sustain increased magnitudes of exercise. Aerobic capacity declines with aging because of a cumulative effect of age-related functional changes in the heart as well as muscle mass loss caused by disuse or disease. The higher the O_2max value (measured in milliliters of oxygen used per kilogram of body weight per minute), the greater the person's aerobic capacity, or aerobic fitness. A higher aerobic capacity will allow an individual to exercise more comfortably and will also permit the older individual to complete activities of daily living without fatigue. Thus, functional ability is improved when aerobic fitness is improved.

Up to age thirty, VO_2max declines about 1 percent per year. Once adults reach middle age, the loss of VO_2max is accelerated unless regular aerobic exercise is undertaken. Between forty-five and fifty-five years of age, O_2max will be lost at a rate of 9 to 15 percent. Other accelerated losses occur between the ages of sixty-five to seventy-five and from seventy-five to eighty-five years of age. However, regular participation in aerobic exercise can slow or even reverse this decline. When middle-aged or older individuals participate regularly in aerobic exercise, they can expect a 10 to 25 percent improvement in VO_2max. This can mean the difference between being functionally impaired, on one hand, and gaining back independent-living skills and sports participation, on the other.

Individuals can have their aerobic capacities determined with an exercise stress test administered by a team of medical professionals, including a cardiologist, a nurse, and an exercise physiologist. An aerobic exercise training program that elicits 50 to 70 percent of one's O_2max would be sufficient to improve an older individual's aerobic capacity. Examples of aerobic exercise are walking, swimming, cycling, skiing, and dancing. Exercise of moderate intensity—enough to cause an increase in breathing and heart rate but not so much that it prevents one from being able to carry on a conversation—is sufficient for most people to gain health benefits. The experience of pain is a cue to stop exercise and reevaluate the exercise intensity level.

THE CARDIOVASCULAR AND RESPIRATORY SYSTEMS

The primary purpose of the cardiovascular and respiratory or pulmonary systems (also referred to collectively as the cardiopulmonary or cardiorespiratory system) is to deliver oxygen and nutrients to the tissues while removing carbon dioxide and waste products from the tissues.

With aging, lung tissue loses elasticity, the chest wall becomes more rigid, and respiratory muscle strength is lost. This causes a loss of ventilatory (breathing) efficiency, making the mechanics of breathing harder for the aged. With exercise, the demand for more oxygen requires more frequent and deeper breaths. Since the aged pulmonary system is compromised, pulmonary ventilation is decreased during maximal exercise as well as during recovery after exercise. Even with aging limitations, in the absence of pulmonary disease, the resting tissues still have an adequate oxygen supply to carry out daily functional and recreational activities. The oxygen deficit and higher respiratory work is not noticed until vigorous exercise puts a demand on the system for more oxygen, challenging the ventilatory capacity of the lungs. Although the total amount of blood flow increases as aerobic capacity increases, this does not result in an improvement in gaseous diffusion in the aged. In fact, gas exchange of oxygen and carbon dioxide in the tissues decreases with aging, and exercise training appears to have little impact on this function. On the other hand, forced vital capacity (FVC), the maximum amount of air that can be expelled after a maximal inhalation, is one of the few pulmonary volumes influenced by both aging and exercise training. With aging, FVC declines approximately 4 to 5 percent per decade in the average individual. However, research studies that tracked aerobically trained individuals over twenty or more years found that their FVCs at age forty-five were the same as their FVCs at age twenty. This maintenance may be because of the mechanical stressing of the respiratory muscles afforded by regular aerobic exercise.

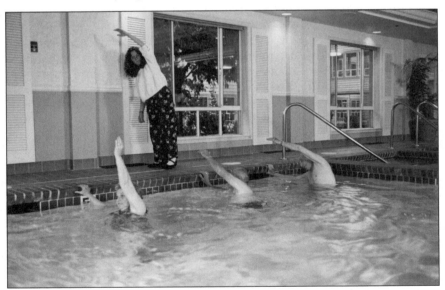

Elderly individuals may find low-impact exercise, such as swimming, to be a safer and easier way to stay fit. (PhotoDisc)

As with the pulmonary system, resting cardiovascular function experiences only moderate changes, whereas the cardiovascular response during exercise declines substantially with aging. The major reason that maximal aerobic capacity declines with aging is because of the decrease in maximal heart rate. Maximal heart rate (the highest heart rate attainable) declines approximately 6 percent per decade. Using the mathematical formula to estimate maximal heart rate (220 minus age equals heart rate in beats per minute), it can be seen that the estimated maximal heart rate of a seventy-year-old (150 beats per minute) is significantly less than that of a twenty-year-old (200 beats per minute). Heart rate is under the control of both the parasympathetic and sympathetic nervous systems. The parasympathetic nervous system is responsible for keeping the heart rate lower at rest. The sympathetic nervous system takes over during exercise so that heart rate can be increased in order to meet the increased oxygen demand. The decline in maximal heart rate is caused by the aging heart becoming less sensitive to sympathetic nervous system stimulation, thereby decreasing the heart's maximal contractile capabilities. This results in the inability of the heart to attain the higher maximal values that were possible during youth. No amount of exercise training can alter this. Submaximal exercise is also more strenuous for an older adult. Exercise sessions that were once easy during youth cause higher heart rates and longer recovery times when one is older. This reflects the heightened need of the aging heart to work harder in order to meet the increased oxygen demands of the exercising tissues.

Regular exercise participation lowers resting heart rate (the number of times the heart beats per minute) and improves stroke volume (the volume of blood ejected with each beat of the heart) in both the young and the old. Even though cardiac contractility and total blood volume in older individuals are less and the ventricular walls are less compliant, regular aerobic exercise training increases total blood volume and tone of the peripheral vessels, thereby reducing vascular resistance and increasing the volume of blood flow back to the heart. This enables the heart to eject more blood with each beat. In aerobically trained individuals, stroke volume is improved not only during exercise but also at rest. The lower resting heart rates commonly seen in trained individuals is partially caused by the improved stroke volume. Since the heart is able to deliver more blood with each beat of the heart, the heart does not need to work as hard to deliver oxygen. In addition, regular aerobic exercise enhances the heart's parasympathetic activity. Therefore, the combined effect of improved parasympathetic activity and improved stroke volume explains the bradycardia (a heart rate below 60 beats per minute) commonly observed in healthy, aerobically trained individuals.

Even though the cardiovascular parameters that determine aerobic fitness all decline with the aging process, participation in regular aerobic exercise has been shown to improve maximal stroke volume and cardiac output (the volume of blood pumped by the heart each minute, equal to heart rate minus stroke volume) by as much as 25 percent. Maximal cardiac output is increased because of the increase in stroke volume, since maximal heart rate does not increase. The types of exercise training employed, as well as the person's initial level of fitness, influence the magnitudes of these increases. Aerobic exercise, not strength training, is the type of exercise required to improve cardiovascular function. Those who are more severely deconditioned will be able to accomplish greater gains simply because they have more room for improvement.

ANAEROBIC POWER

Converse to aerobic capacity, anaerobic power is not dependent upon the replenishment of oxygen to the cells. The fuel source used to power anaerobic movement is retrieved from energy stores located within the cell. Quick, explosive movements characterize anaerobic activities. In most athletic events, the ability to generate anaerobic power will have a direct effect upon athletic success. It is also important in daily living when one encounters an emergency situation demanding a quick, powerful response. A few examples of anaerobic activities include sprinting, throwing the discus, and lifting heavy objects.

The sports-related "anaerobic response" includes a sharp rise in lactic acid accumulation in the muscles and blood, a sharp increase in pulmonary ventilation, and a drop in the blood pH, giving rise to a more acidic state. Lactic acid accumulates with high-intensity or maximal exercise because of a combination of an increased production rate and a reduced rate of removal. The recruitment of fast-twitch muscle fibers (those fibers responsible for performing quick, explosive movements) also triggers the production of lactic acid. In addition, the need for more oxygen at maximal exercise stimulates the metabolic pathways to speed up. This results in an increase in glycolysis. Glycolysis is the energy pathway responsible for the initial breakdown of blood glucose (blood sugar) so that energy (adenosine triphosphate, or ATP) can be created to perform work. At the end of glycolysis, if enough oxygen is not available, excess lactic acid will be formed. An abundance of lactic acid quickly causes muscle fatigue, and exercise soon stops.

Data on aging suggest that anaerobic power, mechanical power, and mechanical capacity peak by age forty, then decline thereafter. Several factors may explain this decline. First, older adults have reduced blood glucose stores (glycogen) in the muscle tissue, which results in a decrease in glycolysis. A decrease in glycolysis will decrease energy production. Second, with aging, fewer fast-twitch muscle fibers are available because of atrophy (shrinkage from disuse). Third, the enzyme lactate dehydrogenase (LDH), which is responsible for lactic acid production when fast-twitch muscle fibers are activated, decreases with aging. Even though the anaerobic processes decline with aging, participation in anaerobic-type activities is still possible as long as the health and fitness status of the older adult is carefully considered.

THE NERVOUS AND MUSCULOSKELETAL SYSTEMS

With aging, the nervous system is unable to receive, process, and transmit messages as quickly as it did in youth. The clinical outcome is slower reaction and movement times. This is an important issue, as many aspects of functional independence require an individual to be able to react quickly in certain situations to prevent potential injury, such as when driving a car or regaining one's balance to prevent a fall. Older individuals who exercise regularly have demonstrated better reaction times, balance, and coordination in comparison to their sedentary peers. Research investigating older adults who play tennis regularly has demonstrated that active older adults can maintain and perhaps improve their motor skills with continued use. Blood flow to the brain also increases during exercise. Short-term, immediate improvements in performance of memory tasks have been demonstrated immediately following aerobic exercise. Whether there is a long-term increase in cerebral blood flow because of regular exercise participation is a question subject to continued research.

Beginning in middle age, muscular strength declines because of a combination of factors, such as muscle mass loss, decreased motor unit activation, and a decreased ability of the muscles to contract forcefully. This decline is selective as well, with some muscle groups losing substantially more strength than others. For instance, leg and trunk muscle strength appears to decline at a faster rate than arm strength. The decline in muscle mass occurs in phases. From twenty-five to fifty years of age, only about 10 percent of muscle mass is lost. However, by age eighty, almost 40 percent of muscle mass is lost because of atrophy. This "wasting away" of muscle tissue commonly seen in the elderly is known as sarcopenia. Weakened respiratory muscles will result in limited aerobic capabilities. Weakened lower-extremity muscles give rise to balance problems and increased risk for falls. Insufficient strength to carry out activities of daily living or functional tasks results in a loss of independent living. Although the age-related loss of muscle mass and strength cannot be totally eliminated, it can be reduced. Aging does not impair the ability of skeletal muscles to respond to exercise training. Progressive strength training programs have demonstrated that older adults can achieve gains in muscle mass (hypertrophy) and muscle strength similar to what has been observed in young individuals.

Exercise has been shown to be beneficial in reducing bone mass loss (osteoporosis). Both weight-bearing aerobic training and strength training have been found to be beneficial in improving bone mass. However, the modest improvements shown to occur with bone mass because of exercise conditioning is not great enough to prevent a fracture caused by a fall. Rather, exercise training will help to reduce the risk of falls by strengthening the ambulatory musculature. Research studies indicate that aerobic training and strength training improve neuromuscular functioning, gait, and balance, all of which are important variables in the risk profile for falls.

Psychosocial Benefits of Exercise

Psychological well-being includes components such as self-esteem, self-efficacy, depression, and anxiety. The majority of research studies investigating these factors in older individuals agree that participation in regular exercise is associated with improved psychological well-being. The benefits are greater and more consistent if the individual participates in an exercise program for at least ten weeks. Either aerobic training or strength training will work well, but very light or very vigorous exercise is not as effective as moderate-intensity exercise.

It is often cited that older individuals benefit from group activities—group interactions alleviate feelings of loneliness often encountered with aging. While this may be true for some, home-based exercise may be preferable to the class setting for certain groups of older adults. Many older adults remain very active and are unable to fit a regularly scheduled exercise class into their own tight schedule. Others are unable to get to the exercise site because of transportation problems or physical disabilities but are still capable of performing some type of exercise or physical activity at home. A safe, moderately paced home program would better meet their needs.

Health Benefits

It has been demonstrated that participation in regular exercise can assist with weight management and body-fat reduction, lower blood pressure for those with mild hypertension (elevated blood pressure), reduce blood triglyceride and low-density lipoproteins (LDL, or "bad cholesterol"), and improve high-density lipoprotein levels (HDL, or "good cholesterol"). Both aerobic and strength training programs can promote a loss of calories and therefore reduce fat deposits and encourage muscle maintenance or growth throughout the life span. However, only aerobic training has been proven to be effective in improving the lipoprotein profiles and lowering blood pressure in older individuals.

The risk of glucose intolerance increases as one ages because of insulin resistance. "Glucose intolerance" is a term used to describe the body's inability to regulate its glucose (blood sugar) level. This causes the blood glucose level to be chronically elevated, which can lead to diabetes. Insulin is a hormone that helps to regulate blood glucose levels. It is released when the blood glucose levels are elevated, such as after eating a meal or during high-intensity exercise. Therefore, the role of insulin is to reduce the blood glucose level. However, sometimes the body cannot utilize its insulin properly. This creates a condition known as insulin resistance. The result is an overload of blood glucose in the system, which again predisposes the individual to diabetes. Physical inactivity and obesity compound the problem. Regular participation in either aerobic exercise or strength training has been shown to be equally effective for improving glucose balance and the body's ability to use insulin in older adults.

RISKS AND GUIDELINES

There are many exercise options available for the older adult, depending on specific goals and health status. Even though exercise is associated with a variety of health benefits, it is also associated with such health risks as worsening existing medical problems, muscle and joint injuries, and, in some cases, heart attack. Therefore, exercise programs should be designed to maximize the benefits and minimize the potential risks.

Regardless of age, the Report of the Surgeon General recommends that everyone should participate in moderate exercise for at least thirty minutes on all or most days of the week for optimal health and fitness. This should be accomplished gradually. If one's goal is to improve aerobic fitness, blood pressure, cholesterol level, mood, or glucose tolerance or to reduce body fat, moderate aerobic exercise should be done at least three times per week. This requires activities that are rhythmic in nature, involve the use of larger muscle groups, and can be sustained for at least fifteen to twenty continuous minutes. If the goal is to increase muscle mass, muscular endurance, or strength, then a well-rounded strength-training program should be done twice per week, with each session followed by at least one day of rest. If the goal is to maintain or improve bone mass, either weight-bearing aerobic exercise or resistance training could be used. The ideal exercise program includes both aerobic training and strength training.

A healthy older individual can begin a light to moderate exercise program without the need for a medical examination or clinical exercise test. However, if the individual has risk factors for heart disease, is taking medications, or has any medical concerns, he or she should consult with a physician to determine a safe level of exercise participation.

—Bonita L. Marks

See also Aging; Broken bones in the elderly; Cholesterol; Diabetes mellitus; Exercise; Exercise and children; Hypertension; Medications and the elderly; Mobility problems in the elderly; Muscle loss with aging; Osteoporosis; Reaction time and aging; Safety issues for the elderly; Sports injuries among children; Temperature regulation and aging.

FOR FURTHER INFORMATION:
American College of Sports Medicine. *ACSM Fitness Book.* Edited by Susan M. Puhl, Madeline Paternostro-Bayles, and Barry Franklin. 2d ed. Champaign, Ill.: Human Kinetics, 1998. A basic book written by academic and clinical professionals intended to guide adults who wish to begin a low-intensity exercise program.
Ettinger, Walter H., Brenda S. Mitchell, and Steven N. Blair. *Fitness After Fifty.* St. Louis: Beverly Cracom, 1996. A "how-to" book written by experts in the field of aging and epidemiology for middle-aged and older individuals desiring to become physically active.

Hurley, Ben F., and James M. Hagberg. "Optimizing Health in Older Persons: Aerobic or Strength Training?" In *Exercise and Sport Science Reviews*, edited by John O. Hollszy. American College of Sports Medicine Series 26. Baltimore: Williams & Wilkins, 1998. This chapter in a collection of exercise-related papers reviews the facts known about the effects of aerobic exercise and strength training on the physiological processes in the older adult.

Rowe, John W., and Robert L. Kahn. *Successful Aging*. New York: Pantheon Books, 1998. A summary of research results dedicated to determining the effects of aging on the body and maximizing health in older individuals; written for the layperson by renowned gerontologists.

Westcott, Wayne L., and Thomas R. Baechle. *Strength Training Past Fifty*. Champaign, Ill.: Human Kinetics, 1998. An excellent layperson's guide for safe and effective strength training written by leaders in the field of strength and conditioning.

✦ Factitious disorders

Type of issue: Mental health

Definition: Psychophysiological disorders in which individuals intentionally produce symptoms in order to play the role of patient.

Although factitious disorders cover a wide array of physical symptoms and are believed to be closely related to a subset of psychophysiological disorders (somatoform disorders), they are unique in all of medicine for two reasons. The first distinguishing factor is that whatever the physical disease for which treatment is sought and regardless of how serious, the patients who seek its treatment have deliberately and intentionally produced the condition. They may have done so in one of three ways, or in any combination of these three ways. First, patients fabricate, invent, lie about, and make up symptoms that they do not have; for example, they claim to have fever and night sweats or severe back pain that they actually do not have. Second, patients have the actual symptoms that they describe, but they intentionally caused them; for example, they might inject human saliva into their own skin to produce an abscess or ingest a known allergic food to cause the predictable reaction. Third, someone with a known condition such as pancreatitis has a pain episode but exaggerates its severity, or someone else with a history of migraines claims his or her headache to be yet another migraine when it is not.

The second element that makes these disorders unique (and at the same time both fascinating to study and frustrating to treat) is that the sole motivation for causing or claiming the symptoms is for these patients to become and remain patients, to assume the sick role wherein little can be expected from them. These patients are not malingerers, individuals who consciously use actual or feigned symptoms for some other gain (such as claiming a fever so one does not have to go to work or school, or insisting that one's post-traumatic stress is worse than it is to enhance the judgment in a lawsuit). In fact, it is the absence of any discernible external benefit that makes these disorders so intriguing.

Types of Factitious Disorder

Factitious disorders have three subtypes. In the first, patients claim to have predominantly psychological symptoms such as memory loss, depression, contemplation of suicide, the hearing of voices, or false memory of childhood molestation. Characteristically, the symptoms worsen whenever the patients know themselves to be under observation. In the second, patients have predominantly physical symptoms that at least superficially suggest some general medical condition. In a more extreme form called Münchausen syndrome, individuals will have spent much of their lives getting admitted to medical facilities and, once there, remaining as long as possible. While common complaints include vomiting, dizziness, blacking out, generalized rashes, and bleeding, the symptoms can involve any organ and seem limited only to the individuals' medical knowledge and experience with the medical system. The third subtype combines both psychological and physical complaints in such a way that neither predominates.

Factitious disorders are difficult to diagnose. Usually, the diagnosis is considered when the course of treating either a medical or a mental illness becomes atypical and protracted. Often, the person with a factitious disorder will present in a way which seems odd to the experienced clinician. The person may have an unusually extensive history of traveling, much familiarity with medical procedures and terminology, a complex medical and surgical history, few visitors during the hospitalization, behavioral disruptions and disturbances while hospitalized, exacerbation of symptoms while under observation, and/or fluctuating illness with new symptoms and complications arising as the workup proceeds. When present, these traits along with others make suspicion of factitious disorders reasonable.

No one knows how many people suffer with factitious disorders, but the condition is generally regarded as uncommon. It is certainly rarely reported, but this in part may be attributable to the difficulties in determining the diagnosis. While brief episodes of the condition occur, most people who claim a factitious disorder have it chronically, and they usually move on to another physician or facility when they are confronted with the true nature of their illness. It is therefore likely that some individuals are reported more than once by different hospitals and providers.

THE QUESTION OF CAUSE

There is little certainty about what causes factitious disorders. This is true in large measure because those who know the most about the subject—patients with the disorder—are notoriously unreliable in providing information about their psychological state and often seem only dimly aware of what they are doing to themselves. It may be that they are generally incapable of putting their feelings into words. They are unaware of having inner feelings and may not know, for example, that they are sad or angry. It is possible that they experience emotions more physically, behaviorally, and concretely than do most others.

Another view suggests that people learn to distinguish their primitive emotional states through the responsivity of their primary caretaker. A normal, healthy parent responds appropriately to an infant's differing affective states, thereby helping the infant, as he or she develops, to distinguish, define, and eventually name what he or she is feeling. When a primary caretaker is, for any of several reasons, incapable of responding in consistently appropriate ways, the infant's emotional awareness remains undifferentiated and the child experiences confusion and emotional chaos.

TREATING FACTITIOUS DISORDERS

Internists, family practitioners, and surgeons are the specialists most likely to encounter patients with factitious disorder, although psychiatrists and psychologists are often consulted in the management of these patients. These patients pose a special challenge because in a real sense they do not wish to become well even as they present themselves for treatment. They are not ill in the usual sense, and their indirect communication and manipulation often make them frustrating to treat using standard goals and expectations.

Sometimes mental and medical specialists' joint, supportive confrontation of these patients results in a disappearance of the troubling and troublesome behavior. During these confrontations, the health professionals are acknowledging that such extreme behavior evidences extreme distress in these patients, and as such is its own reason for psychotherapeutic intervention. These patients are not psychologically minded, however; they also have trouble forming relationships that foster genuine self-disclosure, and they rarely accept the recommendation for psychotherapeutic treatment. Because they believe that their problems are physical, not psychological, they often become irate at the suggestion that their problems are not what they believe them to be.

—*Paul Moglia*

See also Münchausen syndrome by proxy.

FOR FURTHER INFORMATION:

American Psychiatric Association. *Diagnostic and Statistical Manual of Mental Disorders.* Rev. 4th ed. Washington, D.C.: Author, 2000.

Feldman, Marc D., and Charles V. Ford. *Patient or Pretender? Inside the Strange World of Factitious Disorders.* New York: John Wiley & Sons, 1994.

Ford, Charles V. *The Somatizing Disorders: Illness as a Way of Life.* New York: Elsevier Biomedical, 1983.

Viederman, M. "Somatoform and Factitious Disorders." In *The Personality Disorders and Neuroses,* edited by Arnold M. Cooper, Allen J. Frances, and Michael H. Sacks. New York: Basic Books, 1986.

✦ FAILURE TO THRIVE

Type of issue: Children's health

Definition: A disorder of early childhood growth that includes disturbances in psychosocial skills and development.

Failure to thrive may be organic or nonorganic; in many children, the etiology is multifactorial. The onset of growth problems may be prenatal as a result of maternal substance abuse, most notably alcohol use, or of maternal infection, particularly with rubella, cytomegalovirus (CMV), or toxoplasmosis. Small size in infants secondary to prematurity resolves by two to three years of age unless there are complications.

Many children with failure to thrive are both stunted (linear growth-affected) and wasted (weight-affected). Assessing which of the two conditions predominates can be done using the body mass index (BMI), which is calculated by dividing weight in kilograms by height in meters squared. A low BMI is a sign of malnutrition. Children with environmental failure to thrive fall into this category.

A child who is small but has an appropriate BMI has short stature rather than failure to thrive. The two leading causes of short stature are familial short stature and constitutional delay.

LEARNING TO THRIVE

The main focus of the medical intervention with failure to thrive is to ensure a nurturing environment and adequate nutrition. Nutritional intervention can be achieved in many ways, such as by securing adequate access to food for the family and offering concentrated formulas, nutritional supplementation, and calorie dense food, depending on the age of the child. Developmental intervention should also be provided if delay is detected. Likewise, family counseling, especially focusing on parenting skills, may be indicated.

The term "failure to thrive" originated in 1933; it replaced the term "cease to thrive," which appeared in 1899. Initially, the condition was reported in institutionalized children, including those in orphanages. In the 1940's, it was recognized as a condition that could also affect children living at home with their biological or adoptive parents.

Although the list of conditions that can cause growth impairment in children is quite extensive, a systematic approach using history and both physical and psychosocial assessment will provide clues to the diagnosis. Intervention ensures an adequate outcome, with improved prospects for physical growth and brain development.

—*Carol D. Berkowitz, M.D.*

See also Children's health issues; Fetal alcohol syndrome; Malnutrition among children; Nutrition and children; Well-baby examinations.

FOR FURTHER INFORMATION:
Garrow, J. S., and W. P. T. James, eds. *Human Nutrition and Dietetics.* Rev. 9th ed. New York: Churchill Livingstone, 1993.
Kreutler, Patricia A., and Dorice M. Czajka-Narins. *Nutrition in Perspective.* 2d ed. Englewood Cliffs, N.J.: Prentice Hall, 1987.
Whitney, Eleanor Noss, and Sharon Rady Rolfes. *Understanding Nutrition.* 6th ed. St. Paul, Minn.: West, 1993.
Winick, Myron, Brian L. G. Morgan, Jaime Rozovski, and Robin Marks-Kaufman, eds. *The Columbia Encyclopedia of Nutrition.* New York: G. P. Putnam's Sons, 1988.

✦ FALLS AMONG CHILDREN

Type of issue: Children's health, prevention
Definition: Episodes of sudden, usually unintentional movement from an erect to a prone position.

Falls may occur at any age in the pediatric population. In the younger age groups, they may be caused by toys, rugs, stairs, unguarded windows, and climbing. In older groups, falls may be related to bicycle riding, climbing, and various risk-taking behaviors.

AFTER TUMBLING

The treatment of falls ranges from nothing at all to immediate intervention, depending on the severity of the resulting injuries. Toddlers often tumble down without adverse consequences. Sprains, fractures, significant bruising, lacerations, or head injury, however, can occur. Any child who falls and is unresponsive needs to be transported to an emergency room for evaluation. Appropriate precautions must always be taken in case of neck injury.

Falls from a moderate height in children under the age of twelve rarely cause fractures. A child who sustains a significant injury from a minor fall should be evaluated for potential child abuse, as should the toddler with a head injury.

PREVENTING FALLS

Especially in the early years, parents need to monitor the child's environment for risk of falls. Stairways should be well lit, and carpet should be tacked down firmly. Throw rugs and scattered toys may lead to falls. If the floors in a home are slippery, parents should provide the child with skid-proof socks or footwear. Stairwells should be closed off with a door or gate. For those living above ground level, windows should have guards to prevent falls. Infant walkers on wheels are associated with falls resulting in serious injuries. The use of these walkers must be monitored closely or avoided if possible.

Children and adolescents should be warned about climbing in hazardous areas. Falls in adolescents may be associated with alcohol or other drug use. Mind-altering substances not only affect balance but also may impede judgment, leading teenagers to take risks that they would not take when sober.

—*Rebecca Lovell Scott*

See also Child abuse; Children's health issues; Drug abuse by teenagers; Falls among the elderly; First aid; Safety issues for children; Sports injuries among children.

FOR FURTHER INFORMATION:

American Academy of Pediatrics. *Playground Safety.* Elk Grove Village, Ill.: Author, 1994. This brochure reviews the safety hazards of playgrounds and offers prevention measures. Free samples of this brochure are available upon request with a self-addressed, stamped envelope to AAP, Dept C-"Playground Safety," 141 Northwest Point Blvd., P.O. Box 927, Elk Grove Village, IL 60009. The phone number of the AAP is (800) 433-9016.

Shelov, Steven P., et al., eds. *Caring for Your Baby and Young Child: Birth to Age Five.* Rev. ed. New York: Bantam Books, 1998. Offers a comprehensive discussion of the accidents that commonly occur with young children, accident-prevention techniques for the home and outdoors, and emergency measures to enact if an accident does take place.

✧ Falls among the elderly

Type of issue: Elder health, prevention
Definition: Falling as a result of imbalance, dizziness, or weakness, which is common among the elderly and which may cause serious injury, particularly hip fractures.

Falls are the most frequent cause of injury among the elderly. Those people over eighty years of age have a mortality rate from falls eight times greater than people sixty years of age. Falls are the major risk factor for hip fractures; approximately 200,000 hip fractures occur each year in the United States, 12 to 20 percent of which lead to death. Only one-fourth of older adults who sustain a hip fracture fully recover. Elderly people who suffer from osteoporosis have a greater chance of sustaining fractures of the hips, wrist, pelvis, and lumbar vertebrae. The loss of skin elasticity and subcutaneous tissue that generally accompanies aging can also lead to bruising and skin tears.

Although most falls occur when a person is descending a stairway, they may be caused by numerous factors in the home, including unstable furniture, loose floor coverings, poor lighting in hallways and bathrooms, clutter, pets, and slick substances on the floor, such as polish, ice, water, or grease. The use of certain medications may also cause the elderly to fall. Some diuretics, sedatives, antibiotics, antidepressants, and antipsychotics can induce drowsiness, confusion, or dizziness. Physical changes that accompany the aging process can also make people more susceptible to sustaining injuries from falls. Vision and hearing may become impaired, leading to changes in perception. Reflexes may become slower. Vertigo and syncope episodes may cause falls. Mental changes, such as depression and inattention, can also cause falls in the elderly.

Prevention and Precautions

Medical experts advise elderly people to take precautions against falls. People who do not have good balance are often advised to wear shoes with a soft sole and a low, broad heel. High heels, loose-fitting slippers, or socks without shoes on stairs or waxed floors should be avoided. In addition, tennis shoes that have good traction can cause people to trip. Elderly people with poor night vision can use bedside lamps or night-lights in case they have to get up in the middle of the night. Those prone to dizziness are advised to stand up slowly to avoid vertigo. Keeping the thermostat at 65 degrees Fahrenheit or above at night can help people avoid the drowsiness that tends to accompany prolonged exposure to cold temperatures.

Another way to prevent falls is to keep walkways free of clutter and to keep electrical and phone cords out of the way. Low furniture can be positioned so it is not an obstacle to people when walking. White paint or white strips on the edges of steps can help elderly people see them better. The risk of falls in the kitchen can be minimized by placing frequently used items in accessible cupboards to avoid reaching, bending, or stooping, and by covering tile or linoleum floors with nonskid wax. In the bathroom, grab bars can be installed on the wall by the tub, shower, and toilet, while nonskid mats or adhesive strips can be placed on all surfaces that can get wet and slippery.

Exercise can also help minimize the risk of injury from falls. Such activities as walking, gardening, and housework can improve gait, posture, and balance. Weight-bearing exercise, such as walking, helps prevent loss of bone mass, as well as stiffness and loss of muscle tone. Lifting small weights can prevent loss of muscle tone and help strengthen hand grip, both of which are important for holding on to railings and properly executing such tasks as getting up from chairs.

Elderly people who fear falling may decrease their activity level, which causes their muscles to deteriorate even more. The fear of falling can also make them clinically depressed, which often shortens their attention span and makes them more likely to fall. This is especially true if they have fallen before and have sustained an injury or fracture.

—Mitzie L. Bryant

See also Aging; Broken bones in the elderly; Canes and walkers; Disabilities; Exercise and the elderly; Falls among children; Foot disorders; Hospitalization of the elderly; Medications and the elderly; Mobility problems in the elderly; Osteoporosis; Reaction time and aging; Safety issues for the elderly; Temperature regulation and aging; Vision problems with aging; Wheelchair use among the elderly.

FOR FURTHER INFORMATION:

DeWit, Susan C. *Essentials of Medical-Surgical Nursing.* 4th ed. Philadelphia: W. B. Saunders, 1998. DeWit provides information on fractures, accidents, and burns in the elderly and how to prevent them.

Murray, Ruth Beckmann, and Judith Proctor Zentner. *Health Assessment and Promotion Strategies Through the Life Span.* 7th ed. Englewood Cliffs, N.J.: Prentice Hall, 2000. Provides insight on contributing factors and prevention of injuries in the elderly.

Rosdahl, Caroline Bunker, ed. *Textbook of Basic Nursing.* 7th ed. Philadelphia: Lippincott Williams & Wilkins, 1999. Discusses the normal physical signs of aging that can be associated with and contribute to injuries.

Solomon, Jacqueline. "Osteoporosis: When Supports Weaken." *RN* 61 (May, 1998). Solomon provides useful information on a condition of the bone common among the aged that causes fractures and weak muscles.

Walker, Bonnie L. "Preventing Falls." *RN* 61 (May, 1998). Walker discusses the likelihood of falls in the elderly and how to minimize the risk.

✧ Fetal alcohol syndrome

Type of issue: Children's health, women's health
Definition: Growth retardation and mental or physical abnormalities in a child resulting from alcohol consumption by the mother during pregnancy.

Fetal alcohol syndrome was first identified in the early 1970's. Whether consumed as beer, wine, or hard liquor, alcohol is a teratogen, a toxic substance that can cause abnormalities in unborn children. The damage ranges from subtle to severe, depending on the quantity consumed and the stage of pregnancy when the exposure occurs. A critical period is in early pregnancy, when a woman may not know that she is pregnant. Even one or two drinks a day by the mother may have an effect on her child.

Effects and Causes of Fetal Alcohol Syndrome

There are three diagnostic criteria for fetal alcohol syndrome: growth retardation, certain facial anomalies, and central nervous system impairment. Growth retardation begins in utero, causing low birth weight. Babies with low birth weight are at risk for delayed growth and development and even death. Growth impairment affects not only the skeleton but also the brain and face. The resulting head and facial abnormalities are characterized by thin lips; small, wide-set eyes; a short, upturned nose; a receding chin; and low-set ears. Fetal alcohol syndrome children have intelligence quotients (IQs) well below the mean of the population because of impaired brain growth that results in irreversible mental retardation. Fetal alcohol syndrome is a leading cause of mental retardation. Abnormalities often originate during the first trimester, when bones and organs are forming. Major organ systems such as the heart, kidney, liver, and skeleton can be impaired.

Less specific problems that result from alcohol damage are clumsiness, behavioral problems, a brief attention span, poor judgment, impaired memory, and a diminished capacity to learn from experience. These symptoms are often labeled "fetal alcohol effects."

Alcohol enters the fetal bloodstream as soon as the mother has a drink. It not only can damage the brain but also may impair the function of the placenta, which is the organ interface between maternal and fetal circulation. The exact mechanism for this damage is not completely understood. The most probable cause is that alcohol creates a glucose or oxygen deficit for the fetus. Because it is not known what dose of alcohol is safe, the best preventive measure is to abstain from alcohol during pregnancy and even when planning a pregnancy.

—Wendy L. Stuhldreher, R.D.

See also Addiction; Alcoholism; Alcoholism among teenagers; Birth defects; Child abuse; Childbirth complications; Drug abuse by teenagers; Genetic diseases; Pregnancy among teenagers; Premature birth; Prenatal care; Screening; Smoking; Tobacco use by teenagers.

FOR FURTHER INFORMATION:

Abel, Ernest L., ed. *Fetal Alcohol Syndrome: From Mechanism to Prevention*. Boca Raton, Fla.: CRC Press, 1996.

Huebert, Kathryn M., and Cindy Raftis. *Fetal Alcohol Syndrome and Other Alcohol-Related Birth Defects*. Edmonton: Alberta Alcohol and Drug Abuse Commission, 1996.

Spohr, Hans-Ludwig, and Hans-Christoph Steinhausen., eds. *Alcohol, Pregnancy, and the Developing Child*. New York: Cambridge University Press, 1996.

Stratton, Kathleen, Cynthia Howe, and Frederick Battaglia, eds. *Fetal Alcohol Syndrome: Diagnosis, Epidemiology, Prevention, and Treatment*. Washington, D.C.: National Academy Press, 1996.

Streissguth, Ann Pytkowicz. *Fetal Alcohol Syndrome: A Guide for Families and Communities*. Baltimore: Paul H. Brookes, 1997.

✧ FETAL TISSUE TRANSPLANTATION

Type of issue: Ethics, medical procedures, treatment
Definition: The controversial use of tissue from aborted human fetuses to replace damaged tissue in patients with diseases in which the patient's own tissue has been destroyed.

Tissues from aborted fetuses have been shown in experimental trials to be an excellent source of replacement tissue for patients whose diseases have destroyed their own vital tissues. Parkinson's, Huntington's, and Alzheimer's diseases (in which regions of the brain deteriorate) or type I diabetes mellitus (in which insulin-secreting cells of the pancreas degenerate) theoretically could be cured with suitable tissue replacement.

Fetal tissues do not induce a full-scale immune response when transplanted. Fetal cells are said to be immunologically naïve since they have not yet acquired the cell surface molecular markers that are recognized by the immune system. When transplanted into a patient, they seem to be invisible to the patient's immune system and are tolerated without the use of immunosuppression.

Other properties add to the suitability of fetal tissue for transplantation. Because it is not yet fully differentiated, fetal tissue is said to be very plastic in its abilities to adapt to new locations. Moreover, once placed in a patient, it secretes factors that promote its own growth and those of the new blood vessels at the site. Tissue from an adult source does not have these properties, and consequently is slow-growing and poorly vascularized. Though growth factors can be added along with the graft, adult tissue is less responsive to these hormones than is fetal tissue.

CONTROVERSY OVER SOURCES OF FETAL TISSUE

It is the source of fetal tissue that has fired such debate over its use for transplantation. Though there has been general acceptance of tissue from spontaneous abortions (miscarriages) or ectopic pregnancies which, because of their location outside of the womb, endanger the life of the mother and must be terminated, these sources are not well suited to transplantation. Spontaneous abortions rarely produce viable tissue, since in most cases the fetus has died two to three weeks before it is expelled. In addition, there are usually major genetic defects in the aborted fetus. In ectopic pregnancies as well, more than 50 percent of the fetuses are genetically abnormal, and most resolve themselves in spontaneous abortion outside a clinic setting. These types of abortions are almost always accompanied by a sense of tragic loss felt by the parents. Many researchers find it unacceptable to request permission from these parents to transplant tissue from the lost fetus.

The alternative source of fetal tissue is elected abortions. One-and-a-half million of these abortions occur in the United States every year. The debate over the ethical correctness of elected abortions has left a cloud of confusion over the issue of using this tissue for transplantation.

When an abortion is performed in a clinic, the tissue is removed by suction through a narrow tube. Normally, the tissue would be thrown away. If it is to be used for transplantation, written permission must be obtained from the woman after the abortion is completed. No discussion of transplantation is to take place prior to the abortion, and no alteration in the abortion procedure, except to keep the tissue sterile during collection, is to be made. The donor may not be paid for the tissue, and both the donor and the recipient of the tissue must remain anonymous to each other.

USES OF FETAL TISSUE TRANSPLANTS

The major focus for fetal tissue transplantation has been the treatment of patients with Parkinson's disease, and results have been encouraging. The drugs used to treat the disorder, dopamine precursors such as L-dopa, produce side effects that cause unrelenting and uncontrolled movement of the limbs, periods in which the patient is completely frozen, and hallucinations. Patients with parkinsonism who have received fetal tissue transplants have shown remarkable improvement and diminished requirements for drug treatment. Even better results have been obtained in patients with induced Parkinson-like symptoms. Because no patient with parkinsonism or Parkinson-like symptoms has yet been cured by a fetal tissue transplant, however, some have considered the results of such experiments to be disappointing. Yet many parkinsonism patients themselves are encouraged, and many have resumed driving and the other tasks of normal daily life.

That transplanted fetal brain tissue can replace damaged brain tissue to any extent has opened the doors of hope for many diseases. For example, Huntington's disease, a genetic disorder that destroys a different set of neurons but in the same region as that affected by parkinsonism, brings a slow death to those carrying the dominant trait. Its severe dementia and uncontrollable jerking and writhing that steadily progress have had no treatment and no cure. In animal studies in which fetal brain tissue was transplanted into rats with symptoms mimicking Huntington's disease, results have been encouraging enough to warrant human trials, and one human trial in Mexico has shown limited success. Researchers are hopeful, though less optimistic, that Alzheimer's disease also may be treatable with fetal tissue transplants. Because the destruction is so widespread, however, it is difficult to determine where the transplants should be placed.

Type I or insulin-dependent diabetes also has been treated with fetal tissue transplants. After animal tests showed a complete reversal of the disease when fetal pancreatic tissue was transplanted into diabetic rats, human trials were initiated with great expectations. Though complete success has not been achieved, the sixteen diabetic patients who were given fetal pancreatic tissue transplants by Dr. Kevin Lafferty between 1987 and 1992 all showed significant drops in the amount of insulin needed to manage their disease. The transplanted tissue continued to pump out insulin.

An unusual variation of such procedures has been to transplant fetal tissue into fetuses diagnosed with severe metabolic diseases. It is more effective to treat the condition while the fetus is still in the womb than to wait until after birth, when damage from the disease may already be extensive. Fetuses with Hurler's syndrome and similar "storage" diseases have been treated in this way. Hurler's syndrome is a lethal condition in which tissues become clogged with stored mucupolysaccharides, long-chain sugars that the body is unable to break down because it lacks the appropriate enzyme. One of the fetuses to receive this treatment was the child of a couple who had lost two children to the disease. With the transplanted tissue, the child lived and by one year of age was producing therapeutic levels of the enzyme. It has been estimated that at least 155 other genetic disorders could be similarly treated by fetal tissue transplants in utero.

Other ailments that fetal tissue transplants may alleviate include sickle-cell disease, thalassemias, metabolic disorders, immune deficiencies, myelin disorders, and spinal cord injuries.

—*Mary S. Tyler*

376 ✧ First aid

See also Abortion; Alzheimer's disease; Diabetes mellitus; Ethics; Genetic diseases; Genetic engineering; Law and medicine; Parkinson's disease; Transplantation.

For Further Information:

Beardsley, Tim. "Aborting Research." *Scientific American* 267, no. 2 (August, 1992): 17-18. An excellent encapsulation of the debate over fetal tissue transplantation and the instances in which it has been used.

Begley, Sharon. "From Human Embryos, Hope for 'Spare Parts.'" *Newsweek,* November 16, 1998, 73. Researchers have teased out clumps of cells from human embryos and induced them to burst into a veritable cellular symphony, forming most of the 210 kinds of cells that constitute the human body. These colonies could revolutionize transplantation medicine.

"Fetal Cell Study Shows Promise for Parkinson's." *The Los Angeles Times,* April 22, 1999, p. 29. The first federally funded trial to study the effectiveness of fetal cell transplants for Parkinson's disease has proved that it works for some patients, mainly those under the age of sixty.

Singer, Peter, H. Kuhse, S. Buckle, K. Dawson, and P. Kasimba, eds. *Embryo Experimentation.* Cambridge, England: Cambridge University Press, 1990. This text provides an excellent discussion of the moral questions raised by the use of fetal tissue for transplantation.

Wade, Nicholas. "Primordial Cells Fuel Debate on Ethics." *The New York Times,* November 10, 1998, p. 1. Two groups of scientists report success in the attempt to grow primordial human cells outside the body, increasing the ethical debate over the use of these cells.

✧ First aid

Type of issue: Medical procedures, public health, treatment
Definition: The immediate evaluation, care, stabilization, and transport of victims suffering sudden and/or acute trauma or illness.

First aid begins when someone recognizes and responds to an emergency. Unusual sounds can mean emergency: moans, cries for help, shattering glass, squealing brakes, or the thud of falling objects. Out-of-the-ordinary sights often indicate emergency: fallen electric wires, overturned vehicles, smoke, spilled medicines, or bleeding. Strong or unrecognizable odors sometimes require quick action: burning smells or the odor of spilled caustic liquids or volatile gases. Children or adults may need help if they are exhibiting unusual behavior: gasping, clutching at the chest, sweating profusely, staggering, turning red or blue, or abruptly losing color or consciousness.

How to Evaluate an Emergency

The *ABCD* survey helps first responders evaluate a situation quickly.

A stands for airway, the path from the mouth or nose to the lungs. Blood, food, mucus, foreign objects, or broken teeth can obstruct a child's flow of air. Removing the obstruction with a finger sweep or an abdominal thrust (the Heimlich maneuver) usually clears the airway and often allows spontaneous breathing.

B stands for breathing. Allergic reactions, electrical shock, drowning, or severe asthma can cause breathing to stop. Tilting the patient's head and performing rescue breathing can cause the victim to begin breathing spontaneously or can provide sufficient oxygen for the patient to survive while awaiting advanced emergency care. Unless the victim has an open airway and can breathe, no other emergency care can succeed.

C stands for circulation. If the victim has no perceptible pulse, then the child has no blood circulating. Body parts, especially the vulnerable brain, can begin to die in four minutes without oxygen. Where no heartbeat exists, first responders can perform rhythmic chest thrusts. "Squeezing" the heart between the center chest and the backbone causes the heart to push blood through the body and can lead to spontaneous resumption of a heartbeat or keep a victim alive until advanced life support becomes available.

Circulation refers to the amount of blood in the victim's venous system as well as to the heartbeat. If bleeding is profuse, the heart can shut down. Bright red, spurting blood means a damaged artery and requires prompt treatment. First responders can apply pressure directly to the wound or fasten a constriction band between the wound and the heart to slow bleeding. Because tourniquets cut off the blood supply to an injured area completely, they pose dangers of their own, including gangrene and/or loss of the wounded limb; tourniquets are usually considered a last resort, when the only alternative is death from blood loss.

Darker red, nonspurting blood means that a vein has been damaged. Applying direct pressure, a constricting band, or a snug and thick bandage or elevating the injured area usually slows the bleeding.

D stands for disability. It includes the victim's level of consciousness and the likelihood of a neck or spinal cord injury. First responders can keep the victim quiet and warm. Pillows, rocks, or branches can immobilize the patient and prevent further damage to the neck or spine.

Tending to Lesser Injuries

The *ABCD* pattern applies only to the rudiments of immediate care, without which the victim might die. Tending to less-threatening injuries and illnesses makes up the rest of first responder care. Pediatric emergencies can include burns, bites, sprains, broken bones, the ingestion of toxic substances, dislocations, snakebites, sunburn, frostbite, splinters, and many other illnesses and injuries. Because children's heads are proportionally smaller and their bones are less dense than those of adults, they can incur greater injuries than adults in similar situations. In addition, children usually lack adult awareness of hygiene, environmental dangers, and their own limitations, so they may require first aid more frequently than do adults.

Any first aid or emergency care involves the complication of later infection or undetected injuries. Both rescuers and victims may suffer emotional trauma or physical problems. Checking with a health care professional benefits everyone involved in first aid.

World wars and assorted disasters have challenged health care professionals to develop better means of triage, treatment, transport, and follow-up. Emergency medical services (EMS) systems in the United States now include air transport, first responder training, trauma centers, burn units, 911 dialing, and an array of lifesaving implements to improve the survival chances for victims.

—Sonya H. Cashdan

See also Allergies; Asthma; Burns and scalds; Children's health issues; Choking; Drowning; Electrical shock; Falls among children; Falls among the elderly; Food poisoning; Broken bones in the elderly; Frostbite; Heat exhaustion and heat stroke; Injuries among the elderly; Meningitis; Poisoning; Poisonous plants; Snakebites; Sports injuries; Suicide; Suicide among children and teenagers; Suicide among the elderly; Sunburns.

FOR FURTHER INFORMATION:
American Red Cross. *First Aid: Responding to Emergencies.* 3d ed. St. Louis: Mosby-Year Book, 1996.
National Safety Council. *Infant and Child CPR.* Sudbury, Mass.: Jones & Bartlett, 1997.
Watson, Sheila, and Elena Bosque. *Safe and Sound: How to Prevent and Treat the Most Common Childhood Emergencies.* Rev. ed. New York: St. Martin's Press, 1997.

✧ FLUORIDATION OF WATER SOURCES

Type of issue: Environmental health, prevention, public health
Definition: The treatment of water with chemicals that release fluoride into a community's water-supply system.

Fluoridation is an example of preventive medicine and was first introduced into the United States in the 1940's in an attempt to reduce tooth decay. Since then, many cities have added fluoride to their public water-supply systems.

Proponents of fluoridation have claimed that it has dramatically reduced tooth decay, which was a serious and widespread problem in the early twentieth century. Opponents of fluoridation have not been entirely convinced of its effectiveness and have been concerned about possible health risks that many be associated with fluoridation. The decision to fluoridate drinking water has generally rested with local governments and communities and has always been a controversial issue.

Fluoride and Tooth Decay

Fluoride is the water-soluble, ionic form of the element fluorine. It is present naturally in most water supplies at low levels, generally less than 0.2 part per million (ppm), and nearly all food contains traces of fluoride. Tea contains more fluoride than most foods, while fish and vegetables also have relatively high levels. Most scientific studies have suggested that water containing a concentration of about 1 ppm fluoride dramatically reduces the incidence of tooth decay.

Tooth decay occurs when food acids dissolve the protective enamel surrounding teeth and create holes, or cavities, in the teeth. These acids are present in food and can also be formed by acid-produced bacteria that convert sugars into acids. Americans have always consumed large quantities of sugar, which is a significant factor in the high incidence of tooth decay. By contrast, studies of people in primitive cultures reveal tooth decay to be less common, which has been attributed to their more natural diets.

Early fluoridation studies between 1930 and 1950 demonstrated that fluoridation of public water systems produced a 50 to 60 percent reduction in tooth decay and that there were no immediate health risks associated with increased fluoride consumption. Consequently, many communities quickly moved to fluoridate their water, and fluoridation was endorsed by most major health organizations in the United States.

Growth of Opposition to Fluoridation

Strong opposition to fluoridation began to emerge in the 1950's as opponents claimed that the possible side effects of fluoride had not been adequately investigated. This concern was not unreasonable, since high levels of ingested fluoride can be lethal. However, it is not unusual for a substance that is lethal at high concentration to be safe at low levels, as is the case with most vitamins and trace elements. Opponents of fluoridation were also concerned on moral grounds because fluoridation represented compulsory mass medication.

Since the 1960's, controversy and heated debate have surrounded the issue of fluoridation across the country. Critics have pointed to the harmful effects of large doses of fluoride, including bone damage and special risks for some people with kidney disease or those who are particularly sensitive to toxic substances. Between the 1950's and 1980's, some scientists suggested that fluoride may have a mutagenic effect—that is, it may be associated with human birth defects, including Down syndrome.

Controversial claims that fluoride can cause cancer were also raised in the 1970's, most notably by biochemist John Yiamouyiannis, who claimed that U.S. cities with fluoridated water had greater cancer death rates than cities with unfluoridated water. Fluoridation proponents were quick to discredit his work by pointing out that he had failed to take other factors into consideration, such as the levels of known environmental carcinogens. Most scientific opinion suggests that the link between cancer and fluoride is a tenuous one. Nevertheless, it is a link that cannot be completely ignored, and a number of respected scientists continue to argue that the benefits of fluoridation are not without potential health risks. A 1988 article in the American Chemical Society publication *Chemical and Engineering News* created considerable attention by suggesting that scientists opposing fluoridation were more credible than had been previously acknowledged. By the 1990's even some fluoridation proponents began suggesting that observed tooth decay reduction as a result of water fluoridation may have been at levels of only around 25 percent. Other factors—such as education, better dental hygiene, and the addition of fluoride to some foods, salt, toothpastes, and mouthwashes—may also contribute to the overall reduction in tooth decay levels.

FLUORIDATION IN THE INTERNATIONAL ARENA

The development of the fluoridation issue in the United States was closely observed by other countries. Dental and medical authorities in Australia, Canada, New Zealand, and Ireland endorsed fluoridation, although not without considerable opposition from various groups. Fluoridation in Western Europe was greeted less enthusiastically, and scientific opinion in some countries, such as France, Germany, and Denmark, concluded that it was unsafe. As a result, few Europeans drink fluoridated water.

While there is little doubt that fluoride does reduce tooth decay, the exact degree to which fluoridated water contributes to the reduction remains unanswered. It also remains unclear what, if any, side effects are involved in ingesting 1 ppm levels of fluoride in water over many years. Although it has been argued that any risks associated with fluoridation are small, these risks may not necessarily be acceptable to everyone.

Since the 1960's and 1970's, concerns over environmental and health issues have been growing, and it has often been difficult, if not impossible, for science to resolve completely the potential hazard of small amounts of chemical substances in the environment. The fact that only about 50 percent of U.S. communities have elected to adopt fluoridation is indicative of people's cautious approach to the issue. In 1993 the National Research

Council published a report on the health effects of ingested fluoride and attempted to determine if the Environmental Protection Agency's maximum recommended level of 4 ppm for fluoride in drinking water should be modified. The report concluded that this level was appropriate but that further research may indicate a need for revision. The report also found inconsistencies in the scientific studies of fluoride toxicity and recommended further research in this area.

—Nicholas C. Thomas

See also Birth defects; Chlorination; Dental problems in children; Dental problems in the elderly; Environmental diseases; Fluoride treatments in dentistry; Preventive medicine; Water quality.

For Further Information:
De Zuane, John. *Handbook of Drinking Water Quality.* 2d ed. New York: Van Nostrand Reinhold, 1997. A good summary of fluoridation.
Hileman, Bette. "Fluoridation of Water." *Chemistry and Engineering News* 66 (August 1, 1988). An easy-to-read article in a readily accessible journal.
Martin, Brian. *Scientific Knowledge in Controversy: The Social Dynamic of the Fluoridation Debate.* Albany: State University of New York Press, 1991. A detailed look at the fluoride debate.
National Research Council. *Health Effects of Ingested Fluoride.* Washington, D.C.: National Academy Press, 1993. Report on fluoridation.
Stewart, John Cary. *Drinking Water Hazards.* Hiram, Ohio: Envirographics, 1989. Another good summary of fluoridation.

❖ Fluoride treatments in dentistry

Type of issue: Children's health, medical procedures, prevention, treatment
Definition: Treatment of the teeth with a fluoride-releasing substance to help the enamel resist tooth decay.

Tooth decay involves the solubility of food during eating. Consumed carbohydrates are oxidized to organic acids, such as lactic acid, by the action of specific bacteria that adhere to the teeth. These acids dissolve tooth enamel, which mainly consists of a mineral called hydroxyapatite and is considered to be the hardest substance in the body. The protection of the enamel, and thus the inner part of the tooth, from decomposition can be achieved through fluoride treatments.

Fluoride treatment involves the ingestion of fluoride ions in drinking water, toothpaste, and other sources to change the nature and composition of hydroxyapatite by producing a new compound called fluorapatite. Because it is less basic than hydroxyapatite, fluorapatite forms a more resistant enamel. Because of its effectiveness in preventing cavities, fluoride is added in the form of sodium fluoride or sodium hexafluorosilicate to the public water supply of many municipalities in the United States in concentrations of about 1 milligram per milliliter, or 1 part per million.

THE BENEFITS OF FLUORIDE

As a result of this so-called fluoridation process, a drastic reduction in dental decay has been observed. In addition, more than 80 percent of all tooth-pastes and gels now sold in the United States contain fluoride, in the form of stannous fluoride, sodium monofluorophosphate, and/or sodium fluoride in concentrations of about 0.1 percent fluoride by weight.

The recommended annual or semiannual dental cleaning by a dentist or oral hygienist removes accumulated plaque and may include further application with a fluoride substance. Generally, only children and teenagers receive such a fluoride treatment, although some adults may also have it.

It must be noted that fluoride ions are toxic in large quantities. As a result, when the fluoride concentration in water is about 2 to 3 parts per million, discoloration (mottling) or damage of the teeth may occur.

—Soraya Ghayourmanesh

See also Children's health issues; Dental problems in children; Fluoridation of water sources; Preventive medicine.

FOR FURTHER INFORMATION:
Foster, Malcolm S. *Protecting Our Children's Teeth: A Guide to Quality Dental Care from Infancy Through Age Twelve*. New York: Insight Books, 1992.
Smith, Rebecca W. *The Columbia University School of Dental and Oral Surgery's Guide to Family Dental Care*. New York: W. W. Norton, 1997.
Woodall, Irene R., ed. *Comprehensive Dental Hygiene Care*. 4th ed. St. Louis: C. V. Mosby, 1993.

❖ FOOD IRRADIATION

Type of issue: Environmental health, industrial practices, public health
Definition: A process that uses nuclear radiation to sterilize foods in order to reduce spoilage and decrease the incidence of illness from contaminated food.

The U.S. Food and Drug Administration (FDA) has certified that irradiation is safe for many foods, including spices, fresh fruit, fish, poultry, and hamburger meat. Opponents of food irradiation focus on the inherent hazards of nuclear technology—especially the production, transportation, and disposal of radioactive materials—and criticize the possible creation of harmful radiation products in foods.

THE PROCESS OF IRRADIATION

The most common radioactive source used for food processing is cobalt 60, which is produced by irradiating ordinary cobalt metal in a nuclear reactor. The shape of the source is typically a bundle of many thin tubes mounted in a rack. The source is kept in a building with thick walls and under 4.6 meters (15 feet) of water for shielding. The food to be irradiated is packaged and put on a conveyor belt. The operator raises the cobalt-60 source out of the water by remote control, while the food packages slowly travel past the source on the moving belt. The typical exposure time is three to thirty minutes, depending on the type of food, the required dose, and the source intensity. Radiation dose is measured in a unit called the kilogray, where 1 kilogray equals 1,000 Grays, and 1 Gray equals 100 radiation absorbed doses (rads). The Gray is named for a British radiation biologist. The rad is an older unit still commonly used in the medical profession. When radiation passes through the food, it interacts with atomic electrons and breaks chemical bonds. Microorganisms that cause food spoilage or illnesses are inactivated so they cannot reproduce.

Fresh strawberries, sweet cherries, and tomatoes have a normal shelf life of only seven to ten days. Research has shown that a radiation dose of 2 kilograys can double their shelf life without affecting the flavor. Trichinosis parasites in fresh pork can be controlled with a dose of 1 kilogray. Doses up to 3 kilograys are used to destroy 99.9 percent of salmonella in chicken meat and *Escherichia coli* in ground hamburger. A dose of less than 0.1 kilogray is sufficient to interrupt cell growth in onions and potatoes to prevent undesirable sprouting in the spring. Larger doses, up to 30 kilograys, are used to eliminate insects, mites, and other pests in spices, herbs, and tea. The American Dietetic Association supports food irradiation as an effective technique to reduce outbreaks of food-borne illnesses, which cause several million cases of sickness and more than nine thousand fatalities annually in the United States.

Irradiated food does not become radioactive. It does not "glow in the dark" as some opponents have claimed. Hundreds of animal feeding studies with irradiated foods have been done since the late 1950's. Irradiated chicken, wheat, oranges, and other foods were fed to four generations of mice, three generations of beagles, and thousands of rats and monkeys. No increase in cancer or other inherited diseases was detected in comparison to a control group eating nonirradiated food. In one experiment, several thousand mice were fed nothing but irradiated food. After sixty generations—about ten years—the cancer rate for the experimental group was no greater than for the control group.

Chemical analyses of irradiated foods have looked for potentially harmful by-products from radiation. Small quantities of benzene and formaldehyde were found. However, canning, cooking, and baking have been shown to create these same by-products even more abundantly. Based on the accumulated evidence, food irradiation has been endorsed by an impressive list of organizations: the American Medical Association, the U.S. Department of Agriculture, the American Diabetic Association, the World Health Organization, the United Nations Food and Agriculture Organization, and the FDA. Astronauts on space missions have eaten irradiated foods since 1972, and many hospitals use irradiated foods for patients with an impaired immune system.

FEARS CONCERNING IRRADIATION

A consumer activist organization called Food and Water, based in Walden, Vermont, connects fear of the atomic bomb with food irradiation by showing a picture of a mushroom cloud hovering over a plate filled with food. The caption says, "The Department of Energy has a solution to the problem of radioactive waste. You're going to eat it." The most serious safety issues relating to food irradiation are in the production of radioactive cobalt; the safety of workers while transporting, installing, and using the source; and the eventual disposal of radioactive waste. Such issues, however, do not have the same impact on consumers as the implied claim that foods may become tainted by irradiation. Commercial food processors have been deterred from installing irradiation facilities by fear of negative publicity and a potential consumer backlash.

The FDA requires that irradiated foods be labeled with a special radura symbol and the statement "treated with radiation." It will be up to consumers to decide if the benefits of a safer food supply outweigh the potential hazards of an expanded nuclear industry.

—Hans G. Graetzer

See also Environmental diseases; Food poisoning; Radiation.

FOR FURTHER INFORMATION:
Gibbs, Gary. *The Food That Would Last Forever: Understanding the Dangers of Food Irradiation.* Garden City Park, N.Y.: Avery Publishing Group, 1993. A critical assessment of irradiation technology.
Massachusetts Institute of Technology. *Technology Review* (November-December, 1997). Contains an informative article quoting both supporters and opponents of food irradiation.
Satin, Morton. *Food Irradiation: A Guidebook.* 2d ed. Lancaster, Pa.: Tech-

nomic, 1996. Description of the application of radiation to food preservation.

Wagner, Henry, and Linda Ketchum. *Living with Radiation: The Risk, the Promise.* Baltimore: The Johns Hopkins University Press, 1989. A good introduction to the uses and hazards of radioactivity.

✧ FOOD POISONING

Type of issue: Environmental health, epidemics, public health
Definition: Food-borne illness caused by bacteria, viruses, or parasites consumed in food and resulting in acute gastrointestinal disturbance that may include diarrhea, nausea, vomiting, and abdominal discomfort.

A person feeling the symptoms of nausea, vomiting, diarrhea, and abdominal discomfort may assume that influenza is to blame, but the presence of a true influenza virus is uncommon. More likely, these symptoms are caused by eating food that contains undesirable bacteria, viruses, or parasites. This is called food-borne illness, or food poisoning. Most food-borne pathogens are colorless, odorless, and tasteless.

COMMON SOURCES OF FOOD POISONING

Certain foods, particularly foods with a high protein and moisture content, provide an ideal environment for the multiplication of pathogens. The foods with high risk in the United States are raw shellfish (especially mollusks), underdone poultry, raw eggs, rare meats, raw milk, and cooked food that another person handled before it was packaged and chilled. In addition, some developing countries could add raw vegetables, raw fruits that cannot be peeled, foods from sidewalk vendors, and tap water or water from unknown sources. Most of the documented cases of food-borne illness are caused by only a few bacteria, viruses, and parasites.

Bacteria known as *Salmonella* are ingested by humans in contaminated foods such as beef, poultry, and eggs; they may also be transmitted by kitchen utensils and the hands of people who have handled infected food or utensils. Once the bacteria are inside the body, the incubation time is from eight to twenty-four hours. Since the bacteria multiply inside the body and attack the gastrointestinal tract, this disease is known as a true food infection. The main symptoms are diarrhea, abdominal cramps, and vomiting. The bacteria are killed by cooking foods to the well-done stage.

The major food-borne intoxication in the United States is caused by eating food contaminated with the toxin of *Staphylococcus* bacteria. Because the toxin or poison has already been produced in the food item that is ingested, the onset of symptoms is usually very rapid (between one-half hour and six hours). Improperly stored or cooked foods (particularly meats, tuna, and potato salad) are the main carriers of these bacteria. Since this toxin cannot be killed by reheating the food items to a high temperature, it is important that foods are properly stored.

Botulism is a rare food poisoning caused by the toxin of *Clostridium botulinum.* It is anaerobic, meaning that it multiplies in environments without oxygen, and is mainly found in improperly home-canned food items. Originally one of the sources of the disease was from eating sausages (the Latin word for which is *botulus*)—hence, the name "botulism." A very small amount of toxin, the size of a grain of salt, could kill hundreds of people within an hour. Danger signs include double vision and difficulty swallowing and breathing.

GROUPS AT HIGH RISK

Though everyone is at risk for food-borne illness, certain groups of people develop more severe symptoms and are at a greater risk for serious illness and death. Higher-risk groups include pregnant women, very young children, the elderly, and immunocompromised individuals, such as patients with acquired immunodeficiency syndrome (AIDS) and cancer.

Bacteria known as *Listeria* were first documented in 1981 as being transmitted by food. Most people are at low risk of becoming ill after ingesting these bacteria; however, pregnant women are at high risk. *Listeria* infection is rare in the United States, but it does cause serious illness. It is associated with consumption of raw (unpasteurized) milk, nonreheated hot dogs, undercooked chicken, various soft cheeses (Mexican style, feta, Brie, Camembert, and blue-veined cheese), and food purchased from delicatessen counters. *Listeria* cause a short-term illness in pregnant women; however, this bacteria can cause stillbirths and spontaneous abortions. A parasite called *Toxoplasma gondii* is also of particular risk for pregnant women. For this reason, raw or very rare meat should not be eaten. In addition, since cats may shed these parasites in their feces, it is recommended that pregnant women avoid cleaning cat litter boxes.

As the protective antibodies from the mother are lost, infants become more susceptible to food poisoning. Botulism generally occurs by ingesting the toxin or poison; however, in infant botulism it is the spores that germinate and produce the toxin within the intestinal tract of the infant. Since honey and corn syrup have been found to contain spores, it is recommended that they not be fed to infants under one year of age, especially those under six months.

The Treatment of Food Poisoning

In cases of severe food poisoning marked by vomiting, diarrhea, or collapse—especially in cases of botulism and ingestion of poisonous plant material such as suspicious mushrooms—emergency medical attention should be sought immediately, and, if possible, specimens of the suspected food should be submitted for analysis. Identifying the source of the food is especially important if that source is a public venue such as a restaurant, because stemming a widespread outbreak of food poisoning may thereby be possible.

In less severe cases of food poisoning, the victim should rest, eat nothing, but drink fluids that contain some salt and sugar; the person should begin to recover after several hours or one or two days and should see a doctor if not well after two or three days.

Thorough Cooking

Cooking foods well means cooking them to a high enough temperature in the slowest-to-heat part and for a long enough time to destroy pathogens that have already gained access to foods. Cooking foods well is only a concern when they have become previously contaminated from other sources or are naturally contaminated.

Recommendations for cooking temperatures are based not only on the temperature required to kill food-borne pathogens but also on aesthetics and palatability. Generally, a margin of safety is built into the cooking temperature because of the possibility of nonuniform heating. Based on generally accepted temperature requirements, cooking red meat until 71 degrees Celsius (160 degrees Fahrenheit) will reach the thermal death point. Hamburger should be well cooked so that it is medium-brown inside. If pressed, it should feel firm and the juices that run out should be clear. Cooking poultry to the well-done stage is done for palatability. Tenderness is indicated when there is a flexible hip joint, and juices should run clear and not pink when the meat is pierced with a fork. Fish should be cooked until it loses its translucent appearance and flakes when pierced with a fork. Eggs should be thoroughly cooked until the yolk is thickened and the white is firm, not runny. Cooked or chilled foods that are served hot (that is, leftovers) should be reheated so that they come to a rolling boil.

Sources of Contamination

There are a number of possible sources of contamination of food products. Coastal water may contaminate seafood. Filter-feeding marine animals (such as clams, scallops, oysters, cockles, and mussels) and some fish (such as anchovies, sardines, and herring) live by pumping in seawater and sifting out organisms that they need for food. Therefore, they have the ability to concentrate suspended material by many orders of magnitude. Shellfish grown in contaminated coastal waters are the most frequent carriers of a virus called hepatitis A.

Contaminated eggs can be another vehicle of food-borne illness. Contamination of eggs can occur from external as well as internal sources. If moist conditions are present and there is a crack in the shell, the fecal material of hens carrying the microorganism can penetrate the shell and membrane of the egg and can multiply. In the early 1990's, *Salmonella enteritidis* began to appear in the intact egg, particularly in the northeastern part of the United States. It is hypothesized that contamination occurs in the oviduct of the hen before the egg is laid. Food vehicles in which *Salmonella enteritidis* has been reported include sandwiches dipped in eggs and cooked, hollandaise sauce, eggs Benedict, commercial frozen pasta with raw egg and cheese stuffing, Caesar salad dressing, and blended food in which cross-contamination had occurred. Foods such as cookie or cake dough or homemade ice cream made with raw eggs are other possible vehicles of food-borne illness.

Milk, especially raw milk, can be contaminated. Sources could be an unhealthy cow (such as from mastitis, a major infection of the mammary gland of the dairy cow) or unclean methods of milking, such as not cleaning the teats well before attaching them to the milker or using unclean utensils (milking tanks). If milk is not cooled fast enough, contaminants can multiply. Modern mechanized milking procedures have reduced but not eliminated food-borne pathogens. Postpasteurization contamination may occur, however, especially if bulk tanks or equipment have not been properly cleaned and sanitized.

AVOIDING CROSS-CONTAMINATION

Cross-contamination occurs when microorganisms are transmitted from humans, cutting boards, and utensils to food. Contamination between foods, especially from raw meat and poultry to fresh vegetables or other ready-to-eat foods, is a major problem. One of the best ways to prevent cross-contamination is simply washing one's hands with soap and water. Twenty seconds is the minimum time span that should be spent washing one's hands. In order to prevent the spread of disease, it is also recommended that the hands be dried with a paper towel, which is then thrown away. Thoroughly washed hands can still be a source of bacteria, however, so one should use tongs and spoons when cooking to prevent contamination. It is especially important to wash one's hands after blowing the nose or sneezing, using the lavatory, diapering a baby, smoking, or petting animals and before cooking or handling food.

Other sources of cross-contamination include utensils and cutting surfaces. If people use the same knife and cutting board to cut up raw chicken for a stir-fry and peaches for a fruit salad, they are putting themselves at great risk for food-borne illness. The bacteria on the cutting board and the knife could cross-contaminate the peaches. While the chicken will be cooked until it is well done, the peaches in the salad will not be. In this situation, one could cut the fruit first and then the chicken, and then wash and sanitize the knife and cutting board. Cleaning and sanitizing is actually a two-step process. Cleaning involves using soap and water and a scrubber or dishcloth to remove the major debris from the surface. The second step, sanitizing, involves using a diluted chloride solution to kill bacteria and viruses.

Wooden cutting boards are the worst offenders in terms of causing cross-contamination. Since bacteria and viruses are small, they can adhere to and grow in the grooves of a wooden cutting board and spread to other foods when the cutting board is used again. Use of a plastic or acrylic cutting board prevents this problem.

PREVENTING BACTERIAL GROWTH

The danger zone in which bacteria can multiply is a range of 4.4 degrees Celsius (40 degrees Fahrenheit) to 60 degrees Celsius (140 degrees Fahrenheit). Room temperature is generally right in the middle of this danger zone. The danger zone is critical because, even though they cannot be seen, bacteria are increasing in number. They can double and even quadruple in fifteen to thirty minutes. Consequently, perishable foods such as meats, poultry, fish, milk, cooked rice, leftover pizza, hard-cooked eggs, leftover re-fried beans, and potato salad should not be left in the danger zone for more than two hours. Keeping hot foods hot means keeping them at a temperature higher than 60 degrees Celsius. Keeping cold foods cold means keeping them at a temperature lower than 4.4 degrees Celsius.

Other rules are helpful for preventing contamination. When shopping, the grocery store should be the last stop so that foods are not stored in a hot car. When meal time is over, leftovers should be placed in the refrigerator or freezer as soon as possible. When packing for a picnic, food items should be kept in an ice chest to keep them cold or brought slightly frozen. Much serious illness and death could be prevented if such food safety rules were followed.

OVERSEEING FOOD SAFETY IN THE UNITED STATES

An important role of government and industry is to ensure a safe food supply. In the United States, setting and monitoring of food safety standards are the responsibility of the Food and Drug Administration (FDA) under the auspices of the U.S. Department of Health and Human Services and the Food Safety and Inspection Service (FSIS) under the auspices of the U.S. Department of Agriculture (USDA). The FDA is responsible for the wholesomeness of all food sold in interstate commerce, except meat and poultry, while the USDA is responsible for the inspection of meat and poultry sold in interstate commerce and internationally.

Food poisoning is a worldwide problem. In developing countries, diarrhea is a factor in child malnutrition and is estimated to cause 3.5 million deaths per year. Despite advances in modern technology, food-borne illness is a major problem in developed countries as well. In the United States, an estimated 24 million cases of food-borne diarrheal disease occur each year, which means that about one out of ten people experience a food-associated illness in a given year.

—Martha M. Henze, R.D.; updated by Maria Pacheco

See also Antibiotic resistance; Epidemics; Food irradiation; Genetically engineered foods; Lead poisoning; Mad cow disease; Parasites; Pesticides; Poisoning; Poisonous plants; Ulcers; Zoonoses.

For Further Information:

Gaman, P. M. *The Science of Food: An Introduction to Food Science, Nutrition, and Microbiology.* 4th ed. New York: Pergamon Press, 1996. An easy-to-read book dealing with food composition and microbiology. Includes good bibliographical references and an index.

Hobbs, Betty C. *Food Poisoning and Food Hygiene.* London: Edward Arnold, 1993. A nontechnical handbook of the causes of food poisoning and other food-borne diseases for those in the fields of food microbiology and food hygiene. Emphasis is given to the main aspects of hygiene necessary for the production, preparation, sale, and service of safe and palatable food.

Jay, James Monroe. *Modern Food Microbiology.* 6th ed. New York: Van Nostrand Reinhold, 2000. This excellent textbook summarizes the current state of knowledge of the biology and epidemiology of the microorganisms that cause food-borne illness.

Longree, Karla, and Gertrude Armbruster. *Quantity Food Sanitation.* 5th ed. New York: John Wiley & Sons, 1996. An excellent reference guide on food safety for quantity cooking in institutions such as hospitals and restaurants.

Ray, Bibek. *Fundamental Food Microbiology.* Boca Raton, Fla.: CRC Press, 1996. A comprehensive text on the basic principles of food microbiology. Includes bibliographical references and an index.

✦ Foot disorders

Type of issue: Elder health, women's health

Definition: Problems associated with the feet such as flat feet, neuromas, Achilles tendinitis, plantar fascitis, and heel spurs.

Each foot contains twenty-six bones, including fourteen phalanges (toe bones), five metatarsals (instep bones), and seven tarsals (ankle bones). The thirty-three joints in each foot are stabilized by more than a hundred ligaments, with their movements governed by nineteen muscles and their tendons. All these structures must work together in precise harmony during gait. When the delicate biomechanical action of one or both feet is upset and compensatory movements are made, abnormal compensations and pain often occur.

It is estimated that the average American takes approximately nine thousand steps per day and walks the equivalent of three and a half times around the equator in a lifetime. Recreational and competitive sports enthusiasts who previously had well-functioning feet often develop foot health problems at around age fifty, by which time the average foot has ambulated more than seventy-five thousand miles. Even less-active people in midlife and later are prone to foot disorders that can have serious consequences for mobility, even loss of the ability for independent living.

FLATFEET AND NEUROMAS

Chronic foot problems are often caused by excessive pronation (rotation of the midtarsal medial bones inward when walking, so that the foot comes down on its inner margin) of the rearfoot at the subtalor joint between the heel bone (calcaneus) and the wedge-shaped talus bone directly above it. Also called overpronation or fallen arches, flatfeet involve a flattening of the medial longitudinal arch, resulting in the middle of the ankle joint rolling in toward the midline of the body and a calcaneus that often appears to turn out laterally when viewed from the back. The big toe may also point up more than it should during weightbearing, causing the medial part of the foot to be more unstable. Calluses may build up under the second or third toes, indicating a lack of propulsion during the toe-off phase of running.

A neuroma, essentially a benign tumor of the nerves, involves the classic signs of aching, burning, numbness, and shooting sensations in the forefoot, often occurring during the latter half of prolonged activities. Excessive foot pronation is often the culprit, as rotation of the metatarsal heads tends to pinch the nerve running between the third and fourth toes. Chronic pinching inflames and enlarges the nerve sheath, causing increasing pain as the enlarged sheath becomes squeezed even more.

CHRONIC HEEL PROBLEMS

The most common disorder of the heel is plantar fasciitis, evidenced by pain and fatigue on the sole, arch swelling, and inflammation of dense fibrous connective tissue called fascia on the plantar (bottom) surface of the foot. When the foot flattens and becomes unstable during stance, the plantar fascia stretches excessively, possibly even pulling away from its attachment onto the calcaneus. The discomfort is particularly evident while pushing off with the toes, as this motion further stretches the inflamed fascia. When fascia begins to tear away from the bone, the bone often attempts to compensate by laying down more calcium and creating more bone, thus forming a heel spur that can been seen on an X ray. Plantar fasciitis and heel spurs that go untreated often cause an alteration in stride mechanics, with these additional compensatory actions causing even more damage.

Muscle and Tendon Injuries

The Achilles tendon connects the calcaneus to both the lateral and medial heads of the gastrocnemius muscle (which crosses the knee, ankle, and subtalor joints) and the soleus (an important balance muscle underneath the gastrocnemius that does not cross the knee). Nagging inflammation of the Achilles tendon often takes months to heal, with the biggest contributor to chronic tendinitis being ignoring the pain and continuing heavy activity during its early stages. The Achilles tendon is not protected by a true tendon sheath as are many other tendons, and it does not possess a rich blood supply to enhance healing. It is highly recommended that, if the Achilles tendon is feeling sore, one should reduce activities that aggravate it immediately. Sudden increases in exercise level and movement up and down hills greatly aggravate Achilles tendon problems.

Some runners attempt to combat chronic Achilles tendinitis by wearing excessive heel cushioning such as huge air-filled soles, but this action may actually increase the ongoing damage. Wearing shoes that provide inappropriately large shock absorption causes the heel to sink lower as the shoe attenuates the shock, thus rapidly stretching the already-tender tendon more than necessary with every step. Prolonged, gentle stretches to both the calves and the hamstrings are important prior to any lower extremity workout; repeated, short, and bouncy stretches, however, are the primary cause of tendinitis.

Shoe Selection

Distance walking and running for people of all ages is best done in shoes designed predominantly for forward running, whereas court sport shoes (such as tennis shoes) are designed more to provide stability during lateral movements in addition to forward movement. Court sport shoes generally do not have enough heel elevation to make them effective running shoes. Running shoes have a slightly elevated heel to reduce stress to the Achilles tendon, although this design does reduce lateral stability and can contribute to ankle sprains. The feet of distance runners generally come into contact with the ground heel first for a majority of the race, until the sprint to the finish, and are thus designed appropriately. Shoes for sprinting are constructed for more forefoot contact upon footstrike.

The useful life of athletic shoes is approximately 350 to 550 miles, depending greatly on the ground surface. Shoes should be purchased at the end of the average day because the feet will be somewhat larger. The heel counter should be vertical, and pressing down vertically with the end of a pencil in the middle of the heel can determine shoe stability. The area of highest flexibility of a running shoe should occur approximately 40 percent of the way from the toe of the shoe to the heel.

ORTHOTIC INSERTS AND HEEL LIFTS

Orthotic inserts placed within the shoe can be made of soft, semiflexible, or rigid material. They can be customized via computer-aided construction or with casts made of each foot. Orthotic inserts improve function and efficiency of foot motion by keeping the subtalar joint in neutral at midstance and balancing the rear part of the foot to both the forefoot and the ground. Orthotics are often specifically designed to prevent the foot from excessive pronation during midstance and to maintain stability so the foot can function as a rigid lever during push-off. An orthotic device only exerts its influence when the foot comes into contact with the ground, and often, but not always, creates an arch within the foot. Orthotic inserts can be designed to support or restrict range of motion in specific foot joints, dissipate body weight over a larger contact area and thus decrease shearing force on the bottom of the foot, redistribute weightbearing to stronger parts of the foot, and eliminate contact on weaker areas. Semiflexible orthotics, constructed from rubber, plastic, or leather, are generally first used to determine if the expense of individualized computer-constructed orthotics is necessary.

Heel lifts essentially bring the ground up to the foot and save the individual from having to compensate continually by slapping the foot to the ground. They are effective in alleviating a variety of orthopedic problems, including leg length discrepancies and loss of the fat pad beneath the heel. Leg length discrepancies should be corrected gradually by increasing the heel lift height over several months. Instantly overcorrecting foot problems will quickly redistribute the weight of the body over a relatively smaller and weaker area of the foot and possibly cause more problems than before.

DIAGNOSIS AND TREATMENT

Foot abnormalities can only be diagnosed specifically during a clinical evaluation by a physician, physical therapist, or podiatrist. Most active older adults do not make the effort to see a physician or physical therapist for foot problems until knee pain develops. Examination of the feet and also shoes worn for at least 300 miles can help identify many foot disorders. The skin

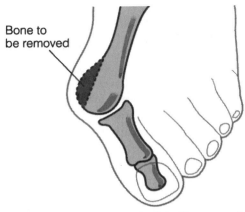

Bone to be removed

A bunion, a bony overgrowth of the big toe, can be removed surgically by cutting off the excess segment of bone, thus reshaping the foot. (Hans & Cassidy, Inc.)

of the foot should be thick in areas where an increase in weightbearing normally occurs, such as the heel, the lateral border, and just medial to the base of the first and fifth toes at the metatarsal heads. Bunion deformities are common in older women who wear dress shoes with high heels and pointed toes. Shoes worn by flatfooted individuals will generally have broken medial counters, whereas persons with toe-in gait will cause excessive wear on the shoe's lateral sole. The absence of a significant crease across the forefoot area indicates a reduction in toe-off at the end of stance phase.

Rehabilitation after even a relatively minor foot injury caused by either overuse or trauma can become a long and frustrating process if not conducted properly. Balance, coordination, strength, and overall posture during various types of movements are the major focus of clinical treatment. Foot pain can often be alleviated at home by superficial heat and cold application, stretching the muscles and fascia, and stimulating the feet using various types of massage.

—Daniel G. Graetzer

See also Broken bones in the elderly; Canes and walkers; Exercise and the elderly; Mobility problems in the elderly; Wheelchair use among the elderly; Women's health issues.

For Further Information:

Hertling, Darlene, and Randolph M. Kessler. *Management of Common Musculoskeletal Disorders: Physical Therapy Principles and Methods.* Philadelphia: Lippincott, 1996. An often-referenced physical therapist text on the evaluation and treatment of orthopedic disorders.

Lorimer, Donald L., Gwen French, and Steve West, eds. *Neal's Common Foot Disorders: Diagnosis and Management.* 5th ed. New York: Churchill Livingstone, 1997. A general clinical guide to foot disorders and diseases and their treatment. Includes a bibliography and an index.

Magee, David J. *Orthopaedic Physical Therapy Assessment.* Philadelphia: W. B. Saunders, 1997. Discusses physical therapy assessment and treatment of various orthopedic conditions affecting the middle aged and elderly.

✧ FROSTBITE

Type of issue: Environmental health, public health
Definition: An injury or destruction of skin and underlying tissues as a result of the freezing of extremities.

Frostbite generally occurs in people who exercise at high altitudes (such as athletes or mountain climbers), those who are at risk for diabetes, and those who are required to take particular care of their fingers and toes in cold situations. Frostbite can occur in anyone, however, upon exposure to extreme cold (below 0 degrees Celsius or 32 degrees Fahrenheit) and wind.

The first symptom of frostbite is a pins-and-needles sensation, followed by complete numbness. The skin turns white, cold, and hard before becoming red and swollen. Frostnip, a mild form of frostbite, affects the cheeks or nose, turning them white and numb. Blisters can develop in more serious cases, and the skin then hardens gradually or turns black, or gangrenous, indicating that the tissue has died as a result of ischemia (insufficient blood supply). This is followed by swelling and aching of the underlying tissue. If the injury is superficial, the dead tissue peels off in a few months. In severe cases, muscles, bone, and tendon can be frozen and the affected parts become swollen, mottled, blue or grey, although without any blisters or immediate pain.

Iatrogenic frostbite is caused by the excessive use of ethyl chloride sprays as local anesthesia for relief of muscle and tendon strains.

PREVENTION AND TREATMENT

To guard against frostbite, it is essential that children and adults wear proper clothing and never venture out in extremely cold weather. Frostnip should be treated immediately by warming the affected part with a warm hand or glove until blood circulation returns to normal and the color of the skin is restored.

In more severe cases, hospital treatment is necessary. The affected part is thawed through repeated applications of warm air or water for twenty-minute periods. Movement or massage of the affected areas is not helpful, and exposure to open fire is dangerous. Generalized warming of the whole body may be required by way of hot drinks or the use of a sleeping bag. If gangrene has set in, amputation of an affected part is necessary.

—Keith Garebian

See also Environmental diseases; First aid; Injuries among the elderly; Safety issues for children; Safety issues for the elderly.

For Further Information:
Calvert, John H., Jr. "Frostbite." *Flying Safety* 54, no. 10 (October, 1998): 24-25.
Phillips, David. "How Frostbite Performs Its Misery." *Canadian Geographic* 115, no. 1 (January/February, 1995): 20-21.
Tilton, Buck. "The Chill That Bites." *Backpacker* 28, no. 7 (September, 2000): 27.
Wilkerson, James A., ed. *Medicine for Mountaineering.* 4th ed. Seattle: The Mountaineers, 1992.

✦ Gene therapy

Type of issue: Medical procedures, treatment
Definition: A procedure that attempts to cure a condition by adding specific genes to cells; the expression of these genes results in the production of specific proteins.

Gene therapy is a technology that holds great promise for treating a variety of illnesses. Its major goal is to transfer genes into cells that will be of therapeutic use. Where defective genes are responsible for causing inherited diseases such as cystic fibrosis, it is hoped that the defective gene can be replaced by a corrected copy of the gene. Where a disease state, such as cancer or acquired immunodeficiency syndrome (AIDS), could be improved by delivering therapeutic substances to specific sites, it is hoped that genes coding for therapeutic products could be transferred to specific cells at specific sites. The cells that are being targeted for gene therapy are somatic cells, body cells other than those that give rise to eggs or sperm. This ensures that the therapy does not affect future generations.

THE MECHANICS OF GENE THERAPY

Inserting copies of genes into cells can be done in a variety of ways, typically using cloning vectors. A vector is anything that will deliver a copy of the gene to the cells. Viruses are often used as vectors because of their ability to bring genetic material into a cell with great efficiency, infecting as many as 100 percent of the cells to which they are exposed. Since viruses are normally pathogens, however, they must first be engineered so that they can no longer multiply or cause disease. This is done by removing certain viral genes before inserting the gene of choice into the virus. Retroviruses and adenoviruses are two types that are often used. A retrovirus inserts its genetic material directly into the host cell's genome, making the inserted genes stable. A retrovirus will infect only dividing cells and, by inserting its genes into the cell's genome, may interfere with normal cell function. An adenovirus infects both dividing and nondividing cells but does not insert its genetic material into the host cell's genome. The advantage of using adenoviruses is that they do not carry the risk of interfering with normal gene function. The genetic material brought into the cell, however, is less stable and can easily be lost.

Nonviral vectors can also be used to deliver genes to their target cells. One of the more successful methods is to use lipids to envelop the gene. Nonviral vectors are less efficient than viral vectors, infecting as few as one in every ten thousand cells; however, they do not carry some of the risks involved in using viruses. A more direct method, in which naked DNA is injected directly into a tissue, has yielded results as well, although how the cells take up the DNA is not known.

When gene therapy is being delivered, treatment can be either in vivo, in which the viral or nonviral vector is introduced directly into the patient's body, or ex vivo, in which the target cells are removed from the patient, treated, and then returned to the patient's body. Ex vivo methods allow the selection of cells that have incorporated the therapeutic gene and their growth in culture to increase cell number greatly before returning them to the patient.

POTENTIAL USES

Gene therapy is being investigated as a tool for treating a number of disorders. By the end of the twentieth century, however, no patient had been cured of a disease using gene therapy, despite more than one hundred clinical trials involving more than two thousand patients. Nevertheless, there was a report of success in using gene therapy to cause the growth of new blood vessels around blocked blood vessels. This use of gene therapy—in which genes are added to cells not to replace a faulty gene product but to cause the production of a substance such as a growth factor in a selected location—greatly increases the possible applications beyond the correction of inherited genetic disorders.

Initially, it was thought that gene therapy would first be used to cure a number of disorders caused by defects in a single gene. By 1990, candidates for the earliest gene therapies included beta-thalassemias, severe combined immunodeficiency syndrome (SCID), hemophilia types A and B, familial hypercholesterolemia, inherited emphysema, cystic fibrosis, Duchenne muscular dystrophy, and lysosomal storage disease. By 1995, gene therapies for most of these diseases were in clinical trials, but without any clear successes. By then, however, added to this list of disorders in clinical trials were a number in which treatment was aimed not at correcting a single gene but at delivering a gene product to a specific site. Among these were gene therapies for rheumatoid arthritis, AIDS, and cancer. By 1997, about 50 percent of all gene therapy research was focused on cancer, with the next largest group of studies, about 10 percent, focused on AIDS.

The first authorized human gene therapy was performed on a four-year-old girl, Ashanti DeSilva, who had adenosine deaminase (ADA) deficiency. Without treatment, this genetic deficiency leads to a fatal malfunctioning of the immune system. In 1990, a correct version of the ADA gene packaged in a retroviral vector was delivered by injection to the young girl. Several other young patients were treated afterward, but DeSilva was the only patient to show marked improvement in her condition. In all cases, however, the more traditional treatment, in which a synthetic version of ADA is administered in the form of PEG-ADA, was continued, indicating that the gene therapy did not cure the condition completely.

Cystic fibrosis is another disease that has been thought to be potentially curable through gene therapy. Several characteristics make it a promising candidate. Since correcting the gene CFTR in as few as 6 percent of the cells of an affected organ can produce normal function, not all cells would need to incorporate a functional gene. Also, the cells in most critical need of correction are those lining the airways of the lungs, cells that are easily accessible for in vivo treatment. Most trials have involved using an adenovirus as a vector to carry the CFTR gene, since these viruses normally infect human airways—they are the viruses that produce the common cold. The engineered viruses carrying the CFTR gene are delivered through an aerosol spray. Although patients show partially corrected chloride ion transport, the effect is short lived because most of the cells incorporating the corrected gene are short lived. Consequently, the gene therapy must be repeated every few months, but this method soon becomes ineffectual. Because the adenovirus stimulates an immune response, with repeated treatment the patient's immune system soon destroys the viral vector. Therefore, nonviral vectors are being tried in order to avoid an immune response.

A number of gene therapies that have entered clinical trials have been aimed at cancer. Among these are therapies designed to make tumor cells incorporate genes for substances such as interleukin-2 that will stimulate or augment an immune system attack against the cancer. In other approaches, genes dubbed "suicide" genes, which cause cell death, are being incorporated into tumor cells. Other trials have been aimed at trying to correct the genes that have caused the cells to become cancerous. An alternative approach has been to introduce the multidrug resistance (MDR) gene into normal bone marrow cells in order to increase their resistance to the toxic effects of the chemotherapy used to kill cancer cells.

Quite a different use of gene therapy has been to insert genes into highly accessible cells, such as muscle or skin fibroblasts, to turn them into protein factories for particular components that normally would be produced elsewhere—for example, to produce clotting factors, normally produced in the liver, that are missing in hemophiliacs.

—*Mary S. Tyler*

See also AIDS; AIDS and children; AIDS and women; Arthritis; Cancer; Genetic diseases; Genetic engineering.

FOR FURTHER INFORMATION:

Bank, Arthur. "Human Somatic Cell Gene Therapy." *BioEssays* 18 (December, 1996): 999-1007. A sophisticated discussion of clinical trials in gene therapy, focusing primarily on cancer.

Clark, William R. *The New Healers: The Promise and Problems of Molecular Medicine in the Twenty-first Century*. New York: Oxford University Press, 1999. Clark's background as a teacher of immunology helps him initiate readers into the realm of molecular biology and gene therapy, the likely linchpin in eradicating most of the four thousand genetic disorders within the next fifty years.

Felgner, Philip L. "Nonviral Strategies for Gene Therapy." *Scientific American* 276 (June, 1997): 102-106. Explains how lipoplexes (DNA surrounded by lipids) rather than viruses could be used as a method of delivering genes.

Friedmann, Theodore. "Overcoming the Obstacles to Gene Therapy." *Scientific American* 276 (June, 1997): 96-101. Discusses in vivo and ex vivo methods of gene therapy and the advantages and disadvantages of different gene delivery systems.

Ho, Dora Y., and Robert M. Sapolsky. "Gene Therapy for the Nervous System." *Scientific American* 276 (June, 1997): 116-120. Predicts ways in which gene therapy might be used to combat neurological disorders such as Parkinson's disease and stroke.

✧ GENETIC COUNSELING

Type of issue: Children's health, ethics, mental health, prevention
Definition: The use of biochemical and imaging techniques, as well as family histories, to provide information about genetic conditions or diseases in order to help individuals make medical and reproductive decisions.

Genetic counseling is a process of communicating to a couple the medical problems associated with the occurrence of an inherited disorder or birth defect in a family. Included in this process is a discussion of the prognosis and treatment of the problem. Specific reproductive options include abortion of an ongoing pregnancy, birth control or sterilization to prevent additional pregnancies, artificial insemination, the use of surrogate mothers, embryo transplantation, and adoption.

Genetic Disorders

The two major categories of medical problems covered in genetic counseling are birth defects and genetic diseases. The first group includes Down syndrome and spina bifida, while the latter includes hemophilia, sickle-cell disease, and Tay-Sachs disease. Although the distinction between these two categories can sometimes blur, the key difference involves the clear pattern of inheritance shown by the genetic diseases.

A genetic disease can occur when deoxyribonucleic acid (DNA) changes in structure, which is also known as a mutation. A mutation can lead to the production of a defective protein that cannot carry out its normal function, thus causing a physiological defect. As with all genetic diseases, such mutations are relatively rare. Certain diseases may, however, be more prevalent within certain ethnic groups; for example, African Americans have a high incidence of sickle-cell disease, and Ashkenazic Jews have a high incidence of Tay-Sachs disease.

Humans have two of each kind of chromosomes; one set of twenty-three is inherited from the mother and another set inherited from the father. Thus, each person has two copies of each gene. Many types of defects, such as sickle-cell disease, require that both genes have mutations in order to have an effect. Individuals who have one normal gene and one mutated gene are normal but carry the disease; they can pass the mutation to the next generation in their eggs and sperm. This type of disease is called a recessive genetic disease.

Since it is equally likely for each parent to pass on the normal gene in eggs or sperm as to pass on the mutation, the laws of probability predict that, on the average, one-fourth of such a couple's offspring should have the disease. One of the major tasks of genetic counseling is to advise couples of these probabilities if the diagnoses and family histories suggest that they are carriers. Since the laws of genetics involve random occurrences, however, it is possible that in a family with three or four children, all the children will be normal, or that in another family, all the children will have the disease.

Other diseases, such as Huntington's disease or chorea, are dominant, which means that an individual needs to inherit only one mutated gene in order to have the disease. Unlike recessive diseases that can disappear from a family for generations, a dominant mutation can be inherited only from a person who has the disease. In most cases, such a person has one normal gene and one with the mutation, which means that there is a 50 percent chance that the gene will be passed on. Huntington's chorea is a particularly insidious genetic disease, because the symptoms usually begin to show only in middle age, often after childbearing decisions have been made. Thus, the children of an afflicted parent must decide whether they will marry and have children before they know whether they have inherited the mutation from their parents.

The Screening Controversy

One of the more controversial aspects of genetic counseling is the procedure of screening, in which at-risk individuals are tested for a mutation. Screening can let people know whether they have a disease or whether they are carriers. Screening can be extended to all individuals, regardless of family or ethnic history. For example, in the United States, most states require that all newborn infants undergo a test for phenylketonuria (PKU). Although the costs of this screening are not insignificant, the benefit is that those infants found to have the disease can be treated immediately by being placed on a special diet.

Other screening procedures are targeted at specific groups. In the United States, a screening program for Tay-Sachs disease focuses on ethnic Jewish populations. This successful, voluntary program has reduced the incidence of the disease significantly. The key to success was the money spent to educate the targeted group. Because of the much-larger potential group at risk, similar efforts to screen African American populations for sickle-cell disease have been much less successful. Ethical concerns about the motivations behind government-sponsored or government-encouraged screening of minority populations make these programs difficult to implement. In addition, in mandatory programs, concerns about confidentiality and information release become major obstacles.

Collecting and Interpreting the Data

Genetic counseling usually begins when a couple or an individual seeks the advice of a family physician or obstetrician regarding the medical risks associated with having a child. Motivating this request may be a previous birth of a child with a defect, a general uneasiness on the part of a couple worried about environmental exposure to potentially harmful agents, a family history of genetic disease, or advanced maternal age. If pregnant already, the woman may undergo a prenatal diagnostic procedure that could include ultrasound, blood tests, amniocentesis, and chorionic villus sampling.

The counselor's task is to take the diagnostic results and interpret them in the context of the medical history and particular family situation. The counselor must point out the options available, both for further diagnosis to confirm or rebut less-sensitive preliminary tests and to discuss potential medical interventions such as the special diets available for children born with PKU. In cases in which no medical intervention is possible, the severity of the problem should be discussed honestly so that the parents can choose either to continue or to abort the pregnancy. Other options, including adoption, artificial insemination, and embryo transplants, can also be evaluated. Finally, the risk of recurrence of the problem in future pregnancies should be discussed.

Compounding the tasks of the counselor is the fact that, in many cases, exact diagnoses are not yet possible. Sometimes, only the relative risks associated with another pregnancy can be determined. Different couples will perceive risks very differently depending on their own religious and moral backgrounds, as well as on the expected severity of the defect. In the case of a genetic disease such as Tay-Sachs, which is 100 percent fatal and requires extensive hospitalization of the child, a modest risk may be considered unacceptable. In the case of a birth defect such as Down syndrome, whose severity cannot be predicted, a modest risk may be considered quite differently.

THE FUTURE OF GENETIC COUNSELING

The need for centers specializing in genetic counseling arose when it became clear that certain diseases and birth defects had a hereditary component. Many families request the services of counselors from these centers, and the centers are also involved in both voluntary and mandatory screening programs. In the United States, about 4 percent of all newborns suffer from a defect that is recognized either at birth or shortly thereafter. This group includes 0.5 percent who have a chromosomal abnormality that results in an obvious medical problem, 0.5 to 1 percent who have classical genetic diseases, and 2 percent who suffer from a birth defect that may have a heritable component. Estimates vary, but more than one-third of all children in pediatric hospitals are there because of some association with a genetic disease.

Genetic counseling clinics usually employ a range of specialists, including clinicians, geneticists, laboratory personnel for performing diagnostic testing, and public health and social workers. Today, most large counseling programs at medical centers use specially trained personnel. In rural areas, however, family physicians are still a primary source of counseling; thus, genetic training is an important component of basic medical education.

As DNA tools become more widely available, counseling will become a more integral part of preventive medicine. A DNA diagnostic procedure for a heritable form of breast cancer is available that allows women who have the mutation to monitor their health closely in order to receive prompt, lifesaving medical intervention. An important ethical issue here is that some women who have been diagnosed as having the mutation are undergoing preventive mastectomies without having developed any growths in order to ensure that they will not develop cancer. This radical therapy carries with it considerable emotional stress and should be undertaken only after consultation with a physician.

As DNA-based diagnostic procedures, perhaps coupled with mandatory screening, become more commonplace, concerns about the release of this information to potential employers or health insurers will become more critical.

—Joseph G. Pelliccia

See also Abortion; Amniocentesis; Birth defects; Breast cancer; Disabilities; Down syndrome; Ethics; Gene therapy; Genetic diseases; Genetic engineering; Mastectomy; Phenylketonuria (PKU); Prenatal care; Preventive medicine; Screening; Spina bifida.

FOR FURTHER INFORMATION:

Filkins, Karen, and Joseph F. Russo, eds. *Human Prenatal Diagnosis.* 2d rev. ed. New York: Marcel Dekker, 1990. An advanced sourcebook that describes the procedures of prenatal diagnosis in great detail. Contains information on risk, reliability, cost, and so forth.

Harper, Peter S. *Practical Genetic Counselling.* 5th ed. London: Wright, 1998. A good overview of all aspects of genetic counseling, including a discussion of the types of diagnoses, treatments, risks, and emotional strains associated with counseling. Also gives a history of counseling as a discipline.

Mange, Arthur P., and Elaine J. Mange. *Genetics: Human Aspects.* 2d ed. Sunderland, Mass.: Sinauer Associates, 1990. An excellent advanced high school or college text that introduces most of the concepts relevant to genetic counseling, from basic theory to practical applications.

Pierce, Benjamin A. *The Family Genetic Sourcebook.* New York: John Wiley & Sons, 1990. Good background reading on genetics and genetic diseases. The book gives short, clear descriptions of a number of genetic diseases, along with their diagnosis and treatment.

U.S. Congress. Office of Technology Assessment. *Genetic Counseling and Cystic Fibrosis Carrier Screening: Results of a Survey-Background Paper.* OTA-BP-BA-97. Washington, D.C.: Government Printing Office, 1992. Genetic screening is a controversial subject. This source discusses the problems and successes associated with one such effort.

✧ GENETIC DISEASES

Type of issue: Children's health, public health
Definition: A variety of disorders transmitted from parent to child through chromosomal material.

Genetic diseases are inherited as a result of the presence of abnormal genes in the reproductive cells of one or both parents of an affected individual. There are two broad classifications of genetic disease: those caused by defects in chromosome number or structure and those resulting from a much smaller flaw within a gene. Within the latter category, four predominant mechanisms exist by which the disorders can be transmitted from generation to generation: autosomal dominant inheritance, autosomal recessive inheritance, X-linked chromosomal inheritance, and multifactorial inheritance.

TYPES OF GENETIC DISEASES

Errors in chromosome number include extra and missing chromosomes. The most common chromosomal defect observed in humans is Down syndrome, which is caused by the presence of three copies of chromosome 21, instead of the usual two. Gross defects in chromosome structure include duplicated and deleted portions of chromosomes and broken and rearranged chromosome fragments. Prader-Willi syndrome results from a deletion of a small portion of chromosome 15. Children affected with this disorder are mentally retarded, obese, and diabetic. Cri du chat (literally, cat cry) syndrome is associated with a large deletion in chromosome 5. Affected infants exhibit facial abnormalities, are severely retarded, and produce a high-pitched, kittenlike wail.

Manifestation of an autosomal dominant disorder requires the inheritance of only one defective gene from one parent who is afflicted with the disease. Inheritance of two dominant defective genes, one from each parent, is possible but generally creates such severe consequences that the child dies while still in the womb or shortly after birth. An individual who bears one copy of the gene has a 50 percent chance of transmitting that gene and the disease to his or her offspring. Among the most common autosomal dominant diseases are hyperlipidemia, hypercholesterolemia, and Huntington's disease. The onset of the symptoms is usually in adulthood, frequently after the affected individual has had children and potentially transmitted the faulty gene to them.

Autosomal recessive genetic diseases require that an affected individual bear two copies of a defective gene, inheriting one from each parent. Usually the parents are simply carriers of the defective gene; their one normal copy masks the effect of the one flawed copy. If two carriers have offspring, 25 percent will receive two copies of the flawed gene and inherit the disease, and 50 percent will be asymptomatic carriers. Autosomal recessive disorders in the United States include cystic fibrosis, which occurs at a rate of about one in two thousand live births among Caucasians, and sickle-cell disease, the most common genetic disease among African Americans.

X-linked genetic diseases are transmitted by faulty genes located on the X chromosome. Females need two copies of the defective gene to acquire such a disease, and in general women carry only one flawed copy, making them asymptomatic carriers of the disorder. Males, having only a single X chromosome, need only one copy of the defective gene to express an X-linked disease. Half of the male offspring of a female carrier will inherit the defective gene and develop the disease. In the rare case of a female with two defective X-linked genes, 100 percent of her male offspring will inherit the disease gene, and, assuming that the father does not carry the defective gene, 50 percent of her female offspring will be carriers. More than 250 X-linked disorders exist; some of the more common are Duchenne muscular dystrophy, hemophilia, and red-green color blindness.

Multifactorial inheritance is caused by the complex interaction of one or more genes with each other and with environmental factors. This group of diseases includes many disorders which, anecdotally, run in families. Representative disorders include cleft palate, spina bifida, anencephaly, and some inherited heart abnormalities. Other diseases appear to have a genetic component predisposing an individual to be susceptible to environmental stimuli that trigger the disease, such as cancer, hypertension, diabetes, schizophrenia, alcoholism, depression, and obesity.

DIAGNOSIS AND DETECTION

Most, but not all, genetic diseases manifest their symptoms immediately or soon after the birth of an affected child. Rapid recognition of such a medical condition and its accurate diagnosis are essential for the proper treatment and management of the disease by parents and medical personnel. In many cases, testing of the fetus occurs prior to birth. In addition, tests are available that determine the carrier status of an individual for many autosomal recessive and X-linked diseases. These test results are used in conjunction with genetic counseling of individuals and couples who are at risk of transmitting a genetic disease to their offspring. Thus, such individuals can make informed decisions when planning their reproductive futures.

Defects in chromosome number and structure can be identified in a fetus using amniocentesis and chorionic villus sampling. Errors in chromosome number and structure can be detected in an individual by analyzing his or her chromosomes. A small piece of skin or a blood sample is taken, the cells in the sample are grown to a sufficient number, and the chromosomes within each cell are stained with special dyes so that they may be viewed with a microscope. A picture of the chromosomes, called a karyotype, is taken, and the patient's chromosome array is compared with that of a normal individual. Extra or missing chromosomes or alterations in chromosome structure are determined, thus identifying the genetic disease. Karyotyping is the method used to determine the presence of Down, Prader-Willi, and cri du chat syndromes, among others.

IDENTIFYING GENETIC ERRORS

The majority of hereditary disorders, however, are caused by gene flaws that are too small to see microscopically. For many of these diseases, diagnosis is available through either biochemical testing or deoxyribonucleic acid (DNA) analysis. Many genetic disorders cause a lack of a specific biochemical which is necessary for normal metabolism. These types of disorders are frequently referred to as inborn errors of metabolism. Many of these errors can be detected by the chemical analysis of fetal tissue.

For example, galactosemia is a disease which results from the lack of galactose-1-phosphate uridyl transferase. Infants with this disorder cannot break down galactose, one of the major sugars in milk. If left untreated, galactosemia can lead to mental retardation, cataracts, kidney and liver failure, and death. By analyzing fetal cells obtained from amniocentesis or chorionic villus sampling, the level of this important chemical can be assessed, and if necessary, the infant can be placed on a galactose-free diet immediately after birth.

DNA analysis can be used to determine whether a genetic disease has been inherited when the chromosomal location of the gene is known, when the chemical sequence of the DNA is known, and/or when particular DNA sequences commonly associated with the gene in question, called markers, are known. Direct analysis of the DNA of the individual suspected of carrying a certain genetic disorder is possible in many cases. For example, in sickle-cell disease, it is known that a change in a single DNA chemical element leads to the disorder. To test for this disease, a tissue sample is obtained from prenatal sources. The DNA is isolated from the cells and analyzed with highly specific probes that can detect the presence of the defective gene which will lead to sickle-cell disease. Informed action may be taken regarding the future of the fetus or the care of an affected child.

Evaluating Risk Factors

Individuals who come from families in which genetic diseases tend to occur can be tested as carriers. In this way, they will know the risk of passing a certain disease to offspring. DNA samples from the potential parents can be analyzed for the presence of a defective gene.

Many of the gene flaws of multifactorial diseases, those that interact with environmental factors to produce disease, have been identified and are testable. Individuals armed with the knowledge of having a gene which puts them at risk for certain disorders can incorporate preventive measures into their lifestyle, thus minimizing the chances of developing the disease.

The Future of Genetic Disease Research

Recombinant DNA revolution spawned the development of the DNA tests for genetic diseases and carrier status. Knowledge of what a normal gene product is and does is exceptionally helpful in the treatment of genetic diseases. For example, Duchenne muscular dystrophy is known to be caused by the lack of a protein called dystrophin. This suggests that a possible treatment of the disease is to provide functional dystrophin to the affected individual.

Ultimately, medical science seeks to treat genetic diseases by providing a functional copy of the flawed gene to the affected individual. While such gene therapy would not affect the reproductive cells—the introduced gene copy would not be passed down to future generations—the normal gene product would alleviate the genetic disorder.

—*Karen E. Kalumuck*

See also Alzheimer's disease; Amniocentesis; Attention-deficit disorder (ADD); Autism; Birth defects; Breast cancer; Cancer; Colon cancer; Diabetes mellitus; Down syndrome; Dyslexia; Environmental diseases; Gene therapy; Genetic counseling; Genetic engineering; Lactose intolerance; Learning disabilities; Mental retardation; Phenylketonuria (PKU); Schizophrenia; Screening.

FOR FURTHER INFORMATION:

Bellenir, Karen, ed. *Genetic Disorders Sourcebook: Basic Information About Heritable Diseases and Disorders Such as Down Syndrome, PKU, Hemophilia, and Von Willebrandt Diseases.* New York: Omnigraphics, 1996. This nontechnical sourcebook offers basic information about lifestyle expectations, disease management techniques, and current research initiatives for the most common types of genetic disorders, including a resource list of three hundred genetic disorders and related topics.

Gormley, Myra Vanderpool. *Family Diseases: Are You at Risk?* Reprint. Baltimore: Genealogical Publishing, 1999. The author, a certified genealogist and syndicated columnist, explores the relationship between family trees and genetic diseases. Written in popular language, this book gives instruction on how to assess a family's genetic risk, information on the latest scientific breakthroughs, and direction for obtaining further information.

Maxon, Linda, and Charles Daugherty. *Genetics: A Human Perspective.* Dubuque, Iowa: Wm. C. Brown, 1992. This textbook, designed for persons with no science background, thoroughly covers the background information on cells and genetics needed for an informed understanding of human genetic disease. The discussion of scientific advances in the understanding,treatment, and diagnosis of genetic disease is a strong point of the text.

Millunsky, Aubrey, ed. *Genetic Disorders of the Fetus: Diagnosis, Prevention, and Treatment.* Baltimore, Md.: Johns Hopkins University Press, 1998. This source treats a number of issues, from fetal cells in the maternal circulation to ethical issues surrounding a misdiagnosis, in chapters written by experts in the field. Recommended for clinicians in training and scientists working on the laboratory side of prenatal genetic testing.

Tropp, Burton E. *Biochemistry: Concepts and Applications.* Belmont, Calif.: West/Wadsworth, 1997. This book presents the basic concepts of biochemistry, including proteins and their functions, genetic information, and recombinant DNA technology. A good source for basic biochemical information.

✧ GENETIC ENGINEERING

Type of issue: Ethics, medical procedures
Definition: The use of recombinant deoxyribonucleic acid (DNA) technology to create DNA carrying specific genes or parts of genes that can be transferred from one organism to another to alter an organism's genetic makeup.

Genetic engineering relies foremost on the ability of the scientist to cut and rejoin DNA molecules and to increase the ability of bacteria to take up DNA from a culture solution. One type of enzyme that cuts a linear DNA molecule into fragments is called a restriction endonuclease or restriction enzyme. Restriction enzymes cut DNA into predictable, reproducible-sized fragments by cutting at specific nucleotide sequences.

Recombinant DNA molecules made by combining fragments of DNA from different sources such as bacteria and humans rely on the fact that restriction enzymes leave the same type of ends on every fragment they generate. Therefore, fragments can be rejoined in almost any desirable combination. The types of DNA fragments that are commonly joined by genetic engineers include a DNA fragment containing a gene of interest, such as the human insulin gene, and a special DNA fragment which will allow that gene to propagate and be expressed in bacteria. Once the appropriate fragments are combined, the recombinant DNA molecule must be inserted into the bacteria. Because inserting new genetic information into a bacterium will change or transform its genetic makeup, this procedure is called transformation.

BENEFITS FOR DIABETICS AND DIALYSIS PATIENTS

One of the greatest potential uses of genetic engineering technology is in the diagnosis and treatment of human disease. The first genetically engineered product, approved by the Food and Drug Administration in 1982, was marketed by the Eli Lilly company under the product name of Humulin—a human form of insulin for the treatment of diabetes mellitus.

Patients suffering from diabetes must take injections of insulin daily. The traditional source of insulin has been beef and pork pancreas, but there are associated problems. The methods of extraction can be tedious and costly and provide a relatively small amount of insulin from a large amount of animal tissue. Also, a common problem among diabetics is allergic reactions to impurities in the insulin preparation and resistance to the insulin itself. Genetic engineering has provided a way to obtain pure, human insulin in large quantities.

In normal human cells, an insulin precursor is synthesized as a single protein chain and then split into two pieces, which remain held together by strong chemical bonds. Scientists can engineer separate genes into bacteria to produce each of the two pieces that compose insulin. Each segment is purified from the bacteria and then combined chemically to form active insulin. Although the insulin is produced by bacteria, the genetic instructions used are human in origin, and the insulin protein is indistinguishable from insulin actually produced in human cells.

Another useful protein that can be genetically engineered is erythropoietin, which stimulates the production of red blood cells, or erythrocytes, the oxygen-carrying cells in the blood. The kidneys normally help remove toxic substances from the body. Sufferers of kidney disease can undergo a treatment known as dialysis that substitutes for this cleansing function. Dialysis is a much safer alternative for most patients than kidney transplantation. Because the kidneys also normally produce erythropoietin, however, patients with diseased kidneys often have a low number of red blood cells and suffer from severe anemia. This anemia can be alleviated with blood transfusions, but transfusions carry the risk of blood-borne diseases. Fortunately, genetically engineered erythropoietin is available to stimulate red blood cell production in dialysis patients.

Vaccines and Gene Therapy

Another medical use of genetic engineering involves the creation of safe and effective vaccines for viral diseases. Vaccines work by presenting a harmless protein from the virus or a noninfectious or nonpathogenic strain of the virus to the immune system. One way to produce a vaccine for human immunodeficiency virus (HIV) might be to engineer bacteria genetically to synthesize a viral protein. The protein could then be purified and injected into a human. The person's immune system would make antibodies to the HIV protein, and, if he or she were ever exposed to the virus, the immune system would be able to combat the virus before an infection could be established. Unfortunately, purified proteins cannot always serve as effective vaccines. Another approach might be to engineer the HIV viral protein genetically into a relatively harmless virus and intentionally infect people with that virus. The harmless virus would present the HIV protein to the immune system so that antibodies could be created for protection against HIV infection.

Genetic engineering is also being applied to human cells in attempts to treat cancer and genetic diseases. Medical treatments using genetic engineering are called human gene therapies. In gene therapy, genes may be added, deleted, or altered to change the properties of certain cells within the body. Human gene therapy may succeed in providing cures for some of the more than three thousand known genetic diseases.

One particularly severe disease is readily amenable to gene therapy.

Adenosine deaminase (ADA) deficiency results when an individual's own cells are unable to produce the enzyme ADA. The most harmful effect of this deficiency is the lack of an effective immune system to fight disease. Consequently, the individual must live in an almost entirely sterile environment to avoid potentially harmful bacteria, fungi, and viruses. Bone marrow cells could be extracted from an ADA-deficient person, however, and a new ADA gene could be inserted into the cells. When the bone marrow cells are replaced, they should function normally.

THE ETHICAL QUESTIONS

Human gene therapy brings up several important ethical questions. First, do humans have the moral and ethical right to alter the genetic makeup of themselves or others? A more critical question is whether one has the right to alter the genetic makeup of future generations. Gene therapy of normal body cells that will die when the individual dies is called somatic cell gene therapy. Most people see little ethical problem with such techniques. Yet the potential also exists to alter genetically sperm and egg cells, the germ cells, so that future progeny will all carry the alterations. Many individuals argue against the development of such germ cell gene therapy.

Scientists involved in the early development of recombinant DNA methodology saw the danger of reckless experimentation. In fact, in 1974, those scientists called for a worldwide moratorium on genetic engineering until they could discuss the safety concerns. In 1975, the scientists met at Asilomar, California, and developed a set of guidelines under which they would conduct their research. In 1976, the National Institutes of Health (NIH) stepped in and issued formal guidelines based on those recommended at the Asilomar conference. Since the initial NIH guidelines, concern about the potential risks of genetic engineering has subsided. Most experiments are now performed in an open laboratory environment with little containment other than that used for handling normal bacteria or viruses.

In addition to those concerned about the issues of safety, opponents of genetic engineering include those who question the ethics and morality of altering the genetic makeup of organisms, especially humans. Genetic recombination takes place every day in the natural world, but this recombination is usually limited to members of the same species. When organisms reproduce, groups of genes from each parent are recombined to form progeny. Yet scientists have taken the process one step further, developing the ability to recombine genes from different organisms. Many people, including some scientists, believe that genetic engineering goes against the laws of nature or is playing God; they call for a halt to genetic engineering. Many others, scientists and laypersons alike, believe that genetic engineering mimics natural events such as viral infections and evolution and that the potential benefits—scientific, social, and medical—are too great to stop genetic engineering.

—*Gary J. Lindquester*

See also Cancer; Chemotherapy; Diabetes mellitus; Ethics; Fetal tissue transplantation; Gene therapy; Genetically engineered foods; Hormone replacement therapy.

FOR FURTHER INFORMATION:

Frank-Kamenetskii, Maxim D. *Unraveling DNA—The Most Important Molecule of Life.* Rev. ed. Reading, Mass.: Addison-Wesley, 1997. This very readable book provides an excellent history of the discovery of DNA. Also describes the nature of DNA and discusses genetic engineering and the ethical questions that surround its use.

McHughen, Alan. *Pandora's Picnic Basket: The Potential and Hazards of Genetically Modified Foods.* New York: Oxford University Press, 2000. McHughen offers a balanced, informed look at the new technology of genetically modified foods. He easily imparts a basic understanding of the molecular genetics required to understand genetic modification and the controversy it sparks.

Nicholl, Desmond. *Introduction to Genetic Engineering.* Cambridge, England: Cambridge University Press, 1994. A valuable textbook for the nonspecialist and anyone interested in genetic engineering. It provides an excellent foundation in molecular biology and builds on that foundation to show how organisms can be genetically engineered. Particularly useful is the glossary of terms.

Wilmut, Ian, Keith Campbell, and Colin Tudge. *The Second Creation: Dolly and the Age of Biological Control.* New York: Farrar, Straus and Giroux, 2000. Science writer Tudge helps the scientists responsible for cloning the sheep Dolly tell their story. Discusses the groundwork laid by others and the scientific methodology they employed in cloning the first mammal from the cell of an adult of its species.

✧ GENETICALLY ENGINEERED FOODS

Type of issue: Environmental health, industrial practices, public health
Definition: Foods that are derived from living organisms that have been modified by gene-transfer technology.

Humans rely on plants and animals as food sources and have long used microbes to produce foods such as cheese, bread, and fermented beverages. Conventional techniques such as cross-hybridization, production of mutants, and selective breeding have resulted in new varieties of crop plants or improved livestock with altered genetics. However, these methods are relatively slow and labor intensive, are generally limited to intraspecies crosses, and involve a great deal of trial and error.

Recombinant deoxyribonucleic acid (DNA) techniques developed in the 1970's enable researchers to rapidly make specific, predetermined genetic changes. Since the technology also allows for the transfer of genes across species and kingdom barriers, an infinite number of novel genetic combinations are possible. The first animals and plants containing genetic material from other organisms (transgenics) were developed in the early 1980's. By 1985 the first field trials of plants engineered to be pest resistant were conducted. In 1990 the U.S. Food and Drug Administration (FDA) approved chymosin as the first substance produced by engineered organisms to be used in the food industry for dairy products such as cheese. That same year the first transgenic cow was developed to produce human milk proteins for infant formula. The well-publicized Flavr Savr tomato obtained FDA approval in 1994.

The Goals of Genetic Engineering

By the mid-1990's, more than one thousand genetically engineered crop plants were approved for field trials. The goals for altering food crop plants by genetic engineering fall into three main categories: to create plants that can adapt to specific environmental conditions to make better use of agricultural land, increase yields, or reduce losses; to increase quality, nutritional value, and flavor; and to alter transport, storage, and processing properties for the food industry. Many genetically engineered crops are also sources of ingredients for processed foods and animal feed.

Herbicide-resistant plants such as the Roundup Ready soybean can be grown in the presence of glyphosphate, a herbicide that normally destroys all plants with which it comes in contact. Beans from these plants have been approved for food-industry use in several countries, but there has been widespread protest by activists such as Jeremy Rifkin Jeremy and organizations such as Greenpeace. Frost-resistant fruit containing a fish antifreeze gene, insect-resistant plants with a bacterial gene that encodes for a pesticidal protein (*Bacillus thuringiensis*), and a viral disease-resistant squash are examples of other genetically engineered food crops that have undergone field trials. Scientists have also created plants that produce healthier unsaturated fats and oils rather than saturated ones, coffee plants whose beans are caffeine-free without processing, and tomatoes with altered pulp content for improved canned products.

Animals can also be genetically engineered food sources. Transgenic research in animals is technically more difficult than with plants, although the technology used to clone Dolly the sheep in 1997 was a significant advancement. Animal rights issues, vegetarian and religious objections to animal-based components in food, and concerns over infectious agents that could be transferred to humans have all hindered developments in this field. The most notorious application of genetic engineering in animals involves the bovine growth hormone (BGH; also known as BST) synthesized by bacteria containing the bovine BGH gene. When BGH is given to cows as a supplement, milk production can increase up to 20 percent, but concerns over the health of treated cows and the safety of the milk have made this practice controversial.

Genetically engineered microbes are used for the production of food additives such as amino acid supplements, sweeteners, flavors, vitamins, and thickening agents. In some cases, these substances previously had to be obtained from slaughtered animals. Altered organisms are also used for improving fermentation processes in the food industry.

AREAS OF CONTROVERSY

Applications of genetic engineering in agriculture and the food industry could increase world food supplies, reduce environmental problems associated with food production, and enhance the nutritional value of certain foods. However, these benefits are countered by food-safety concerns, the potential for ecosystem disruption, and fears of unforeseen consequences resulting from altering natural selection.

Food safety and quality are at the center of the genetically engineered food controversy. Concerns include the possible introduction of new toxins or allergens into the diet and changes in the nutrient composition of foods. Proponents argue that food sources could be designed to have enhanced nutritional value.

A large percentage of crops worldwide are lost each year to drought, temperature extremes, and pests. Plants have already been engineered to exhibit frost, insect, disease, and drought resistance. Such alterations would increase yields, allow food to be grown in areas that are currently too dry or infertile, and positively impact the world food supply.

Environmental problems such as deforestation, erosion, pollution, and loss of biodiversity have all resulted, in part, from conventional agricultural practices. Use of genetically engineered crops could allow better use of existing farmland and lead to a decreased reliance on pesticides and fertilizers. Critics fear the creation of "superweeds"—either the engineered plants or new plant varieties formed by the transfer of recombinant genes conferring various types of resistance to wild species. These weeds, in turn, would compete with valuable plants and have the potential to destroy ecosystems and farmland unless stronger poisons were used for eradication. The transfer of genetic material to wild relatives (outcrossing, or "genetic pollution") might also lead to the development of new plant diseases. As with any new technology, there may be other unpredictable environmental consequences.

Despite the risks, genetic engineering may be required to develop food sources that can survive rapidly changing environmental conditions. Pollution, global climate change, and increased ultraviolet irradiation result in stress conditions for living organisms, and all impact agriculture. The processes of natural selection and adaptation may be too slow to maintain required food supplies.

—*Diane White Husic*

See also Food irradiation; Genetic engineering.

For Further Information:

Engel, Karl-Heinz, Gary R. Takeoka, and Roy Teranishi, eds. *Genetically Modified Foods: Safety Issues.* Washington, D.C.: American Chemical Society, 1995. A thorough overview of the technology, applications, and risks associated with genetically engineered foods.

Rissler, Jane, and Margaret Mellon. *The Ecological Risks of Engineered Crops.* Cambridge, Mass.: MIT Press, 1996. Discusses the potential environmental impact of this technology.

❖ Hair loss and baldness

Type of issue: Elder health, men's health, social trends
Definition: The loss of hair as a result of aging or illness.

In 1999, more than thirty million men in the United States were bald or going bald, mostly from the condition known as androgenetic alopecia, or male pattern baldness. This condition usually starts with a receding hairline at the forehead and temples and often is accompanied by a hairless spot at the crown of the head—the "monk's tonsure." Finally, the hairless areas join over the skull until the individual is left only with a fringe over the ears and collar.

The Nature of Hair and Types of Loss

Hair is an accessory organ of the skin and consists primarily of two parts: the hair shaft, which protrudes above the skin surface, and the root, which lies below the skin. The hair follicle surrounds the root and it is here, in the follicle, where blood vessels provide nourishment for the growing hair. The hair shaft—which is combed, brushed, pomaded, shampooed, dyed, and "nourished" by a variety of nostrums—is a thread of keratinized cells, dead material similar to fingernails and toenails.

The average number of human scalp hairs is between 100,000 and 150,000. Individual scalp hairs may persist for three to five years and then are shed in a cycle that includes growth, a resting stage, shedding, and another growth period. Balding occurs when the number of hairs shed in the cycle exceeds the number that grow.

Dermatologists, medical specialists in the study and treatment of diseases of the skin, recognize three main forms of alopecia, or baldness. Alopecia areata refers to the loss of hair in patches that vary in size; although it usually affects the scalp, hair loss may involve the beard or other body hair. If the follicles are not compromised, regrowth of the hair usually occurs. Alopecia totalis occurs when all the scalp hair is lost and the scalp remains totally bare, smooth, and shiny. Other body hair such as the eyebrows, pubic hair, and beard usually is not involved. Alopecia universalis is the most extreme form of hair loss. Not only is the scalp hair lost, but the pubic hair, underarm hair, eyebrows, and leg and arm hair is lost as well. The affected individuals undergo both the psychological trauma of the hair loss and the physical trauma of the loss of the protective qualities of the hair. Perspiration that usually is trapped by the eyebrows may now trickle directly into the eyes. Dust, pollen, and other airborne particles freely enter the nasal passages in the absence of nose hair.

GENETICS AND BALDNESS

About 95 percent of male pattern baldness is hereditary and is passed on by both the male as well as the female line. As the name suggests, it affects mostly men, although some older women undergo a general thinning of scalp hair with actual bald spots. Male pattern baldness usually begins at puberty or the early twenties, although it may not make an appearance until the forties. By middle age, the degree of baldness is usually known.

Male pattern baldness appears to run in families on either the mother's or the father's side. As has long been suspected, the tendency toward this condition is influenced by the male sex hormone, testosterone. Testosterone is produced by the primary male sex glands, the testes. The hormone is responsible for the secondary sexual characteristics in males, including facial hair, a deepened voice, and a more robust body build. Testosterone begins to exert its influence at puberty, the time of sexual maturation. It is not the testosterone itself that is the culprit in androgenetic alopecia; it is its derivative, dihydrotestosterone (DHT). As testosterone circulates through the blood, it is converted by an enzyme to DHT, which attaches to hair follicle cells. If there is a large amount of DHT, the follicles begin sprouting hair that is progressively thinner in diameter. Finally, the follicles no longer produce hair and in turn waste away. It is the production of more or less amounts of the enzyme, and thus DHT, not the production of testosterone, that determines the retention or loss of an individual's head of hair.

Baldness Cover-Ups and Surgical Restoration

Some steps can be taken by the balding individual. One alternative is to do nothing about the hair loss and to accept the inevitable as a natural part of the aging process. Some men allow one side of the hair that remains in the fringe to grow long and fashion it in a variety of loops and swirls over the balding center of the scalp. A variation of accepting the inevitable is to remove the remaining hair by shaving the entire scalp. Another option is to buy and wear a hairpiece (toupee) or a wig. A good one is expensive, however, and regardless of how much is paid for it, a hairpiece is detectable in bright light or when the wearer is in close proximity to others.

A number of surgical techniques have been developed to put hair on the balding scalp. One technique is hair weaving, in which anchoring stitches are sewn into the bald scalp and new hair is woven and knotted into the anchors. In the hands of a skilled technician, hair weaving can be a satisfactory prosthesis. The wearer can swim, shower, shampoo, blow dry, and style, as well as be windblown, almost as though the hair was his own natural growth. Periodic tightening of the knots is required, however, and there is always the danger of irritation or infection from the anchoring stitches.

Hair transplantation has worked well for some men. In this technique, skin plugs containing dense hair from the back or sides of the individual's head are transplanted into prepared holes in the bald areas. The success of the procedure depends greatly on the skill of the physician. A skillful surgeon can achieve a natural-looking hairline and a fair-to-good coverage of hair if the donor sites are good. The procedure may take many weeks to months, depending on the area of scalp to be covered. Not all hair transplants "take," and there is also the danger of infection. Women usually are not good candidates for hair transplantation because their hair loss is diffuse, involving almost the entire scalp. Thus, good donor sites generally are not available.

A more radical approach to covering the balding scalp with the individual's own hair is scalp reduction surgery. This involves removing a large section of the hairless scalp and stitching the edges together. The looseness and stretch of the human scalp makes this technique possible. Another radical surgical procedure is one in which a flap of hair-bearing scalp is moved from the sides or back of the head to replace a section of hairless scalp. Unfortunately, the flap technique involves bleeding, infection, and scarring.

Regrowing Hair

The search for a magic bullet to cure male pattern baldness and restore a healthy head of hair to the afflicted individual seemed to have ended with the development and availability of minoxidil (Rogaine). This prescription drug had been developed and prescribed for high blood pressure (hypertension). Researchers discovered that a lotion form of the drug applied to the scalp grew some hair in some men.

Clinical trials of a 2 percent solution of minoxidil among a group of men nineteen to forty-nine years of age with varying degrees of male pattern baldness produced varying results. Approximately 26 percent of the men reported moderate-to-dense regrowth of hair. This is compared to 11 percent of the men of the control group who applied only the liquid part of the solution minus the active ingredient. About 33 percent of the men achieved what was considered minimal regrowth of hair, while 31 percent of the control group also achieved minimal regrowth of hair. In each group, the experimental and the control, a sizable portion of men experienced no regrowth of hair, either with the drug or with the placebo.

The lotion is available in a 2 percent solution form without a prescription. It must be applied twice daily for at least four months before any new hair growth can be expected. If no new hair develops after one year, the user is advised to stop applying the product and consult a physician. The product works best on men under fifty years of age with bald spots no larger than 3 to 5 inches in diameter. Once favorable results are obtained, the user must continue to apply the lotion or the new hair will be lost.

Some cautions are associated with the use of minoxidil. It should not be used if there is no family history of hair loss, if the individual is less than eighteen years old, or if scalp irritation is present. Users should consult their physicians if they experience chest pain, rapid heartbeat, dizziness or fainting, or swelling of the feet or hands. Clearly, the magic bullet has not yet been found.

—Albert C. Jensen

See also Aging; Cosmetic surgery and aging.

FOR FURTHER INFORMATION:

Hanover, Larry. "Hair Replacement: What Works, What Doesn't." *FDA Consumer* 31 (April, 1997). Discusses the use of minoxidil, surgical techniques such as transplants, and cover-ups, including wigs and toupees.

Mayhew, John. *Hair Techniques and Alternatives to Baldness.* New York: Oweni Trado-Medic Books, 1963. A review of hair dressing, care and hygiene of the hair, and alternatives to baldness, including transplantation.

Sadick, Neil S., and Donald C. Richardson. *Your Hair and Helping to Keep It.* Yonkers, N.Y.: Consumer Reports Books, 1991. An authoritative review of baldness, its causes, and what to do about it. Includes a discussion of human hair growth and hair care.

SerVaas, Cory. "Early Male Pattern Baldness." *Saturday Evening Post* 266 (March/April, 1996). In a question-and-answer format, SerVaas offers four suggestions for coping with this condition, including wait and see, application of minoxidil, surgery (including transplantation), and, if necessary, a hairpiece.

Thompson, Wendy, and Jerry Shapiro. *Alopecia Areata: Understanding and Coping with Hair Loss.* Baltimore: The Johns Hopkins University Press, 1996. Provides a guide to the diagnosis and treatment of hair loss with reliable information from two medical professionals.

✧ Hazardous waste

Type of issue: Environmental health, industrial practices, public health
Definition: Products of industrial society that pose dangers to human health and the environment; in the United States they are legally defined as materials that have ignitable, corrosive, reactive, or toxic properties.

In the early 1990's approximately 97 percent of all hazardous waste in the United States was produced by 2 percent of the waste generators. Remediation and cleanup of these wastes involve substantial economic cost. Since the 1970's the United States and other Western democracies have tried to regulate hazardous waste disposal. Hazardous wastes are also a serious problem in the former Soviet Union and other Eastern European nations.

Improper disposal of hazardous waste can lead to the release of chemicals into the air, surface water, groundwater, and soil. High-risk wastes are those known to contain significant concentrations of constituents that are highly toxic, persistent, highly mobile, or bioaccumulative. Examples include dioxin-based wastes, polychlorinated biphenyls (PCBs), and cyanide wastes. Intermediate-risk wastes may include metal hydroxide sludges, while low-risk wastes are generally high-volume, low-hazard materials. Radioactive waste is a special category of hazardous waste, often presenting extremely high risks, as do biomedical and mining wastes.

Degrees of Risk

Hazardous waste presents varying degrees of health and environmental hazards. When combined, two relatively low-risk materials may pose a high risk. Factors that affect the health risk of hazardous waste include dosage received; age, gender, and body weight of those exposed; and weather conditions. The health effects posed by hazardous waste include cancer, genetic defects, reproductive abnormalities, and central nervous system disorders.

Environmental degradation resulting from hazardous waste can render various natural resources, such as cropland or forests, useless and can harm animal life. For example, chemicals can leach out of improperly stored waste and into groundwater. Hazardous wastes may generate long-lasting air and water pollution or soil contamination. Because the amount of waste produced in any period is based on the amount of natural resources used, the generation of both hazardous and nonhazardous waste poses a threat to the sustainability of the economy.

Because there were no standards for what constituted a hazardous waste in the past, such materials were often buried or stored in unattended drums or other containers. This situation created a threat to the environment and human health when the original containers began to leak or the material leached into the water supply.

The technology for dealing with hazardous solid and liquid waste continues to evolve. Several solutions have had positive impacts on the environment and consumption of natural resources. One solution is to reduce the volume of the waste material by generating less of it. The second approach is to recycle hazardous material as much as possible. A third means of dealing with hazardous waste is to treat it to render it less harmful and often reduce its volume. The least-preferred solution is to store the waste in landfills. The Environmental Protection Agency (EPA) has established standards for responsibility and tracking of hazardous wastes, based on the principle that waste generators are responsible for their waste "from cradle to grave." This principle has involved extensive record-keeping by waste generators and disposal sites.

The U.S. Congress's 1984 Resource Conservation and Recovery Act (RCRA) revisions involved a thorough overhaul of hazardous waste legislation. Previously exempt sources that generated between 100 and 1,000

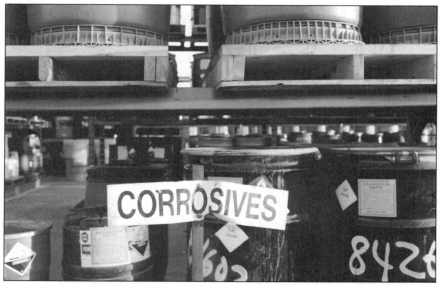

Controversy has surrounded how to store hazardous waste safely to avoid human contamination and illness. (PhotoDisc)

kilograms of hazardous waste per month were brought under the RCRA provisions. Congress further tried to force the EPA to adopt a bias against the landfilling of hazardous waste with a "no land disposal unless proven safe" provision. Congress also added underground storage tanks for gasoline, petroleum, pesticides, and solvents to the list of sources to be regulated and remediated. In addition to the RCRA, Superfund (from the Comprehensive Environmental Response, Compensation, and Liability Act of 1980) provides for the cleanup of all categories of abandoned hazardous waste sites except for radioactive waste. Several other statutes (and ensuing EPA regulations) deal with these aspects of the hazardous waste problem.

The costs for the cleanup and remediation of hazardous waste are substantial and are likely to continue to grow. This situation is particularly true in Eastern Europe and the former Soviet Union, where the magnitude of past dumping of hazardous materials is slowly becoming apparent. Meanwhile, less industrialized nations are ignoring the hazardous waste issue and are therefore setting themselves up for future difficulties.

The waste minimization philosophy expressed in the RCRA is a sound long-range strategy for dealing with hazardous waste. However, some materials will continue to be deposited in landfills. Incineration offers some solutions to the problem of volume of material but poses issues of air quality and highly toxic ash. As some firms have found, minimizing their waste stream affords them economic benefits while conserving natural resources. Household waste, which is not regulated by the RCRA, often includes small quantities of hazardous materials such as pesticides. Most of this waste was still being landfilled in the late 1990's. The cleanup of existing sites will continue to be a troubling problem, while the cleanup and disposal of radioactive waste will be a major issue for the future.

—John M. Theilmann

See also Environmental diseases; Mercury poisoning; Occupational health; Pesticides; Poisoning; Radiation; Water quality.

For Further Information:
Gerrard, Michael B. *Whose Backyard, Whose Risk.* Cambridge, Mass.: MIT Press, 1994. A helpful work.
Grisham, Joe, ed. *Health Aspects of the Disposal of Waste Chemicals.* New York: Pergamon Press, 1986. Another helpful work.
LaGrega, Michael D., Philip L. Buckingham, and Jeffrey C. Evans. *Hazardous Waste Management.* New York: McGraw-Hill, 1994. Useful discussions of various aspects of hazardous waste.
Wildavsky, Aaron. *But Is It True?* Cambridge, Mass.: Harvard University Press, 1995. More discussions of various aspects of hazardous waste.

✦ HEADACHES

Type of issue: Mental health, public health
Definition: A general term referring to pain localized in the head and/or neck, which may signal mere tension or a serious disorder.

In 1988, an ad hoc committee of the International Headache Society developed the current classification system for headaches. This system includes fourteen exhaustive categories of headache with the purpose of developing comparability in the management and study of headaches. Headaches most commonly seen by health care providers can be classified into four main types: migraine, tension-type, cluster, and "other" acute headaches.

MIGRAINES

Migraine headaches have been estimated to affect approximately 12 percent of the population. The headaches are more common in women and tend to run in families; they are usually first noticed in the teen years or young adulthood. For the diagnosis of migraine without aura ("aura" refers to visual disturbances or hallucinations, numbness and tingling on one side of the face, dizziness, or impairment of speech or hearing—symptoms that occur twenty to thirty minutes prior to the onset of the headache), the person must experience at least ten headache attacks, each lasting between four and seventy-two hours with at least two of the following characteristics: The headache is unilateral (occurs on one side), has a pulsating quality, is moderate to severe in intensity, or is aggravated by routine physical activity. Additionally, one of the following symptoms must accompany the headache: nausea and/or vomiting, or sensitivity to light or sounds. The person's medical history, a physical examination, and (where appropriate) diagnostic tests must exclude other organic causes of the headache, such as brain tumor or infection. Migraine with aura is far less common.

Migraines may be triggered or aggravated by physical activity, by menstruation, by relaxation after emotional stress, by ingestion of alcohol (red wine in particular) or certain foods or food additives (chocolate, hard cheeses, nuts, fatty foods, monosodium glutamate, or nitrates used in processed meats), by prescription medications (including birth control pills and hypertension medications), and by changes in the weather. Yet the precise pathophysiology of migraines is unknown. It had been posited that spasms in the blood vessels of the brain, followed by the dilation of these same blood vessels, cause the aura and head pain; however, studies using sophisticated brain and cerebral blood-flow scanning techniques indicate that this is likely not the case and that some type of inflammatory process may be involved related to the permeability of cerebral blood vessels and the resultant release of certain neurochemicals.

Tension Headaches

Tension-type headaches are the most common type; the prevalence is approximately 79 percent. Tension-type headaches are not hereditary, are found more frequently in females, and are first noticed in the teen years of young adulthood, although they can appear at any time of life. For the diagnosis of tension-type headaches, the person must experience at least ten headache attacks lasting from thirty minutes to seven days each, with at least two of the following characteristics: The headache has a pressing or tightening (nonpulsating) quality, is mild or moderate in intensity (may inhibit but does not prohibit activities), is bilateral or variable in location, and is not aggravated by physical activity. Additionally, nausea, vomiting, and light or sound sensitivity are absent or mild. Furthermore, the patient's medical history and physical or neurological examination exclude other organic causes for the headache apart from the following: oral or jaw dysfunction, muscular stress, or drug overuse. Tension-type headache sufferers describe these headaches as a bandlike or caplike tightness around the head, and/or muscle tension in the back of the head, neck, or shoulders. The pain is described as slow in onset with a dull or steady aching.

Tension-type headaches are believed to be precipitated primarily by emotional factors but can also be stimulated by muscular and spinal disorders, jaw dysfunction, paranasal sinus disease, and traumatic head injuries. The pathophysiology of tension-type headaches is controversial. Historically, tension-type headaches were attributed to sustained muscle contractions of the pericranial muscles. Studies indicate, however, that most patients do not manifest increased pericranial muscle activity and that pericranial muscle blood flow and/or central pain mechanisms might be involved in the pathophysiology of tension-type headaches. It is also believed that muscle contraction and scalp muscle ischemia play some role in tension-type headache pain.

Cluster Headaches

Cluster headaches are the least frequent of the headache types and are thought to be the most severe and painful. Cluster headaches are more common in males, with estimates of 0.4 to 1.0 percent of males being affected. Traditionally, these headaches first appear at about thirty years of age, although they can start later in life. There is no genetic predisposition to these headaches. For the diagnosis of cluster headaches, the person must experience at least ten severely painful headache attacks, typically on one side of the face and lasting from fifteen minutes to three hours. One of the following symptoms must accompany the headache on the painful side of the face: a bloodshot eye, tearing, nasal congestion, nasal discharge, forehead and facial sweating, contraction of the pupils, or drooping eyelids. Physical and neurological examination and imaging must exclude organic causes for the headaches, such as tumor or infection. Cluster headaches often occur once or twice daily, or every other day, but can be as frequent as ten attacks in one day, recurring on the same side of the head during the cluster period. The temporal "clusters" of these headaches give them their descriptive name.

A cluster headache is described as a severe, excruciating, sharp, and burning pain through the eye. The pain is occasionally throbbing but always unilateral. Radiation of the pain to the teeth has been reported. Duration can range from ten minutes to three hours, with the next headache in the cluster occurring sometime the same day. Cluster headache sufferers are often unable to sit or lie still and are in such pain that they have been known, in desperation, to hit their heads with their fists or to smash their heads against walls or floors.

Cluster headaches can be triggered in susceptible patients by alcohol consumption, subcutaneous injections of histamine, and sublingual use of nitroglycerine. Because these agents all cause the dilation of blood vessels, these attacks are believed to be associated with dilation of the temporal and ophthalmic arteries and other extracranial vessels. There is no evidence that intracranial blood flow is involved. Cluster headaches have been shown to occur more frequently during the weeks before and after the longest and shortest days of the year, lending support for the hypothesis of a link to seasonal changes. Additionally, cluster headaches often occur at about the same time of day in a given sufferer, suggesting a relationship to the circadian rhythms of the body. Vascular changes, hormonal changes, neurochemical excesses or deficits, histamine levels, and autonomic nervous system changes are all being studied for their possible role in the pathophysiology of cluster headaches.

ACUTE HEADACHES

Acute headaches, using the International Headache Society's classification scheme, constitute many of the headaches not mentioned above. Distinct from the other headache types, which are often considered to be chronic in nature, acute headaches often signify underlying disease or a life-threatening medical condition. These headaches can display pain distribution and quality similar to those seen in chronic headaches. The temporal nature of acute headaches, however, often points to their seriousness.

Acute headaches of concern are usually the first or worst headache the patient has had or are headaches with recent onset that are persistent or recurrent. Other signs that cause a high index of suspicion include an unremitting headache that steadily increases without relief, accompanying weakness or numbness in the hands or feet, an atypical change in the quality or intensity of the headache, headache upon exertion, recent head trauma, or a family history of cardiovascular problems. Such headaches can point to hemorrhage, meningitis, stroke, tumor, brain abscess, hematoma, and infection, which are all potentially life-threatening conditions. A thorough evaluation is necessary for all patients exhibiting the danger signs of acute headache.

Treatment Options for Headaches

A number of pharmacological treatments are available for stopping migraine headaches. Ergotamine tartrate is effective in terminating migraine symptoms by either reducing the dilation of extracranial arteries or in some way stimulating certain parts of the brain. Isomethaptine is a combination of chemicals that stimulates the sympathetic nervous system, provides analgesia, and is mildly tranquilizing. Another class of medications for migraines are nonsteroidal anti-inflammatory drugs (NSAIDs); these drugs work on the principle that inflammation is involved in migraine. Both narcotic and nonnarcotic pain medications are often used for migraines, primarily for their analgesic properties. Antiemetic medications, which prevent or arrest vomiting, have been used in the treatment of migraines. Sumatriptan, a vasoactive agent that increases the amount of the neurochemical serotonin in the brain, shows promise in treating migraines that do not respond to other treatments.

Preventive treatments for migraines include beta-blockers, methysergide, and calcium channel blockers, which are believed to interfere with the dilation or contraction of extracranial arteries by acting on the sympathetic nervous system or on the central nervous system itself. Antidepressants have also been found to prevent migraine attacks; there appears to be an analgesic effect from certain antidepressants that is effective for chronic migraines. Antiseizure medications have been found to be useful for some migraine patients, although the mechanism of action is unknown. NSAIDs have also been used as a preventive measure for migraines.

Several nonpharmacological treatments for migraines are also available, including stress management, relaxation training, biofeedback, psychotherapy, and the modification of headache-precipitating factors, such as avoiding certain dietary triggers.

The treatment options for tension-type headaches include narcotic and nonnarcotic analgesics. More often with tension-type headaches, the milder over-the-counter pain medications (such as aspirin or acetaminophen) are used. NSAIDs, simple muscle relaxants, or antianxiety drugs can also be helpful. Muscle relaxants and antianxiety drugs are believed to relax smooth muscles, reducing scalp muscle ischemia and therefore head pain.

Preventive treatments for tension-type headaches include antidepressants, narcotic and nonnarcotic analgesics, muscle relaxants, and antianxiety drugs. Occasionally, "trigger-point injections" are used to relieve tension-type headaches. Trigger points are areas within muscles, primarily in the upper back and neck, that are hypersensitive; when stimulated, they can cause headaches. These trigger points can be injected with a local anesthetic or steroid to decrease their sensitivity or to eliminate possible inflammation in the area.

Nonpharmacological treatment of tension-type headaches is similar to that for migraines and includes stress management, relaxation training, biofeedback, and psychotherapy. Other self-management techniques include taking a hot shower or bath, placing a hot water bottle or ice pack on the head or back of the neck, exercising, and sleeping.

For cluster headaches, the most common treatment is administering pure oxygen to the patient for ten minutes. The exact mechanism of action is unknown, but it might be related to the constriction of dilated cerebral arteries. Ergotamine tartrate or similar alkaloids given orally, intramuscularly, or intravenously can also abort the attack in some patients. Nasal drops of a local anesthetic (lidocaine hydrochloride) or cocaine have been used to interrupt the activity of the trigeminal nerve that is believed to be involved in cluster attacks. The efficacy of these treatments is inconclusive.

Preventive treatment of this headache type is crucial. Ergotamine, methysergide, calcium channel blockers, antiseizure medications, and steroidal anti-inflammatory medications have been used with some success in the prevention of cluster attacks. The mechanism of action for these medications is unknown. Lithium carbonate, a drug commonly prescribed for bipolar disorder, has been found to be effective for some cluster patients. This medication is believed to affect certain regions of the brain, possibly the hypothalamus.

While no nonpharmacological treatment strategies are routinely offered to cluster headache patients, surgery is an option in severe cases, particularly if the headaches are resistant to all other available treatments. One such surgical procedure destroys the trigeminal nerve pathway, the chief nerve pathway to the face. Modest successes have been found with this extreme treatment option.

The total economic costs of headaches are staggering. Headaches constitute approximately 1.7 percent of all visits to physician offices. Of visits to hospital emergency rooms, 2.5 percent are for headaches. The expenses associated with advances in assessment techniques and routine health care have risen rapidly. The cost in lost workdays adds to this economic picture. Thirty-six percent of headache sufferers in one study reported missing one or more days of work in the previous year because of headaches. The scientific study of headaches is necessary to understand this prevalent illness.

—*Oliver Oyama*

See also Pain management; Stress.

FOR FURTHER INFORMATION:
Blanchard, Edward B., and Frank Andrasik. *Management of Chronic Headaches: A Psychological Approach.* New York: Pergamon Press, 1985. The authors

review the evaluation and treatment of headaches from a psychological perspective. Alternative, nonpharmacological treatments for headaches are described in detail. The chapters are practical and offer a guide for managing headaches derived from the authors' experiences at a headache clinic.

Diamond, Seymour. "Migraine Headaches." *The Medical Clinics of North America* 75, no. 3 (May 1, 1991): 545-566. Diamond is one of the world's authorities on headaches. His article is well organized and comprehensively addresses the subject of migraines in a readable and interesting format. A practical guide to treating the headache patient.

Rapoport, Alan M., and Fred D. Sheftell. *Headache Relief.* New York: Simon & Schuster, 1991. The book takes the often-complicated theory, evaluation, and treatment of headaches and explains each area in very understandable terms for the layperson. The authors describe a "how-to" approach to treating headaches.

Raskin, Neil H. *Headache.* 2d ed. New York: Churchill Livingstone, 1988. A review of headaches from a technical perspective. The reader looking for a thorough resource study of headaches will find this text useful. The review of common headache types is comprehensive and reflects the research on headaches in the mid-1980's.

Saper, Joel R., et al., eds. *Handbook of Headache Management: A Practical Guide to Diagnosis and Treatment of Head, Neck, and Facial Pain.* 2d ed. Baltimore: Williams & Wilkins, 1999. A manual for doctors with patients complaining of headache pain.

✦ Health insurance

Type of issue: Economic issues, public health, social trends
Definition: Insurance to cover medical care.

Medical insurance in the United States began in the 1850's when insurance companies began offering policies protecting railroad passengers against injury. Health maintenance organizations (HMOs) were first implemented in the 1930's, with the 1970's seeing increased HMO proliferation due to higher health care costs and increased competition between growing numbers of physicians. The Health Maintenance Organizations Act of 1973 provided federal grants and loans for HMOs and required many employers to offer HMO membership to employees as a health insurance alternative.

The HMO concept served as a means to control costs by discouraging physicians from performing unnecessary and costly procedures, meet the increased demand for health insurance particularly in medically underserved areas, and foster preventive medicine. Financial incentives are, in theory, the major force behind personal freedom of choice, containment of costs, and assurance of quality. Preferred provider organizations (PPOs) appeared in the 1980's as a flexible alternative to standard HMOs, with many health insurers such as Blue Cross and Blue Shield exerting control over their daily operations.

Medicare and its companion program Medicaid are federally administered programs begun in the 1960's that guarantee medical insurance coverage for elderly and low-income American citizens. Other government medical insurance plans cover armed forces personnel, veterans, American Indians, and federal employees. Social Security pays disability benefits to covered persons and their dependents, whereas workers' compensation pays medical expenses and covers income losses for workers injured on the job. Medical insurance plans can be generally divided into medical expense insurance, income loss insurance, and accidental death and dismemberment coverage.

PRIVATE MEDICAL INSURANCE PROGRAMS

Private insurance companies provide a majority of the medical insurance plans in the United States. Some are for-profit stock companies or mutual companies owned by their policyholders. Nonprofit hospital associations such as Blue Cross and medical associations such as Blue Shield also provide insurance for hospitalization and surgical expenses, respectively.

Hospitalization insurance generally covers the cost of hospital room and board and expenses such as X rays, blood tests, and medications required as an inpatient. A deductible often applies before the insurer begins to pay benefits, with coverage often also limited to a specified number of days per illness. Hospitalization insurance generally does not cover general physician or surgeon fees, with many policies dictating a specified amount per clinic visit or surgical procedure. Prescription drugs, rehabilitation costs, and items such as prostheses are also often covered as stated in the policy.

Major medical insurance has a much higher maximum benefit limit, often over one million dollars and sometimes unlimited. A larger deductible generally applies, with the insurer often paying 80 percent of the expenses over the deductible. Comprehensive major medical policies often do not have an initial deductible and require the insurer to pay all expenses up to a stated amount, with the insurer paying 80 percent of all expenses over that amount.

Disability insurance protects against loss of income resulting from accidental injury or illness, with benefits often structured to pay approximately 40 to 60 percent of earnings up to the maximum total amount. Accidental injury cases may receive payments beginning with the day of injury, whereas illness benefits may not be paid until the insured person has been unable to work for a specified period of time.

Accidental death or dismemberment insurance, commonly advertised in vending machines at transportation centers such as airports, provides benefits in the event of death or loss of organs or limbs as a result of travel.

Health Maintenance Organizations (HMOs)

HMOs provide medical insurance to groups and individuals for an established, prepaid monthly premium. Generally, an HMO attempts to provide care at a lower cost than traditional fee-for-service insurance programs by transferring financial risk to physicians through capitation and other incentives. The result is that patients often have to accept fewer choices in treatment options and specialist providers. Preferred providers are physicians and other health care providers and hospitals who choose to provide health care on a reduced-cost basis to subscribers of an HMO. HMOs function in a dual role as both a health insurance company and a provider of health services, roles that were previously separated within American health care.

HMOs are often organized by employers, physician groups, unions, consumer groups, insurance companies, or for-profit health care agencies. They were originally formed from one, or a mixture of, the following practice models: point of service, staff, group, and independent practice association. A point-of-service model HMO, also called an open-ended HMO, includes an option that allows subscribers to seek medical care outside the established network and receive partial reimbursement, with all remaining expenses paid out of pocket. A staff model HMO is directly controlled at its headquarters locations, with all physicians and other health care workers being direct, full-time salaried employees. A group model HMO is organized by physicians whereby a private professional corporation is established that then individually contracts with an HMO to provide services exclusively for its subscribers. An independent practice association model HMO provides a flexible arrangement created by office physicians and administrators designed to compete with the classic HMOs; several office physicians in a community form a networked professional corporation that seeks group contracts among local employers and provides all medical care for a capitated rate per client per month to subscribers who often choose a personal primary care physician.

The term "managed care" describes the techniques by which an HMO, a health insurance carrier, or a self-insuring employer makes certain that the health care services it endorses are high quality and cost effective. An HMO will also furnish services from other health care providers, such as physical and occupational therapists, pharmacists, and mental health professionals.

HMOs are attractive to employers because the annual medical bill for the average subscriber-patient has consistently proven to be approximately 30 percent less than that of conventional insurers. Advantages of HMO membership include that all medical expenses, from routine and emergency care to hospitalization, are covered within a single, fixed monthly premium and that presenting an HMO membership card at the time of services with a small copayment requires no forms to fill out, deductibles to pay, or bills to submit. Disadvantages include that subscribers often cannot keep a trusted physician that they have had for years, providers become extremely busy when they are assigned five hundred or more patients in exchange for a fixed fee, and subscribers often have to accept fewer choices in treatment options.

Each client is assigned to a "primary care gatekeeper," a physician who is expected to provide most care in his or her private office for limited fees. When a referral to a specialist, laboratory, or hospital is necessary, authorization is required from the headquarters of the managed care organization. Hospitals contract with these organizations to limit their charges and follow established rules about economical care and prompt discharge. The managed care organization reviews utilization by physicians and hospitals, attempts to correct wasteful practices, and subsequently drops health care providers with expensive and/or poor practice styles.

POINT-OF-SERVICE PLANS

In contrast to more traditional HMOs, point-of-service plans have emerged that enable clients to have freedom of choice with respect to providers and some treatment options but that require them personally to pay the balance for their chosen higher-priced services. If a patient goes to physicians, hospitals, and other providers within the network and follows rules about utilization and authorization, the out-of-pocket financial costs are minimal. The patient retains the option to go to an out-of-plan provider, pay the bill in full, and then be reimbursed for the limited amount established in the individual plan. The employer's group contract with the managed care organization provides for limited and predictable premiums. The considerable costs of out-of-plan services thus are shifted from the group contract to the individual patient.

Managed care plans will continue to monitor closely the treatment patterns of physicians and encourage them to prescribe cheaper medications, develop standards that physicians are expected to follow in the treatment of various diseases, and have utilization review panels that examine patient records and decide which treatments a patient's health plan will cover and which it will not. Many states have passed comprehensive managed care laws as a result of numerous consumer complaints about the decisions of case managers who often have no medical training. Legislation has focused on issues such as adopting measures to ban physician gag clauses, establish consumer grievance procedures, require disclosure of financial incentives for physicians to withhold care, conduct external reviews of an HMO's internal decision to deny care, and grant the ability to sue an HMO for malpractice.

The largest looming question regarding the future of HMOs is whether physicians and other health care workers and client subscribers will continue to enroll in and thus support the system. Managed care necessarily adds substantial administrative overhead, with the ongoing question of whether the final result is greater efficiency for the entire system or just for the subscribing employers. An organization that will exert considerable influence on future HMO developments is the American Association of Retired Persons (AARP), a large nonprofit advocacy group for Americans over the age of fifty with more than thirty million members. AARP has begun giving endorsements to HMOs that meet its standards of quality and price.

MEDICARE AND MEDICAID

In 1965, amendments to the Social Security Act of 1935 that established Medicare and Medicaid were enacted. Medicare went into effect in 1966 and authorized compulsory health insurance for American citizens aged sixty-five and older who were entitled to receive Social Security or railroad retirement benefits. Medicaid was established by the 1965 amendments as a means-tested entitlement program to provide medical assistance to low-income persons who were aged, blind, disabled, pregnant, or members of families with dependent children, as well as other groups of needy children.

The establishment of Medicare and Medicaid followed considerable heated political debate over the feasibility of a national health care program, stimulated by a 1963 government survey that revealed only about 50 percent of elderly American citizens had health insurance. Many older Americans could not afford private coverage, and the elderly who attempted to pursue coverage were often denied on the basis of age or preexisting conditions. Passage of Medicare and Medicaid guaranteed insurance coverage for elderly and low-income Americans and initiated numerous major changes involving private financing relationships between physician and patient, physician training, insurance industry growth, and expansion of hospital-only coverage to extended care. The late 1960's saw these programs become substantially more expensive than originally anticipated, with amendments in 1972 being the first major attempts to limit expenditures.

Medicare's basic benefits package, which includes part A (hospital insurance) and part B (supplemental medical insurance), has changed little since its inception, with the only major variation being that many services are now delivered beyond traditional acute care settings. Part A is an earned benefit for most Americans and requires no premium upon eligibility, whereas part B is voluntary for a monthly premium. Nearly all older and disabled beneficiaries elect to participate in part B. Part A benefits include inpatient hospital care coverage for the first sixty days, less a deductible for each period of acute illness; inpatient psychiatric care; skilled nursing care or rehabilitation associated with recuperation for up to one hundred days following hospitalization; home health care as prescribed by a physician; and hospice care for the terminally ill. Not covered are outpatient prescription drugs, routine physical examinations, nonsurgical dental services, hearing aids and eyeglasses, and most long-term care in nursing facilities, in the community, or at home. In 1972, Medicare coverage was extended to persons of any age with end-stage renal (kidney) disease, those receiving Social Security Disability Insurance for at least two years, and persons aged sixty-five and older who are otherwise not eligible but elect to enroll by paying a monthly premium.

In the late 1990's, Medicare accounted for 28 percent of all hospital payments in the U.S. health care system and 20 percent of all physician payments. Medicare covered 45 percent of overall health care spending for the elderly but a lower percentage for the very elderly, particularly those requiring full-time nursing home care.

The Medicare Catastrophic Coverage Act of 1988 attempted to require Medicare beneficiaries to pay the full cost of expanded benefits through an income-related tax surcharge and a flat premium. Elderly citizens organized groups in intense opposition to premium funding, leading to the repeal of the act one year later. Beginning in 1984, Congress made amendments to Medicaid to require individual states to cover all infants and pregnant women below the poverty level, with their eligibility determined by an index based on income level and family size. The Catastrophic Coverage Act gave states the option of covering those below 185 percent of the poverty line and required the states to pay Medicare cost sharing for all poor elderly and disabled Medicare beneficiaries. These provisions were retained when the act was repealed.

OTHER GOVERNMENT MEDICAL INSURANCE PROGRAMS

Numerous other programs exist at various levels of government to help Americans pay medical expenses and meet income losses. The federal government provides medical insurance for armed forces personnel and their dependents, veterans, American Indians, and federal employees. Social Security pays disability benefits to covered workers and their dependents until the individual recovers and returns to work, dies, or reaches age sixty-five, when retirement benefits are received. Workers' compensation pays medical expenses and covers income losses for workers injured on the job.

—Daniel G. Graetzer

See also HMOs; Hospice; Hospitalization of the elderly; Nursing and convalescent homes.

FOR FURTHER INFORMATION:

Brink, Susan, and Nancy Shute. "Are HMOs the Right Prescription?" *U.S. News and World Report* 123, no. 4 (October 13, 1997): 60-65. Covered in this well-researched article is the growing dissatisfaction of subscribers with the quality of health care received, with a rating of the best HMOs in the United States.

Gold, M. "Health Maintenance Organizations: Structure, Performance, and Current Issues for Employee Health Benefits Design." *Journal of Occupational Medicine* 33, no. 3 (1991): 288-296. From an occupational medicine viewpoint, this manuscript reviews numerous health benefit plans designed for large and small company employees by examining consumer satisfaction, quality of health care, and analysis of the cost-benefit ratio.

National Academy on Aging. *Facts on Medicare: Hospital Insurance and Supplemental Medical Insurance.* Washington, D.C.: Author, 1995. Contains current information and answers to frequently asked questions about Medicare. Current information can also be obtained from Medicare's Web site: http://epn.org/aging/agmedi.html.

✧ HEARING AIDS

Type of issue: Elder health, treatment
Definition: Mechanical devices that counteract the effects of hearing loss by amplifying soundwaves as they enter the ear.

In the United States, about 10 percent of the population have some degree of hearing loss. Hearing loss tends to worsen with aging, and, as the proportion of people living past sixty-five years of age increases, so will the percentage of those who develop hearing loss. The causes of hearing loss are many and must be pinpointed in individual cases before any treatment can be initiated.

TYPES OF HEARING LOSS

There are three general types of hearing loss, classified according to what structures of the ear may be involved. All types of hearing loss are not equally amenable to improvements with the use of hearing aids. In conductive hearing loss, changes have occurred in the outer and middle ear. Sensorineural hearing loss involves the inner ear. In the third type, damage involves both conductive and sensorineural aspects, resulting in a mixed loss. It is not unusual to find the mixed type of hearing loss among the elderly.

The causes of the different types of hearing loss are varied. In some cases of conductive damage, the loss may be caused by an infection and may be effectively treated by medication. Surgery may be recommended in those cases where the hearing loss is a result of a problem in the middle ear. In the condition known as otosclerosis, a bony growth forms at the base of the stapes and prevents the proper movement of the small, bony ossicles in the middle ear so that normal transmission of the sound wave cannot occur. Otosclerosis is the most common cause of conductive deafness in adults. The condition can usually be corrected by surgically removing the stapes and replacing it with a plastic or metal device.

Hearing aids may be of considerable benefit to most people who have sensorineural hearing loss. However, people with severe sensorineural hearing loss (commonly known as nerve deafness) who do not gain any benefit from hearing aids may use cochlear implants, which allow the auditory nerve to be directly stimulated.

Presbycusis, or age-related deafness, is the most common cause of sensorineural hearing loss among those individuals sixty-five years of age and older. By the age of sixty-five, nearly 20 percent of the population suffers from presbycusis, which results from changes in the inner ear and in the auditory nerve. The inner ear contains hair cells that are, in fact, nerve cells that respond to stimuli, including sound vibrations.

At birth, there are twenty thousand to thirty thousand hair cells in the ear; as they gradually wear out and die during the course of a lifetime, people experience a loss of their ability to hear high-pitched sounds. A person might have difficulty hearing all the words produced by some women and children. Since individuals suffering from presbycusis have trouble hearing only certain things from certain people, they may not be aware of the deterioration in hearing and may not realize that the situation might be improved through use of a hearing aid. The loss of hearing also may affect a person's ears unequally. If the imbalance is severe enough, a person may experience difficulty in localizing sound, which may lead to disorientation.

This condition tends to get progressively worse with age, and certain families are at higher risk than others. Factors that contribute to presbycusis are many, and it is difficult to determine how these factors interact with those "normal" changes that accompany aging. Without a doubt, occupational noise and other everyday noises are major contributors to presbycusis. There is wide variation in the rate of decline in hearing among individuals as they age.

TYPES OF HEARING AIDS

Hearing aids fall into four general types: those worn on the body, those that are part of an eyeglass frame, those worn behind the ear, and those worn in the ear. Some types are effective only for mild hearing loss, whereas other models may be required for more severe hearing impairments. Continued advances in technology have increased the ability of hearing aids to help improve even severe hearing loss. The different types of hearing aids are not used in equal numbers. Relatively few people use the body-worn type or the eyeglass unit. Used somewhat more frequently is the behind-the-ear aid. However, the majority of hearing-impaired people use some form of the in-the-ear type. Like any product, the useful life of a hearing aid will vary, but they should last, on the average, four to five years.

All hearing aids function in a similar manner. A battery furnishes the operational power source. The size of the battery depends on the size of the aid and the amount of power required to carry out its specific function. The life of a battery is related to the length of time the aid is used and the power needs of the hearing aid. Zinc-air batteries usually maintain performance until they go completely dead, whereas other types, such as mercury batteries, tend to weaken before they are entirely drained. Batteries may last three weeks or less, and it is prudent to always have a supply on hand.

Hearing aids work by picking up sound waves with a microphone and converting them into electrical energy. An amplifier unit controls the volume by increasing the strength of the electrical energy. The receiver then converts the electrical signal back into sound waves. One final, but critical, component of the behind-the-ear hearing aid, the body aid, and the eyeglass aid is the earmold, which connects the hearing aid to the ear. Earmolds must be fitted or molded to individual ears. Since the earmold governs the amount and quality of the sound that passes from the aid into the ear, it not only must match the physical characteristics of each ear but also must be chosen on the basis of the type of hearing loss. Once a person begins to wear a hearing aid, it is essential that hearing and the hearing aid be checked regularly. The checkup usually includes an examination of the earmold, since the shape and size of the ear may change over time. A hearing aid is an extremely sensitive instrument that must be carefully adjusted for the individual who is using it.

The Invisible Handicap

Although the nature and cause of an individual's hearing loss may have been determined and a proper hearing aid may have been decided upon, it does not necessarily mean that a person's hearing problem has been solved. Hearing loss is often referred to as the "invisible handicap." Many people are slow to recognize that their hearing is deteriorating, others are slow to do anything about it, and many go into a period of denial. Individuals may have problems adjusting to wearing hearing aids because they feel embarrassed or do not want to "stand out." Learning to hear with hearing aids also requires a period of adjustment. However, once a hearing-impaired person has overcome these obstacles, a return to a near-normal life, with all its personal and social benefits, follows.

—Donald J. Nash

See also Aging; Disabilities; Hearing loss; Noise pollution.

FOR FURTHER INFORMATION:

American Association of Retired Persons. *A Report on Hearing Aids: User Perspectives and Concerns.* Washington, D.C.: Author, 1993.

Dugan, Marcia P. *Keys to Living with Hearing Loss.* New York: Barron's Educational Service, 1997.

Pope, Anne. *Solutions, Skills, and Sources for Hard of Hearing People.* New York: Dorling Kindersley, 1997.

Wayner, Donna A. *Hear What You've Been Missing.* Minneapolis: Chronimed, 1998.

_____. *The Hearing Aid Handbook: User's Guide for Adults.* Washington, D.C.: Gallaudet University Press, 1990.

✧ HEARING LOSS

Type of issue: Elder health, occupational health, public health
Definition: Loss of sensitivity to sound pressure changes as a result of congenital factors, disease, traumatic injury, noise exposure, or aging.

In the truest sense, hearing loss is any reduction in threshold sensitivity for any frequency, including those below or above the range for the normal hearing of speech. The real issue, however, is whether minor changes in sensitivity create significant problems in understanding speech and other information-bearing acoustic signals. For example, it is known that loss of threshold sensitivity below 300 hertz and above 4,000 hertz has a minimal affect on understanding speech information. It is when hearing loss exists within this critical frequency range that an individual may experience appreciable difficulty in understanding intended messages. The question becomes, then, what conditions cause a permanent or temporary loss of hearing and how such a loss is managed by medical, surgical, or rehabilitative intervention.

CONDUCTIVE HEARING LOSS

Any barrier or impedance that keeps sound from reaching the cochlea of the human auditory system at its intended loudness is termed conductive hearing loss. A very common cause of conduction loss is a buildup of earwax (cerumen) in the external ear canal. Normally, earwax will migrate out of the ear. It is when the earwax accumulates to an amount sufficient to block sound from entering the ear that something needs to be done. In most cases, earwax can be removed by irrigation. A physician washes out the earwax using a special liquid solution that does not damage the tissue of the ear canal or the eardrum itself.

Another cause of conductive hearing loss is a hole (perforation) in the eardrum, which can be created by a number of conditions, including injury. Depending on the size and location of the hole, surgery (tympanoplasty) is often successful in restoring normal hearing function. For some persons, otosclerosis, a disease causing hardening and fixing of the three small bones in the middle-ear space, results in significant conductive hearing impairment. Otosclerosis prevents these tiny bones from moving efficiently as the eardrum moves, and hearing sensitivity is reduced. Advances in surgical procedures have allowed the surgeon to replace the stapes bone with a suitable prosthesis, reinstating relatively normal activity of the ossicles and greatly improving hearing ability.

A frequently occurring cause of conductive pathology is otitis media. Otitis media may refer to inflammation involving the middle-ear space or to a disorder in which the middle ear is filled with a watery fluid. In some cases, the fluid may harbor bacteria, creating significant medical problems if this condition is not treated early. Such middle-ear effusions are more common in children than in adults. If fluid is present in the middle ear, its mass will restrict the movement of the ossicles and create hearing impairment. Generally, patients with otitis media can be successfully treated through medical or surgical intervention.

Conductive pathology does not affect the behavior of inner-ear structures. If the conductive pathology is eliminated by appropriate treatment, normal hearing will be restored. Severity of the condition may prevent the restoration of hearing, however, even if an aggressive treatment program is followed.

SENSORINEURAL HEARING LOSS

There are two types of hearing loss within this classification. One is a sensory loss which involves the destruction of nerve cells (hair cells) in the cochlea. The other is a neural loss which involves neural cells in the ascending auditory pathway from the cochlea to the brain. It is possible to experience one type of loss without the other. Some examples of sensory loss include loss of nerve cells resulting from traumatic injury to the cochlea (such as from whiplash, sharp blows to the head, or sudden, brief, and intense noises); loss of sensory cells from viral infections such as measles; loss of sensory cells caused by ototoxic drugs as those in the mycin group (such as streptomycin or kanamycin); congenital problems associated with a lack of embryonic development; and exposure to loud and continuous noise, a common cause of hearing loss in adults. This last type of impairment is different from traumatic injury resulting from sudden, intense noise because it may take months or years for hearing loss caused by long-term noise to manifest itself. Research has also established a clear correlation between the normal aging process and sensory hearing impairment.

When sensory hearing impairment occurs, it is permanent. At the moment, there is no way of regenerating sensory tissue after the cell body has died. The only exception is found in those patients suffering from Ménière's disease, which is characterized by vertigo, dizziness, vomiting, and hearing loss. In the initial stages, however, the loss of sensitivity to sound is the result of changes in cellular physiology rather than of death of the nerve cells.

Examples of neural hearing loss are found among those hearing-impaired individuals with tumors, acoustic neuromas (benign tumors), cysts, and other anomalous conditions affecting the transmission of nerve impulses from the cochlea to the brain. Depending on the magnitude of the disorder, neural hearing loss has a much more devastating effect on speech understanding and signal processing than does sensory loss. As with sensory hearing impairment, neural hearing loss is a rather frequent occurrence associated with the aging process. For a sizable portion of those who experience hearing impairment, components of both sensory and neural loss are present. If the cause of the hearing deficit is entirely neural in nature, then the impairment is referred to as a retrocochlear loss.

For some types of neural pathology, medical or surgical intervention can be undertaken successfully. Acoustic neuromas are often removed after they have been confirmed by audiologic, otologic, radiologic, and other diagnostic modalities. The size and location of the neuroma or tumorous growth will often dictate whether hearing can be preserved following surgery.

The Prevalence and Treatment of Hearing Loss

Hearing loss is quite common and affects some twenty million Americans, ranging from infants to the elderly. The primary reason for preserving hearing is to maintain social adequacy in communication skills. Hearing conservation programs have been instituted by public and private schools, industry, military installations, construction organizations, and more recently, the U.S. government. In 1970, the Occupational Safety and Health Act (OSHA) was passed, making it mandatory for employers to provide safe work areas for workers exposed to noise levels exceeding government standards.

For those millions suffering from hearing impairment, it is the loss of speech discrimination ability that is of greatest concern. Thousands of studies have been undertaken to investigate the correlation between the magnitude, type, and length of hearing loss and the degree of speech recognition difficulty. One of the essential findings indicates that hearing loss is more pronounced for the high frequencies (above 1,000 hertz), whether the loss is caused by disease, drugs, noise, or the aging process. Another major finding is that one's ability to identify vowel and consonant information is frequency-dependent. Vowel identification is dependent on frequencies from about 200 hertz to 1,000 hertz, while consonant identification is dependent on frequencies above 1,000 hertz. A listener understands about 68 percent of speech sounds if nothing above 1,500 hertz is heard and about 68 percent of speech if nothing below 1,500 hertz is heard.

For the hearing impaired, understanding of speech is related to the degree of loss and the type of impairment. Because medical or surgical care cannot always ameliorate the loss, rehabilitation programs may take the form of speech or lipreading to improve communication skills. These rehabilitative programs constituted the treatment of choice until the introduction of wearable electric hearing aids. Hearing aids have become the treatment of choice when medical or surgical intervention is not indicated in resolving hearing loss. It is possible not only to control the loudness of the hearing aid sound but also to shape the frequency response of the instrument to match the acoustic needs of the patient. Transistor technology makes it possible to reduce the size of the hearing aid device without sacrificing performance. Computer science has also been used in the design of hearing aids. With digital technology, it is now possible to program electroacoustic characteristics into the hearing aid, which extends its utility.

—*Robert Sandlin*

See also Aging; Disabilities; Hearing aids; Noise pollution; Speech disorders.

For Further Information:
Gerber, Sanford. *Introductory Hearing Science.* Philadelphia: W. B. Saunders, 1974. Somewhat more than a basic text, but one that clearly outlines the various aspects of hearing science, from the measurement of sound and hearing to the use and description of hearing aid devices for the acoustically impaired. Suitable for those readers who have some basic knowledge of how the ear works and the fundamentals of sound, but can be understood by those having little or no previous knowledge of acoustics or the auditory system.
Pascoe, David. *Hearing Aids: Who Needs Them?* St. Louis: Big Bend Books, 1991. This easy-to-read text presents an abundance of data relative to hearing, hearing aid devices, and their use. Answers many questions that may arise concerning hearing aid use in direct and simple terms. One of the most significant aspects of this book is that it explains, in reasonable detail, how to use and evaluate hearing aids.
Yost, William. *Fundamentals of Hearing.* 4th ed. San Diego: Academic Press, 2000. This text describes, in easy-to-understand terms, the organ of hearing and its contribution to an individual's behavior. Simple auditory theory is examined, as is the nature of the ear's response to acoustic energy.

✧ HEART ATTACKS

Type of issue: Elder health, public health
Definition: The sudden death of heart muscle characterized by intense chest pain, sweating, shortness of breath, or sometimes none of these symptoms.

Although varied in origin and effect on the body, heart attacks (or myocardial infarctions) occur when there are interruptions in the delicately synchronized system either supplying blood to the heart or pumping blood from the heart to other vital organs. The heart is a highly specialized muscle with four chambers, two ventricles and two atria. The heart's action involves the development of pressure to propel blood through arriving and departing channels—veins and arteries—that must maintain that pressure within their walls at critical levels.

The efficiency of this process, as well as the origins of problems of fatigue in the heart that can lead to heart attacks and eventual heart failure, is tied to the maintenance of a reasonably constant level of blood pressure. If pulmonary problems (blockage caused by the effects of smoking or environmental pollution, for example) make it harder for the right ventricle to push blood through the lungs, the heart must expend more energy. Similarly, and often in addition to the added work for the heart because of pulmonary complications, the efficiency of the left ventricle in handling blood flow may be reduced by the presence of excessive fat in the body, causing this ventricle to expend more energy to propel oxygenated blood into vital tissues.

Although factors such as these may be responsible for overworking the heart and thus contributing to eventual heart failure, other causes of heart attacks are to be found within the heart, particularly in the coronary arteries. The passageways inside these and other key arteries are vulnerable to the process known as atherosclerosis,, the accumulation of fatty deposits. If these deposits continue to collect, less blood can flow through the arteries. A narrowed artery also increases the possibility of a variant form of heart attack, in which a sudden and total blockage of blood flow follows the lodging of a blood clot.

A symptomatic condition called angina pectoris, characterized by intermittent chest pains, may develop if atherosclerosis reduces blood (and therefore oxygen) supply to the heart. These danger signs can continue over a number of years. If diagnosis reveals a problem that might be resolved by preventive medication, exercise, or recommendations for heart surgery, then this condition, known as myocardial ischemia, may not necessarily end in a full heart attack.

Types of Heart Attack

A full heart attack occurs when, for one of several possible reasons including a vascular spasm suddenly constricting an already clogged artery or a blockage caused by a clot, the heart suddenly ceases to receive the necessary supply of blood. This brings almost immediate deterioration in some of the heart's tissue and causes the organ's consequent inability to perform its vital functions effectively.

Another form of attack and disruption of the heart's ability to deliver blood can come either independently of or in conjunction with an arterially induced heart attack. This form of attack involves a sustained interruption in the rate of heartbeats. The necessary pace or rate of contractions is regulated in the sinoatrial node in the right atrium, which generates its own electrical impulses. There are, however, other so-called local pacemakers located in the atria and ventricles. If these sources of electrical charges begin giving commands to the heart that are not in rhythm with those coming from the sinoatrial node, then dysrhythmic or premature beats may confuse the heart muscle, causing it to beat wildly. In fact, the concentrated pattern of muscle contractions will not be coordinated and instead will be dispersed in different areas of the heart.

The result is fibrillation, a series of uncoordinated contractions that cannot combine to propel blood out of the ventricles. This condition may occur either as the aftershock of an arterially induced heart attack or suddenly and on its own, caused by the deterioration of the electrical impulse system commanding the heart rate. In patients whose potential vulnerability to this form of heart attack has been diagnosed in advance, a heart physician may decide to surgically implant a mechanical pacemaker to ensure coordination of the necessary electrical commands to the heart.

Preventing and Treating Heart Attacks

Medical advances have helped reduce the high death rates formerly associated with heart attacks, many in the field of preventive medicine. The most widely recognized medical findings are related to diet, smoking, and exercise. Although controversy remains, there is general agreement that cholesterol absorbed by the body from the ingestion of animal fats plays a key role in the dangerous buildup of platelets inside arterial passageways. It has been accepted that regular, although not necessarily strenuous, exercise is an essential long-term preventive strategy that can reduce the risk of heart attacks. Exercise also plays a role in therapy after a heart attack. In both preventive and postattack contexts, it has been medically proven that the entire cardiovascular system profits from the natural muscle-strengthening process and general cleansing effects that result from controlled regular exercise.

The domains of preventive surgery and specialized drug treatment to prevent dangerous blood clotting are vast. Statistically, the most important

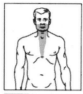

Pain radiating up into jaw and through to back.

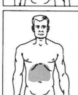

Pain felt in upper abdomen.

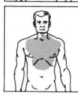

Pressure in the central chest area from mild to severe.

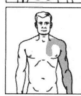

Pain radiating down left arm; may cause sensation of weakness in the arm.

The pain associated with heart attacks can take several different forms. (Hans & Cassidy, Inc.)

and widely practiced operations that were developed in the later decades of the twentieth century were replacement of the aortic valve, coronary bypass, and heart transplantation. Coronary bypass operations involve the attachment of healthy arteries to carry the blood that can no longer pass through the patient's clogged arterial passageways; these healthy arteries are taken by the heart surgeon from other areas of the patient's own body.

Balloon angioplasty held out a major nonsurgical promise of preventing deterioration of the arteries leading to the heart. This sophisticated form of treatment involves the careful, temporary introduction of inflatable devices inside clogged arteries, which are then stretched to increase the space within the arterial passageway for blood to flow. By the 1990's, however, doctors recognized one disadvantage of balloon angioplasty. By stretching the essential blood vessels being treated, this procedure either stretches the plaque with the artery or breaks loose debris that remains behind, creating a danger of renewed clogging. Thus another technique, called atherectomy, was developed to clear certain coronary arteries, as well as arteries elsewhere in the body.

Atherectomy involves a motorized catheter device resembling a miniature drill that is inserted into clogged arteries. As the drill turns, material that is literally shaved off the interior walls of arteries is retrieved through a tiny collection receptacle. Early experimentation, especially to treat the large anterior descending coronary artery on the left side of the heart, showed that atherectomy was 87 percent effective, whereas, on the average, angioplasty removed only 63 percent of the blockage. In addition, similar efforts to provide internal, nonsurgical treatment of clogged arteries using laser beams were being made by the 1990's.

—*Byron D. Cannon*

See also Arteriosclerosis; Cardiac rehabilitation; Cholesterol; Exercise; First aid; Heart disease; Heart disease and women; Hypertension; Obesity; Obesity and aging; Preventive medicine; Resuscitation; Secondhand smoke; Smoking.

FOR FURTHER INFORMATION:

Baum, Seth. *The Total Guide to a Healthy Heart: Integrative Strategies for Preventing and Reversing Heart Disease.* New York: Kensington, 2000. This book brings together the practices of both conventional and alternative approaches to reversing heart disease and maintaining heart health. Offers great insight into why the integrative approach to maintaining a healthy heart will be the medicine of the new millennium.

Gillis, Jack. *The Heart Attack Prevention and Recovery Handbook.* Point Roberts, Wash.: Hartley & Marks, 1995. Using simple, brief explanations, Gillis's text covers essential information that heart attack victims and families need immediately for reassurance and recovery. Presents excellent discussions of emotional effects on patients, medications, and treatments.

McGoon, M. *The Mayo Clinic's Heart Book.* New York: William Morrow, 1993. The most respected text for laypeople on heart disease. Covers all aspects of anatomy, physiology, diagnosis, treatment, and prevention.

Yannios, Thomas A. *The Heart Disease Breakthrough: What Even Your Doctor Doesn't Know About Preventing a Heart Attack.* New York: Wiley, 1999. Yannios, associate director of critical care and nutritional support at Ellis Hospital in Schenectady, New York, describes the smallest components of cholesterol, which can do more damage to the heart than the overall LDL levels that concern so many people.

Zaret, Barry L., Marvin Moser, and Lawrence S. Cohen, eds. *Yale University School of Medicine Heart Book.* New York: Hearst Books, 1992. Discusses the prevention and control of heart disease. Illustrated, with a bibliography and an index.

✧ HEART DISEASE

Type of issue: Prevention, public health
Definition: One of the leading causes of death in many industrialized nations; heart diseases include atherosclerotic disease, coronary artery disease, cardiac arrhythmias, and stenosis.

The heart diseases collectively include all the disorders that can befall every part of the heart muscle: the pericardium, epicardium, myocardium, endocardium, atria, ventricles, valves, coronary arteries, and nodes. The most significant sites of heart diseases are the coronary arteries and the nodes; their malfunction can cause coronary artery disease and cardiac arrhythmias, respectively. These two disorders are responsible for the majority of heart disease cases.

CORONARY ARTERY DISEASE

Coronary artery disease occurs when matter such as cholesterol and fibrous material collects and stiffens on the inner walls of the coronary arteries. This plaque that forms may narrow the passage through which blood flows, reducing the amount of blood delivered to the heart, or may build up and clog the artery entirely, shutting off the flow of blood to the heart. In the former case, when the coronary artery is narrowed, the condition is called ischemic heart disease. Because the most common cause of ischemia is narrowing of the coronary arteries to the myocardium, another designation of the condition is myocardial ischemia, referring to the fact that blood flow to the myocardium is impeded. Accumulation of plaque within the coronary arteries is referred to as coronary atherosclerosis.

As the coronary arteries become clogged and then narrow, they can fail to deliver the required oxygen to the heart muscle, particularly during stress or physical effort. The heart's need for oxygen exceeds the arteries' ability to supply it. The patient usually feels a sharp, choking pain, called angina pectoris. Not all people who have coronary ischemia, however, experience anginal pain; these people are said to have silent ischemia.

The danger in coronary artery disease is that the accumulation of plaque will progress to the point where the coronary artery is clogged completely and no blood is delivered to the part of the heart serviced by that artery. The result is a myocardial infarction (commonly called a heart attack), in which some myocardial cells die when they fail to receive blood. The rough, uneven texture of the plaque instead may cause the formation of a blood clot, or thrombus, which closes the artery in a condition called coronary thrombosis.

Although coronary ischemia is usually thought of as a disease of middle and old age, in fact it starts much earlier. Autopsies of accident victims in their teens and twenties, as well as young soldiers killed in battle, show that coronary atherosclerosis is often well advanced in young persons. Some reasons for these findings and for why the rates of coronary artery disease began to rise in the twentieth century have been proposed. Western societies underwent significant changes in lifestyle and eating habits: high-fat diets, obesity, and the stressful pace of life in a modern industrial society. Further, cigarette smoking, once almost a universal habit, has been shown to be highly pathogenic (disease-causing), contributing significantly to the development of heart disease. In the early and middle decades of the twentieth century, coronary heart disease was considered primarily an ailment of middle-aged and older men. As women began smoking, however, the incidence shifted so that coronary artery disease became almost equally prevalent, and equally lethal, among men and women.

Other conditions such as hypertension or diabetes mellitus are considered precursors of coronary artery disease. Hypertension, or high blood pressure, is an extremely common condition that, if unchecked, can contribute to both the development and the progression of coronary artery disease. Over the years, high blood pressure subjects arterial walls to constant stress. In response, the walls thicken and stiffen. This "hardening" of the arteries encourages the accumulation of fatty and fibrous plaque on inner artery walls. In patients with diabetes mellitus, blood sugar (glucose) levels rise either because the patient is deficient in insulin or because the insulin that the patient produces is inefficient at removing glucose from the blood. High glucose levels favor high fat levels in the blood, which can cause atherosclerosis.

Cardiac Arrhythmias

Cardiac arrhythmias are the next major cause of morbidity and mortality among the heart diseases. Inside the heart, an electrochemical network regulates the contractions and relaxations that form the heartbeat. In the excitation or contraction phase, a chain of electrochemical impulses starts in the upper part of the right atrium in the heart's pacemaker, the sinoatrial or sinus node. The impulses travel through internodal tracts (pathways from one node to another) to an area between the atrium and the right ventricle called the atrioventricular node. The impulses then enter the bundle of His, which carries them to the left atrium and left ventricle. After the series of contractions is complete, the heart relaxes for a brief moment before another cycle is begun. On the average, the process is repeated sixty to eighty times a minute.

This is normal rhythm, the regular, healthy heartbeat. Dysfunction at any point along the electrochemical pathway, however, can cause an arrhythmia. Arrhythmias range greatly in their effects and their potential for bodily damage. They can be completely unnoticeable, merely annoying, debilitating, or frightening. They can cause blood clots to form in the heart, and they can cause sudden death.

The arrhythmic heart can beat too quickly (tachycardia) or too slowly (bradycardia). The contractions of the various chambers can become unsynchronized, or out of step with one another. For example, in atrial flutter or atrial fibrillation, the upper chambers of the heart beat faster, out of synchronization with the ventricles. In ventricular tachycardia, ventricular contractions increase, out of synchronization with the atria. In ventricular tachycardia, ventricular contractions increase, out of synchronization with the upper chambers. In ventricular fibrillation, ventricular contractions lose all rhythmicity and become uncoordinated to the point at which the heart is no longer able to pump blood. Cardiac death can then occur unless the patient receives immediate treatment.

An arrhythmic disorder called heart block occurs when the impulse from the pacemaker is "blocked." Its progress through the atrioventricular node and the bundle of His may be slow or irregular, or the impulse may fail to reach its target tissues. The disorder is rated in three degrees. First-degree heart block is detectable only on an electrocardiogram (ECG), in which the movement of the impulse from the atria to the ventricles is seen to be slowed. In second-degree heart block, only some of the impulses generated reach from the atria to the ventricles; the pulse becomes irregular. Third-degree heart block is the most serious manifestation of this disorder: No impulses from the atria reach the ventricles. The heart rate may slow dramatically, and the blood flow to the brain can be reduced, causing dizziness or loss of consciousness.

HEART VALVE DISORDERS AND HEART FAILURE

Disorders that affect the heart valves usually involve stenosis (narrowing), which reduces the size of the valve opening; physical malfunction of the valve; or both. These disorders can be attributable to infection (such as rheumatic fever) or to tissue damage, or they can be congenital. If a valve has narrowed, the passage of blood from one heart chamber to another is impeded. In the case of mitral stenosis, the mitral valve between the left atrium and the left ventricle is narrowed. Blood flow to the left ventricle is reduced, and blood is retained in the left atrium, causing the atrium to enlarge as pressure builds in the chamber. This pressure forces blood back into the lungs, creating a condition called pulmonary edema in which fluid collects in the air sacs of the lungs. Similarly, malfunctions of the heart valves that cause them to open and close inefficiently can interfere with the flow of blood into the heart, through it, and out of it. This impairment may cause structural changes in the heart that can be life-threatening.

Heart failure may be a consequence of many disease conditions. It occurs primarily in the elderly. In this condition, the heart becomes inefficient at pumping blood. If the failure is on the right side of the heart, blood is forced back into the body, causing edema in the lower legs. If the failure is on the left side of the heart, blood is forced back into the lungs, causing pulmonary edema. There are many manifestations of heart failure, including shortness of breath, fatigue, and weakness.

TREATING HEART DISEASES

The main goals of therapy in treating heart diseases are to cure the condition, if possible, and otherwise help the patient live a normal life and prevent the condition from becoming worse. In coronary artery disease, the physician seeks to maintain blood flow to the heart and to prevent heart attack. Hundreds of medications are available for this purpose, including vasodilators (agents that relax blood vessel walls and increase their capacity to carry blood). Chief among the coronary vasodilators are nitroglycerin and other drugs in the nitrate family. Also, calcium channel blockers are often used to dilate blood vessels. Beta-blocking agents are used because they reduce the heart's need for oxygen and alleviate the symptoms of angina. In addition, various support measures are recommended by physicians to stop plaque buildup and halt the progress of the disease. These include losing weight, reducing fats in the diet, and stopping smoking. The physician also treats concomitant illnesses that can contribute to the progress of coronary artery disease, such as hypertension and diabetes.

Sometimes medications and diet are not fully successful, and the ischemia continues. In a relatively new procedure, the cardiologist can unblock a clogged artery by a procedure called angioplasty. The physician threads a catheter containing a tiny balloon to the point of the blockage. The balloon is inflated to widen the inner diameter of the artery, and blood flow is increased. This procedure is often successful, although it may have to be repeated. When it is not successful, coronary bypass surgery may be indicated. In this procedure, clogged coronary arteries are replaced with healthy blood vessels from other parts of the body.

When coronary artery disease progresses to a heart attack, the patient should be treated in the hospital or similar facility. The possibility of sudden death is high during the attack and remains high until the patient is stabilized. Emergency measures are undertaken to minimize the extent of heart damage, reduce heart work, keep oxygen flowing to all parts of the body, and regulate blood pressure and heartbeat.

Cardiac arrhythmias can be managed by a variety of medications and procedures. Digitalis, guanidine, procainamide, tocanamide, and atropine are widely used to restore normal heart rhythm. In acute situations, the patient's heart rhythm can be restored by electrical cardioversion, in which an electrical stimulus is applied from outside the body to regulate the heartbeat. When a slowed heartbeat cannot be controlled by medication, a pacemaker may be implanted to regulate heart rhythm.

Treatment of heart valve disorders and disorders of the heart wall is directed at alleviating the individual condition. Antibiotics and/or valve replacement surgery may be required. In many cases, valve disorders can be completely corrected. Heart transplantation remains a possible treatment for some heart patients. This is an option for comparatively few patients because there are ten times as many candidates for heart transplants as there are available donor hearts.

—C. Richard Falcon

See also Arteriosclerosis; Cardiac rehabilitation; Cholesterol; Diabetes mellitus; Exercise; Heart attacks; Heart disease and women; Hypertension; Obesity; Obesity and aging; Obesity and children; Secondhand smoke; Smoking; Stress; Tobacco use by teenagers.

FOR FURTHER INFORMATION:

Baum, Seth. *The Total Guide to a Healthy Heart: Integrative Strategies for Preventing and Reversing Heart Disease.* New York: Kensington, 2000. Brings together the practices of both conventional and alternative approaches to reversing heart disease and maintaining heart health. Offers great insight into why the integrative approach to maintaining a healthy heart will be the medicine of the new millennium.

Kowalski, Robert E. *Eight Steps to a Healthy Heart.* New York: Warner Books, 1992. In addition to outlining how to avoid heart disease, this book advises patients with heart disease about how to get the most benefit from their therapy.

Larson, David G., ed. *Mayo Clinic Family Health Book.* 2d ed. New York: William Morrow, 1996. This large reference work was written for the layperson. The sections on the heart diseases are exemplary for clarity and thoroughness.

McGoon, M. *The Mayo Clinic's Heart Book.* New York: William Morrow, 1993. The most respected text for laypeople on heart disease. Covers all aspects of anatomy, physiology, diagnosis, treatment, and prevention.

Yannios, Thomas A. *The Heart Disease Breakthrough: What Even Your Doctor Doesn't Know About Preventing a Heart Attack.* New York: Wiley, 1999. Describes the smallest components of cholesterol, which can do more damage to the heart than the overall LDL levels that concern so many people.

✧ HEART DISEASE AND WOMEN

Type of issue: Prevention, women's health
Definition: Various heart conditions that impair function in female patients.

Coronary artery disease (CAD) is the major form of heart disease that afflicts women in the United States and Canada. CAD is the result of atherosclerosis, a disease that causes plaque to build up in the arterial walls, thereby reducing blood flow to the heart muscle. If complete blockage of the coronary arteries occurs, the result is a myocardial infarction, commonly known as a heart attack. Mitral valve prolapse, a form of heart disease that affects about one-third of all women, is a backflow of blood between the upper and lower chambers of the heart, causing a heart murmur. While this condition is potentially serious, it generally does not interfere with normal daily living. Arrhythmias (irregular heart rhythms) are abnormal electrical conduction patterns in the heart. These abnormal patterns can range from "skipped" beats (premature ventricular contractions, or PVCs) to an accelerated heart rate known as tachycardia.

The mortality rate from heart disease for American women decreased from 305 deaths per 100,000 in 1970 to a rate of 280 deaths per 100,000 in the 1990's. Nevertheless, every year more than 350,000 women die from heart disease in the United States, representing 34.4 percent of all female deaths. While heart disease is the leading cause of death for all women, it primarily affects women after the age of sixty-five (as contrasted to forty-five years and older in men). This twenty-year difference in mortality between men and women is often attributed to the protective effect of female hormones. There is also evidence to suggest that women experience a decreased risk for heart disease, in comparison to men, because of their tendency toward better social cohesion and support.

Diagnosis

The first symptom of heart disease in women is generally angina pectoris, a pain or pressure in the chest and upper body attributable to ischemia, a lack of blood flow to the heart. Angina usually occurs with moderate exertion, such as walking up a flight of stairs. All chest pain or pressure should be reported to a physician immediately and should never be ignored.

The exercise stress test is the first diagnostic tool used to detect CAD. The patient exercises while the physician monitors her electrocardiogram (ECG or EKG) for indications of ischemia. This noninvasive test, however, fails to identify about 20 percent of women with heart disease. If symptoms persist, the next procedure is a thallium exercise test, which involves injecting a radionucleotide into the patient while an X-ray motion picture is taken of the exercising heart. This procedure allows the physician to observe any areas of the heart where blood is not flowing. The definitive diagnostic procedure is heart catheterization, or coronary angioplasty. A tube is inserted through a vein in the leg and threaded to the heart. During a continuous-motion X ray, radioactive isotopes are injected that identify the arteries affected and the extent of coronary artery blockage.

The survival rates for heart disease are dependent on treatment. Women see their doctors more often than men do, but they are less likely to receive the correct diagnosis. This trend may be caused in part by the low rates of heart disease in women before the age of sixty. It may also be the result of physicians mistakenly attributing CAD symptoms to stress. Fortunately, myocardial infarctions that result in sudden cardiac death are less prevalent in women than in men. While women are not always treated for CAD adequately, they do seek medical care more often and are eventually treated, whereas men too often disregard initial symptoms, resulting in more severe outcomes.

Treatment and Survival

Atherosclerotic obstructions in the coronary arteries can be treated by coronary artery bypass graft (CABG) surgery or by balloon angioplasty. CABG involves the removal of veins from the legs and their surgical attachment from the main artery of the body to a point that bypasses the blockage in the coronary arteries. In balloon angioplasty, a catheter with a balloon attachment is inserted into the obstructed artery, and the balloon is expanded, thus opening a channel by compressing the plaque against the arterial walls. Both techniques are effective in improving blood flow to the heart.

Treatments for women after a myocardial infarction are not as effective as they are for men, with generally poorer outcomes such as increased mortality, poorer quality of life, depression, and emotional distress. This finding may be attributable to a higher average age among affected women, making them physically less able to withstand treatment. Another explanation may be that most treatments utilized today are primarily the result of research with male subjects.

Research

CAD afflicts women about twenty years later than men, with the incidence of myocardial infarctions four times higher in men than in women. The greater occurrence of CAD in middle-aged men has drawn most of the attention and research, resulting in a lack of studies that focus on the prevention and treatment of CAD in women. For example, women made up less than 20 percent of apparently healthy subjects and only 4 percent of subjects with preexisting CAD in several major studies that examined methods to lower serum cholesterol.

Compounding the research issue is the perception among women that breast cancer kills more women than CAD when, in reality, more than ten times the number of women die from CAD every year. Fortunately, several major studies on women are underway, such as the Nurses Health Study (with more than 120,000 subjects), the Women's Health Study, and the Women's Health Initiative. These studies are examining the preventive role that physical activity, nutrition, and low-dose aspirin intake may have against CAD in women. Additionally, oral contraceptives, the menopause, and estrogen replacement therapy are being examined to see how each factor affects the rate of CAD in women. The result of these studies on women will provide preventive measures, medications, and treatments for CAD that are appropriate for female populations.

—Chester J. Zelasko

See also Aging; Arteriosclerosis; Cardiac rehabilitation; Exercise; Exercise and the elderly; Heart attacks; Heart disease; Hypertension; Nutrition and women; Preventive medicine; Stress; Women's health issues.

For Further Information:

Baum, Seth. *The Total Guide to a Healthy Heart: Integrative Strategies for Preventing and Reversing Heart Disease.* New York: Kensington, 2000.

Diethrich, Edward, and Carol Cohan. *Women and Heart Disease.* New York: Ballantine Books, 1994.

Helfant, Richard. *The Women's Guide to Fighting Heart Disease: A Leading Cardiologist's Breakthrough Program.* New York: Berkley Publishing Group, 1994.

Rich-Edwards, Janet, JoAnn Manson, Charles Hennekens, and Julie Buring. "The Primary Prevention of Coronary Heart Disease in Women." *New England Journal of Medicine* 332, no. 26 (June 29, 1995): 1758-1766.

Yates, Beverly. *Heart Health for Black Women: A Natural Approach to Healing and Preventing Heart Disease.* New York: Marlowe, 2000.

✧ Heat exhaustion and heat stroke

Type of issue: Environmental health, public health

Definition: Heat-related illnesses in which the body temperature rises to dangerous levels and cannot be controlled through normal mechanisms, such as sweating.

Body temperature in human beings rarely leaves a very narrow range of 36.1 to 37.8 degrees Celsius (97 to 100 degrees Fahrenheit) regardless of how much heat the body produces or what the environmental temperature may be. If internal temperatures rise, brain function becomes slower as important proteins and enzymes lose their ability to operate effectively. Most adults go into convulsions when their temperature reaches 41 degrees Celsius (106 degrees Fahrenheit), and 43 degrees Celsius (110 degrees Fahrenheit) is usually fatal.

A special region of the brain known as the hypothalamus regulates body temperature. The hypothalamus detects blood temperature much like a thermostat detects room temperature. When the body becomes too warm, the hypothalamus activates heat-loss mechanisms. Most excess heat is lost through the skin by the radiation of heat and the evaporation of sweat. Blood vessels in the skin dilate to carry more blood. Heat from the warm blood is then lost to the cooler air. If the increase in blood flow to the skin is not enough, then sweat glands are stimulated to produce and secrete large amounts of sweat. The process, called perspiration, is an efficient means of ridding the body of excess heat as long as the humidity is not too high. At 60 percent humidity, however, evaporation of sweat from the skin stops. When the body cannot dissipate enough heat, heat exhaustion and heat stroke may occur.

HEAT EXHAUSTION AND HEAT STROKE

Heat exhaustion is the most prevalent heat-related illness. It commonly occurs in individuals who have exercised or worked in high temperatures for long periods of time. These people have usually not ingested adequate amounts of fluid. Over time, the patient loses fluid through sweating and respiration, which decreases the amount of fluid in the blood. Because the body is trying to reduce its temperature, blood has been shunted to the skin and away from vital internal organs. This reaction, in combination with a reduced blood volume, causes the patient to go into a mild shock. Common signs and symptoms of heat exhaustion include cool, moist skin that may appear either red or pale; headache; nausea; dizziness; and exhaustion. If heat exhaustion is not recognized and treated, it can lead to life-threatening heat stroke.

Heat stroke occurs when the body is unable to eradicate the excess heat as rapidly as it develops. Thus, body temperature begins to rise. Sweating stops because the water content of the blood decreases. The loss of evaporative cooling causes the body temperature to rise rapidly, soon reaching a level that can cause organ damage. In particular, the brain, heart, and kidneys may begin to fail until the patient experiences convulsions, coma, and even death. Therefore, heat stroke is a serious medical emergency which must be recognized and treated immediately. The signs and symptoms of heat stroke include high body temperature (41 degrees Celsius or 106 degrees Fahrenheit); loss of consciousness; hot, dry skin; rapid pulse; and quick, shallow breathing.

TREATMENT PROCEDURES

As with most illnesses, prevention is the best medicine for heat exhaustion and heat stroke. When exercising in hot weather, people should wear loose-fitting, lightweight clothing and drink plenty of fluids. When individuals are not prepared to avoid heat-related illness, however, rapid treatment may save their lives. When emergency medical personnel detect signs and symptoms of sudden heat-induced illness, they attempt to do three major things: cool the body, replace body fluids, and minimize shock.

For heat exhaustion, the initial treatment should be to place the patient in a cool place, such as a bathtub filled with cool (not cold) water. The conscious patient is given water or fruit drinks, sometimes containing salt, to replace body fluids. Occasionally, intravenous fluids must be given to return blood volume to normal in a more direct way. Hospitalization of the patient may be necessary to be sure that the body is able to regulate body heat appropriately. Almost all patients treated quickly and effectively will not advance to heat stroke. The activity that placed the patient in danger should be discontinued until one is sure all symptoms have disappeared and steps have been taken to prevent a future episode of heat exhaustion.

Heat stroke requires urgent medical attention, or the high body temperature will cause irreparable damage and often death. Reduction of body temperature must be done rapidly. With the patient in a cool environment, the clothing is removed and the skin sprinkled with water and cooled by fanning. Contrary to popular belief, rubbing alcohol should not be used, as it can cause closure of the skin's pores. Ice packs are often placed behind the neck and under the armpits and groin. At these sites, large blood vessels come close to the skin and are capable of carrying cool blood to the internal organs. Body fluid must be replaced quickly by intravenous administration because the patient is usually unable to drink as a result of convulsions or confusion and may even be unconscious. Once the body temperature has been brought back to normal, the patient is usually hospitalized and watched for complications. With early diagnosis and treatment, 80 to 90 percent of previously healthy people will survive.

—*Matthew Berria*

See also Exercise; Exercise and children; Exercise and the elderly; First aid; Resuscitation; Sunburns; Temperature regulation and aging.

FOR FURTHER INFORMATION:
American Red Cross First Aid: Responding to Emergencies. Rev. ed. St. Louis: Mosby Year Book, 1994.
Clayman, Charles B., ed. *The American Medical Association Encyclopedia of Medicine.* New York: Random House, 1989.
Hales, Dianne. *An Invitation to Health.* 9th ed. Belmont, Calif.: Wadsworth Thomson Learning, 2001.
Marieb, Elaine N. *Human Anatomy and Physiology.* 5th ed. Redwood City, Calif.: Benjamin/Cummings, 2000.

✧ Herpes

Type of issue: Epidemics, public health
Definition: A family of viruses that cause several diseases, including infectious mononucleosis, cold sores, genital herpes, and chickenpox.

Herpesviruses that affect humans include herpes simplex virus types 1 and 2, Epstein-Barr virus, varicella-zoster virus, and cytomegalovirus. Herpesviruses cause three types of infections: primary, latent, and recurrent. Most first-time, or primary, infections with herpesviruses cause few or no symptoms in the victim. Following the primary infection, herpesviruses have the unique ability to become latent, or hidden, in the body. Latent infections may persist for the life of the individual with no further symptoms, or the virus may reactivate and cause a recurrent infection.

Although herpesvirus infections are often mild in healthy persons, they can cause potentially fatal infections in immunocompromised patients. Persons in this group include infants, whose immune systems are not fully developed; immunodeficient persons, whose immune systems are lacking some important component; and immunosuppressed patients, such as cancer or transplant patients, whose immune systems are being suppressed by drugs or radiation. Herpesviruses have also been implicated in the causes of certain types of cancer.

HERPES SIMPLEX AND VARICELLA-ZOSTER

Herpes simplex viruses exist in two forms: type 1 (HSV1) and type 2 (HSV2). HSV1 and HSV2 infections cause the formation of painful or itchy vesicular (blisterlike) lesions, which ulcerate, crust over, and heal within a few weeks. The virus is transmitted by direct contact with infected lesions, and the virus enters the recipient through broken skin or mucous membranes.

HSV1 usually causes infections in the mouth, throat, eye, skin, and brain. Gingivostomatitis, the most common form of primary HSV1 infection, is seen mostly in small children and is characterized by ulcerative lesions inside the mouth. Cold sores, the most common recurrent disease caused by HSV1, are characterized by blisters on the outer portion of the lips. HSV1 can also cause infection in any area of the skin where trauma (burns, scrapes, eczema) gives the virus an opening to get in. HSV1 infection of the eye can lead to scarring and blindness, and HSV1 infection of the brain can lead to death.

Genital herpes, a disease transmitted by sexual contact, is most often caused by HSV2. The virus infects the penis in males and the cervix, vulva, vagina, or perineum in females. Two to seven days after infection, painful blisters appear in the genital area that ulcerate, crust over, and disappear in a few weeks. Fever, stress, sunlight, or local trauma may trigger the virus to come out of hiding and cause a recurrent infection, and about 88 percent of persons with an HSV2 genital infection will have recurrences at a frequency of up to five to eight times per year. A severe form of HSV2 infection, neonatal herpes, occurs when a mother suffering from genital herpes passes the virus to her baby as it travels through the birth canal during delivery. This type of infection is usually disseminated, its death rate is high, and its survivors suffer from severe neurological damage.

Varicella zoster virus (VZV) causes two diseases: Chickenpox (varicella) and shingles (zoster). Chickenpox is a highly contagious common childhood disease caused by a primary infection with VZV. The virus is transmitted during close personal contact with an infected patient via airborne droplets that enter the respiratory tract or direct contact with skin lesions. Once inside a person, the virus travels from the respiratory tract to the blood, and then to the skin. Ten to twenty-one days after infection, a typical rash appears on the skin and mucous membranes. On skin, the rash begins as red spots that develop into clear, fluid-filled vesicles that become cloudy, ulcerate, scab over, and fall off in a few days. Mucous membrane lesions in the mouth, eyelid, rectum, and vagina rupture easily and appear as ulcers. Fever, headache, tiredness, and itching may accompany the rash. Recovery from chickenpox confers lifelong immunity to reinfection but not latency. Chickenpox infection in adults is often more severe than in children, and adults run the risk of developing a fatal lung or brain infection.

Individuals with prior varicella infection may later develop shingles, which is caused by the reactivation of latent VZV. More than 65 percent of cases of shingles appear in adults older than forty-five years of age. The mechanism of reactivation is unknown, but recurrence is often associated with physical and emotional stress or a suppressed immune system. Shingles is usually localized to one area of the skin; it begins with pain in the nerves, and then a chickenpox-like rash appears on the skin over the nerves. The pain may be severe for one to four weeks, and recovery occurs in two to five weeks, with pain persisting longer in some elderly patients.

EPSTEIN-BARR VIRUS AND CYTOMEGALOVIRUS

Epstein-Barr virus (EBV) causes infectious mononucleosis, an infection of the lymphatic system. In infected persons, the virus is present in saliva and blood, and thus it is transmitted by intimate oral contact (for example, kissing), sharing food or drinks, or by blood transfusions. Primary infection early in life usually causes no symptoms of disease, whereas primary infection later in life usually causes symptoms of infectious mononucleosis. In countries where sanitation is poor, most people have been infected by the age of five, without symptoms. In contrast, in countries where sanitation is good, primary infection is delayed until adolescence or young adulthood, and thus more than half the people in this age group develop symptoms.

Once the infection begins, the virus grows in the throat and spreads to blood and lymph, invading white blood cells called B lymphocytes. The typical symptoms of infectious mononucleosis are extreme exhaustion, sore throat, fever, swollen lymph nodes, and sometimes an enlarged liver and spleen. The disease is self-limiting, and recovery takes place in four to eight weeks. The virus remains latent in the blood, lymphoid tissue, and throat and can continue to be transmitted to others even when no signs of active infection are present. EBV infection has also been associated with chronic fatigue syndrome and several types of cancer.

The widespread cytomegalovirus (CMV) is responsible for a broad spectrum of diseases. Primary infection by CMV early in life usually results in no symptoms, while primary infection as an adult yields mononucleosis-like symptoms. CMV also causes congenital cytomegalic inclusion disease and is a significant danger to bone marrow transplant patients. The virus is found in body secretions such as saliva, urine, semen, cervical secretions, and breast milk. Babies may acquire the virus from infected mothers during birth or through breast milk. Children in day care may acquire CMV from other children who orally excrete the virus, and parents may get it from their children. CMV may be acquired through sexual transmission and blood transfusions. Patients undergoing transplants, especially bone marrow transplants, are at higher risk for CMV infection, since the virus may be present in the transplanted organs. The mononucleosis-like disease caused by CMV has the same symptoms as EBV-induced mononucleosis except the sore throat, swollen lymph nodes, and enlarged spleen. Congenital cytomegalic inclusion disease causes severe neurological damage, mental retardation, and death in infants; it is a result of primary CMV infection of the mother during pregnancy.

TREATING HERPES SIMPLEX AND VARICELLA-ZOSTER

The major treatment procedure for most mild HSV infections is supportive care. These measures, such as bed rest and medication to relieve itching or pain, treat the symptoms but not the infection. For most infections, the symptoms eventually go away by themselves. For more severe HSV infections, several antiviral drugs have been used. Idoxuridine and trifluridine have been used to treat eye infections. Vidarabine and acyclovir are used to treat encephalitis and disseminated disease; both reduce the severity of the infection but do not reverse any neurological damage or prevent recurrent infections. Acyclovir has also been useful in reducing the duration of primary genital herpes, but not recurrent infection. The use of oral acyclovir to suppress recurrent infection may cause more severe and more frequent infections once the therapy has stopped.

Chickenpox takes care of itself and disappears after a few weeks; therefore, the only treatment needed is supportive care for the patient during that time. Often, drying lotions such as calamine help relieve the itching. It is important to cut the fingernails of young children so that they cannot scratch hard enough to break through the skin and leave themselves susceptible to secondary bacterial infection.

It is extremely important not to give a child aspirin for the fever, because of the association between the use of aspirin during chickenpox and the development of Reye's syndrome. In this syndrome, the patient persistently vomits and exhibits signs of brain dysfunction a few days after the initial infection has receded. Coma and death can follow if the syndrome is not treated. A child with chickenpox may be given acetaminophen if necessary.

Varicella is treated mostly with medication to control the pain. Steroids given early in the infection help reduce the severity of the infection, and acyclovir increases the rate of recovery. Antiviral drugs such as acyclovir, interferon, and vidarabine have been used in the treatment of immunocompromised patients with chickenpox to help reduce the potential severe complications of the disease. Since 1981, varicella-zoster immunoglobin (VZIG) has been available for the prevention and treatment of chickenpox in these patients. VZIG provides a short time of immunity, can lessen symptoms, and is recommended for immunocompromised children exposed to chickenpox, but it has no value once chickenpox has started. A VZV vaccine has been shown to provide protection from infection in children.

TREATING EPSTEIN-BARR VIRUS AND CYTOMEGALOVIRUS

Infectious mononucleosis is a self-limiting disease, which means that it will eventually run its course and go away. Therefore, treatment involves mostly supportive care, such as bed rest and aspirin or acetaminophen for the fever and sore throat. It is also recommended that mononucleosis patients avoid contact sports, to prevent possible rupture of an enlarged spleen. In some severe cases, steroids are administered, and antiviral drugs are in the process of being tested to determine whether they are of any therapeutic value. The best way to prevent an EBV infection is to avoid intimate contact with an infected individual. Unfortunately, many persons shed the virus in their saliva without exhibiting any symptoms.

Mild cases of CMV need no treatment except supportive measures. Antiviral drugs such as interferon, vidarabine, idoxuridine, and cytosine arabinoside as well as CMV immune globin have all been tested for their benefit in severe cases of CMV infections, but none has been successful. The drug ganciclovir has been shown to have some therapeutic value. A CMV vaccine has been developed, but further work is needed. Until better measures are available, it is important to try to avoid infection in immunocompromised patients, especially transplant recipients. The screening of organ donors for the presence of CMV may be helpful in accomplishing this goal. All pregnant women should be tested for CMV antibodies to determine whether they have already been infected; if not, they should avoid contact with small children who might carry CMV.

A PUBLIC HEALTH THREAT

Between 20 and 40 percent of the people in the United States suffer from cold sores, and more than twenty million persons suffer from genital herpes. In addition, HSV1 infection of the eye is the most common cause of corneal blindness in the United States, and HSV2 infection is associated with an increased risk of cervical cancer, which strikes some fifteen thousand women each year. Two hundred babies in the United States die each year, and two hundred more suffer physical or mental impairment caused by HSV infection.

Chickenpox is the second most reported disease in the United States, with more than two hundred thousand cases per year. This number is probably too low, since many cases go unreported. About 100 deaths per year are attributed to chickenpox.

EBV infection is worldwide, and EBV antibodies can be found in more than 90 percent of most adult populations. EBV infection has been shown to be an important factor in the development of Burkitt's lymphoma (a cancer of the jaw) in Africa and nasopharyngeal carcinoma (a fatal cancer of the nose) in China. EBV has also been linked to chronic fatigue syndrome, but the relationship is not conclusive.

CMV infection is worldwide, with 40 to 100 percent of a population possessing antibodies to CMV. Almost all kidney transplant recipients and half of bone marrow recipients get CMV infection. Congenital CMV infection is the cause of severe neurological damage in more than five thousand children born each year in the United States.

—Vicki J. Isola

See also Cervical, ovarian, and uterine cancers; Children's health issues; Chronic fatigue syndrome; Epidemics; Reye's syndrome; Sexually transmitted diseases (STDs).

FOR FURTHER INFORMATION:
Biddle, Wayne. *Field Guide to Germs.* New York: Henry Holt, 1995. This comprehensive book is easily accessible to the nonspecialist and includes a discussion of nearly every virus, bacterium, and fungus known to cause human and nonhuman animal disease. The history of the microbe and the treatment of diseases are included.
Ebel, Charles. *Managing Herpes: How to Live and Love with a Chronic STD.* Research Triangle Park, N.C.: American Social Health, 1998. With 20 percent of the American population now carrying the virus that causes genital herpes, the revised edition of this book, first published in 1994 by a nonprofit organization dedicated to stopping sexually transmitted diseases, is timely and welcome.
Regush, Nicholas. *The Virus Within: A Coming Epidemic.* New York: Dutton, 2000. A virus called HHV-6 (a form of the human herpes virus) is at the heart of a controversy brewing in the scientific community. Scientists are uncovering evidence that it may play a role in serious illnesses such as AIDS and multiple sclerosis. Regush makes a strong case for further research.
Stoff, Jesse A., and Charles Pellegrino. *Chronic Fatigue Syndrome.* Rev. ed. New York: HarperPerennial, 1992. Discusses EBV and its relationship to chronic fatigue syndrome.
Zinsser, Hans. *Zinsser Microbiology.* 20th ed. Edited by Wolfgang K. Joklik et al. Norwalk, Conn.: Appleton and Lange, 1992. The information presented in this textbook is thorough, logical, and supplemented by inter-

esting diagrams, photographs, and charts. Chapter 66, "Herpesviruses," gives a complete description of infections with HSV, VZV, EBV, and CMV.

✧ HIPPOCRATIC OATH

Type of issue: Ethics
Definition: A document, written in the fifth century B.C.E., to offer guidelines for the emerging medical profession, which continues to be the subject of debate in modern practice because of the ethical issues that it addresses.

Western civilization has long held the writings of the fifth century B.C.E. Greek physician Hippocrates, and in particular the Hippocratic oath, as a model of ethical values to be followed in the medical profession. As the nature of Western civilization itself has changed over the centuries, interpretations of the ethical values behind the Hippocratic oath have also changed. The circumstances of modern medical practice and ethical values, however, have ironically made certain elements of the classical Hippocratic tradition even more relevant than they may have appeared in previous eras.

The first part of the oath covers the physician's lifelong commitment to his or her teachers. This commitment extends not only to the symbolic bonds of respect but also to obligation to share one's medical practice and even to provide financial assistance to one's teachers, if requested. Additionally, the physician is committed to train, free of charge, the families of his or her teachers in the art of medicine.

The second part of the Hippocratic oath contains the more general pledges that would contribute to its value as an ethical guide for the medical profession. The physician is bound, in a very general way, to help the sick according to his or her ability and judgment in a manner that can never be interpreted as involving injury or wrongdoing. The physician is bound both to confidentiality concerning direct experiences in the patient-doctor relationship and to extreme discretion to avoid the circulation of professional knowledge that is not appropriate for publication abroad.

In addition to these general precepts, all of which have an ethical timelessness that would survive the centuries, there were two points in the oath that refer to specific issues that cannot be separated from the modern debate over medical ethics. Addressing the questions of euthanasia ("mercy killing") and abortion, Hippocrates stated: "I will give no deadly drug to any, though it be asked of me, nor will I counsel such, and especially I will not aid a woman to procure abortion."

MODERN APPLICATIONS OF THE HIPPOCRATIC OATH

Although neither the original nor edited versions of the Hippocratic oath are applied today as a condition for becoming a doctor, the medical profession in the United States has definitely formalized publication of what it considers to be a necessary code of medical ethics. Evolving versions of this "Code of Medical Ethics" date from the original (1847) text of the American Medical Association (AMA) as revised by specific decisions in 1903, 1912, and 1947.

When the AMA adopted a statement under the title "Guide to Responsible Professional Behavior" in 1980, it assigned to a formal body within its organization, the Council on Ethical and Judicial Affairs, the task of publishing, on a yearly basis, updated paragraphs that reflect ethical guidelines for the profession as a whole. These evolving guidelines are organized under such subheadings as "Social Policy Issues," "Interprofessional Relations," "Hospital Relations," "Confidentiality," and "Fees and Charges."

Thus, in the absence of a specific professional oath with detailed provisions, modern physicians are bound to respect the ethical guidelines provided to them by their professional association. Failure to respect these guidelines is tantamount to breaking one's binding ethical obligations and can lead to expulsion from the medical profession.

Several major changes, both in levels of medical technology and in social attitudes toward issues relating to medical practice, have played key roles in several spheres of an ongoing debate concerning medical ethics. In two cases, those of abortion and euthanasia, debate has focused on the ethics of deciding to end life; in the third, referred to generally as genetic engineering, the central question involves both the living and those yet to be born. In all these spheres, the legal and ethical debates have revolved around potential conflicts between physicians and patients but also in the context of wider social values.

Movement from the historical domain of idealized codes or oaths to the more practical and contemporary realm of changing societal reactions to what constitutes injury or breach of professional ethics in several areas of modern medicine is facilitated by reference to landmark legal decisions that have given a modern and quite different meaning to Hippocratic concepts.

LIFE-SUSTAINING TECHNOLOGY

Two issues, one involving the ethics of sustaining life by means of advanced medical technology and the other involving the "engineering" of lives according to genetic predictions, fall under the provisions of the Hippocratic oath. As one approaches more contemporary statements of professional obligations of medical doctors, such as the "Principles of Medical Ethics" (1957) of the American Medical Association, one finds that, as certain areas of specificity in classical Hippocratic or Christian medical ethics (the illegality of abortions or the administration of deadly potions) tend to decline in visibility, another area begins to come to the forefront; namely, striving continually to improve medical knowledge and skills to be made available to patients and colleagues.

This more modern concern for the application of advancements in medical knowledge, especially in the technology of medical lifesaving therapy, has introduced a new focus for ethical debate: not "lifesaving" but "life-sustaining" techniques, particularly in cases judged to be otherwise terminal or hopeless. The question of a doctor's responsibility to use every means within his or her reach to sustain life, even when there is no hope of a meaningful future for the patient, also reflects a dilemma regarding Hippocratic injunctions. This debate is more important now than in any earlier era because advanced medical technology has made it possible either to extend the lives of aged patients who would die without life-sustaining machines or—in the case of younger persons afflicted by brain damage, for example—to sustain life although the patient remains in a comatose state.

A prototype in the latter case was a 1976 Supreme Court decision that allowed the parents of New Jersey car accident victim Karen Quinlan to instruct her physician to remove life support systems so that their comatose daughter would die. At issue in this complicated case, which also rested on legal discussions of the constitutional right of privacy, was the question of who should decide that inevitable natural death is preferable to prolongation of life by externally administered means. When the Court took this decision away from an appointed court guardian and gave it to those closest to the patient, the question became whose privacy was being protected. To whom does the physician's oath to avoid doing injury actually apply?

GENETIC ENGINEERING

A final area of contemporary debate over medical ethics illustrates how far conceptions of ultimate responsibility for the protection of life have gone beyond frames of reference that might have been familiar not only in Hippocrates' time but also as recently as the generation of doctors trained before the 1980's. Impressive advances in the research field of human genetics by the mid-1980's began to make it possible to predict, through analysis of deoxyribonucleic acid (DNA) structures, the likelihood that certain genetic traits (specifically debilitating chronic diseases) might be transmitted to the offspring of couples under study.

Inherent in the rising debate over the ethics of such studies, which range from the prediction of reproductive combinations (genetic counseling) through actual attempts to detach and splice DNA chains (genetic engineering), was the delicate question of who, if anyone, should hold the responsibility of determining if individuals have ultimate control over their genes. In the most extreme hypothetical argument, a notion of scientific exclusion of certain gene combinations, or planning of desirable gene pools in future generations, began to appear in the 1980's and 1990's. These notions represent potential problems for medical ethics that, because of exponential changes in technological possibilities, surpass the entire realm of Hippocratic principles.

—*Byron D. Cannon*

See also Abortion; Death and dying; Ethics; Euthanasia; Genetic engineering; Law and medicine; Malpractice; Terminal illnesses.

FOR FURTHER INFORMATION:

Casarett, David J., Frona Daskal, and John Lantos. "Experts in Ethics? The Authority of the Clinical Ethicist." *The Hastings Center Report* 28, no. 6 (November/December, 1998): 6-11. This article examines the work of Jurgen Habermas, which provides a basis for a model of clinical ethics consultation in which consensus, grounded in moral theory, assumes a central theoretical role.

Fletcher, John C., et al., eds. *Introduction to Clinical Ethics.* 2d ed. Frederick, Md.: University, 1997. This group of essays by contributing authors addresses the topic of ethics in contemporary medicine. Includes a bibliography.

Gorovitz, Samuel. *Doctors' Dilemmas.* New York: Macmillan, 1982. This book deals with the rising complexity of modern medical practice and moral decisions that increasingly affect doctors' decisions concerning treatment. Also explores issues of public policy making with respect to patient-doctor relations.

Harron, Frank, John Burnside, and Tom Beauchamp. *Biomedical-Ethical Issues.* New Haven, Conn.: Yale University Press, 1983. A collection of key contemporary documents, including court decisions, state and federal laws, and policy statements by a number of professional associations regarding the most-debated ethical issues in medicine.

Jonsen, Albert R., Mark Siegler, and William J. Winslade. *Clinical Ethics: A Practical Approach to Ethical Decisions in Clinical Medicine.* 4th ed. New York: McGraw-Hill, 1998. Discusses the whole range of medical ethics, including legal issues, confidentiality, care of the dying patient, and euthanasia and assisted suicide.

✧ HMOs

Type of issue: Economic issues, social trends

Definition: A company that provides health insurance and services to group and individual clients for an established, prepaid monthly premium and that generally attempts to provide care at a lower cost than traditional fee-for-service insurance programs by transferring financial risk to physicians through capitation and other incentives.

A health maintenance organization (HMO) in a free market economy functions in a dual role as both a health insurance company and a provider of health services, roles that were previously separated within the U.S. health care system. HMOs—also known as competitive medical plans, managed care plans, or alternative delivery systems—are generally organized by an employer, physician group, union, consumer group, insurance company, or for-profit health care agency. They were originally formed from one, or a mixture, of the following models: point of service, staff, group, and independent practice association.

The role of an HMO as an insurer is to seek group contracts with employers and individual clients and to negotiate premiums to be prepaid in exchange for covering preagreed benefits. Its role in service delivery is to affiliate with or hire directly physicians to provide the expected volume of care that is required for all subscribers under contract. An HMO owns or contracts with one or more health centers for ambulatory care and with hospitals for inpatient care. Within its private health center or in contracts with free-standing providers, an HMO will furnish services from other health care providers such as physical and occupational therapy, pharmacy, and mental health care, which are rapidly increasing in their level of responsibility.

HMOs are attractive to employers because the annual medical bill for the average subscriber-patient consistently has proved to be approximately 30 percent less than that of conventional insurers. One advantage of HMO membership is that all medical expenses, from routine and emergency care to hospitalization, are covered within a single, fixed monthly premium. In addition, presenting an HMO membership card at time of services with a small copayment means no forms to fill out, no deductibles to pay, and no bills to submit. Disadvantages include that new subscribers often cannot keep a trusted physician they have had for years, providers become extremely busy when they are assigned hundreds of patients in exchange for a fixed fee, and subscribers often must accept fewer choices in treatment options.

THE PROCESS OF MANAGED CARE

The headquarters of an HMO competitively markets its services to employer groups and individuals and administers the revenue and payments. An HMO generally contracts or directly hires a limited number of physicians in addition to building, staffing, and equipping the necessary number of health centers and hospitals. Its marketing claim is to provide good quality care within the employer's group premium, without seeking further supplements from the employer. Because an HMO and its providers are at personal financial risk, the organization directly imposes financial discipline upon its physicians, hospitals, and other health care providers. The HMO retains a percentage of the premiums paid from employers for its administrative and facility costs and pays a monthly "capitated rate" per client to the providers.

Managed care procedures generally involve the HMO establishing a network of physicians with superior reputations in each region, with these physicians agreeing to bill the carriers according to limited reimbursement rules. Each client is assigned to a "primary care gatekeeper" who is expected to provide most care in his or her private office for limited fees. When a referral to a specialist, laboratory, or hospital is necessary, authorization is required from the headquarters of the managed care organization. Hospitals contract with these organizations to limit their charges and follow established rules about economical care and prompt discharge. The managed care organization reviews utilization by physicians and hospitals, attempts to correct wasteful practices, and subsequently drops health care providers with expensive and/or poor practice styles.

In contrast to more traditional HMOs, point-of-service plans have more recently emerged. These plans enable clients to have freedom of choice with respect to providers and some treatment options but requires them personally to pay the balance for their chosen higher-priced services. If the patient goes to physicians, hospitals, and other providers within the network and follows rules about utilization and authorization, the out-of-pocket financial costs are minimal. The patient retains the option to go to an out-of-plan provider, pay the bill in full, and then be reimbursed for the limited amount established in the individual plan. The employer's group contract with the managed care organization provides for limited and predictable premiums. The considerable costs of out-of-plan services thus are shifted from the group contract to the individual patient.

THE FUTURE OF HMOS

Managed care plans will continue to monitor closely the treatment patterns of physicians and encourage them to prescribe cheaper medications, to develop standards that physicians are expected to follow in treatment of various diseases, and to hold utilization review panels that review patient records and decide which treatments a patient's health plan will cover and which it will not. Because of the numerous consumer complaints that arose from actions resulting from the decisions of case managers, who often do not have medical training, nineteen states had passed comprehensive managed care laws by 1997. In that year alone, states passed a record 182 laws related to managed care, up from 100 in 1996. Legislation has and undoubtedly will continue to focus on issues such as adopting measures to ban physician gag clauses, to establish consumer grievance procedures, to require disclosure of financial incentives for physicians to withhold care, to hold external reviews of internal decisions to deny care, and to ensure the ability to sue an HMO for malpractice.

The largest looming question regarding the future of HMOs is whether physicians and other health care workers, as well as client subscribers, will continue to enroll in and thus support the system. Managed care necessarily adds substantial administrative overhead, with the ongoing question of whether the final result is greater efficiency for the entire system or simply for subscribing employers. Another controversial topic of discussion involves the responsibility of an HMO to provide disability insurance, which becomes necessary when a client incurs loss of income resulting from sickness or an accident that is not covered by workers' compensation.

—Daniel G. Graetzer

See also Ethics; Health care and aging; Health insurance; Law and medicine; Malpractice.

FOR FURTHER INFORMATION:

Borowsky, Steven J., Margaret K. Davis, Christine Goertz, and Nicole Lurie. "Are All Health Plans Created Equal? The Physician's View." *Journal of the American Medical Association* 278, no. 11 (1997): 917-921. This article contains physician ratings of health plan practices with respect to what promoted or impeded delivery of quality care.

Brink, Susan, and Nancy Shute. "Are HMOs the Right Prescription?" *U.S. News and World Report* 123, no. 4 (October 13, 1997): 60-65. Covered in this well-researched article is the growing dissatisfaction of subscribers with the quality of health care received with a rating of the best HMOs in the United States.

Freeborn, D. K., and C. R. Pope. *The Promise and Performance of Managed Care: The Prepaid Practice Model.* Rev. ed. Baltimore: The Johns Hopkins University Press, 1999. This excellent text highlights the evolution of several common promises of HMOs that employ the prepaid practice model and evaluates their performance based on relevant criteria.

Lairson, D. R., et al. "Managed Care and Community-Oriented Care: Conflict or Complement?" *Journal of Health Care for the Poor and Underserved* 8, no. 1 (1997): 36-55. This informative article evaluates models for community health planning and health care reform designed for the medically indigent, including programs that receive support by the U.S. government and programs which do not.

Zelman, W. A. *The Changing Health Care Market Place.* San Francisco: Jossey-Bass, 1996. An excellent evaluation of past trends in HMOs and predictions of what the future might hold.

✧ Holistic medicine

Type of issue: Mental health, social trends
Definition: The practice of medicine to maintain both physical and psychological health as a natural deterrent to disease and as a way of realizing one's highest potential.

Although the phenomenon of holistic medicine gained increased attention in the latter half of the twentieth century, most of the associated principles have appeared in various forms and in various cultures over the centuries.

Ironically, it may have been the progress of medical science generally and the widespread use by doctors of new drugs to treat disease that sparked what some would call holistic medicine's call for a return to basics. For example, some proponents of holism oppose automatic reliance on surgical methods of treating some ailments for not recognizing either their cause or more beneficial modes of treatment. In addition, holists oppose a reliance on drugs not only because they hold certain maladies to be curable (or indeed totally avoidable) without them but also because of possible negative side effects.

PRINCIPLES AND APPROACHES

A number of sophisticated principles could fall under the presumed "basics" of the holistic approach to health. Primary among them is a conviction that—short of obvious conditions involving attacks by viruses and bacteria or chronic debilitation of certain organs of the body—increased awareness of the nature of bodily functions can help maintain a healthy level of balance within the total organism. Essential to the principle of balance is recognition of the importance of the mind in influencing one's reactions, both psychological and physical, to circumstances in the surrounding environment.

Some holists adhere to the Abraham Maslow school of psychology, which places strong emphasis on questions of drive toward "need fulfillment" in both the physical and psychological domains. Certain bodily states can easily be linked to biologically stimulated drives, including hunger and sexuality. Less apparent psychological drives, however, may also trigger physical reactions. Imbalances in fulfilling the natural drives for love or success are held responsible for many forms of physical disorder that could be averted, such as anorexia nervosa, ulcers, and stress.

Several approaches to holistic medicine consider the end goal of good physical health to be not only the avoidance of disease but also the realization of a positive, life-enhancing experience. In some cases, the inspiration for such theories comes from long traditions in Asian philosophies and religions that assume close links between the psychic and the physical realms of life. An assumption that may or may not be shared between such philosophies and holists is that a "true" state of health leads to superior levels of awareness in both spheres.

Physicians interested in holistic medicine need not, however, be tied solely to disease-specific or "consciousness-heightening" aspects of what can be a very general field. Some specialists in geriatrics, for example, adopt holistic approaches to counseling the elderly about natural stages of aging, preparing them to accept, with a minimum of anxiety, the gradual decline that accompanies the end of life. Growing emphasis on hospice care, for the terminally ill or aged, as opposed to hospitalization, is connected with this aspect of holistic medicine.

Although individual physicians may espouse holistic approaches, many persons without formal medical training choose to practice it themselves to maintain their bodies and minds in the healthiest state possible. Such practices may be individual and personal, ranging from exercise and dietary habits to meditation. They may also involve group associations supported by the participation of trained physicians or laypersons. It has become possible to find method-specific holistic centers specializing in a range of techniques. These range from, for example, very general holistic health and nutrition institutes to highly specialized centers that strive to treat those suffering from chronic pain through localized electrical nerve stimulation.

The Future of Holistic Medicine

Two aspects of holistic approaches to health and daily life in the postindustrial world are likely to increase in importance in coming generations: concern over improving dietary habits and exercise patterns. The discovery of the possible long-term harm that can come from poorly balanced diets (particularly those with a high fat content or excessive chemical additives) has made such specialized practices of holists as vegetarianism and fasting more familiar and at least partly attractive to the wider public. Likewise, the holistic emphasis on regular physical exercise for people of all ages has increasingly become part of many general practitioners' standard advice to their patients.

—*Byron D. Cannon*

See also Acupuncture; Aging; Alternative medicine; Biofeedback; Death and dying; Environmental diseases; Exercise; Exercise and children; Exercise and the elderly; Homeopathy; Hospice; Hypnosis; Meditation; Preventive medicine; Stress; Terminal illnesses; Yoga.

For Further Information:
Nordenfelt, Lennart. *On the Nature of Health.* 2d rev. and enlarged ed. Boston: Kluwer, 1995. Deals with the relationship between good health and the welfare of individuals and society as they interact.

Pelletier, Kenneth R. *Holistic Medicine.* New York: Delacorte Press, 1979. A general text that seeks to strengthen the public image of holistic medicine, both for the prevention and for the treatment of disease, while discounting some popular myths.

Salmon, J. Warren, ed. *Alternative Medicines.* New York: Tavistock, 1984. Offers comparative views of Western and Chinese approaches to holistic medicine but also includes other, less widely recognized alternatives, ranging from chiropractic to psychic healing.

Woodham, Anne, and David Peters. *The Encyclopedia of Healing Therapies.* New York: Dorling Kindersley, 1997. This book explains holistic and complementary medicine and offers a guide to well-being. Also contains information on finding practitioners, a directory of associations, a glossary, and a bibliography.

✧ Homeopathy

Type of issue: Medical procedures, social trends, treatment
Definition: A system of medicine based on the principle that an ill patient can be provided effective and nontoxic treatment through the use of weak or very small doses of a substance that would cause similar symptoms in a healthy individual.

Homeopathy is a therapeutic method that consists of prescribing for a patient weak or infinitesimal doses of a substance which, when administered to a healthy person, causes symptoms similar to those exhibited by the ill patient. Homeopathic remedies stimulate the defense mechanisms of the body, causing them to work more effectively and making them capable of curing the individual. While controversial and not accepted by most physicians, homeopathy is not intended to substitute for conventional medicine. Rather, it is a system of therapeutics which is meant to enlarge and broaden the physician's outlook, and in some cases, it might bring about a cure not possible with the usual drugs.

The Principles of Homeopathy

The first and fundamental principle of homeopathy is the selection and use of the similar remedy, based on the patient's symptoms and characteristics and the drug's toxicology and provings. A second principle is the use of remedies in extremely small quantities. The most successful remedy for any given occasion will be the one whose symptomatology presents the clearest and closest resemblance to the symptom-complex of the sick person in question. This concept is formally presented as the Law of Similars, which expresses the similarity between the toxicological action of a substance and its therapeutic action; in other words, the same things that cause the disease can cure it. For example, the effects of peeling an onion are very similar to the symptoms of acute coryza (the common cold). The remedy prepared from *Allium cepa* (red onion) is used to treat the type of cold in which the symptoms resemble those caused by peeling onions. In the same way, the herb white hellebore, which toxicologically produces cholera-like diarrhea, is used to treat cholera.

The homeopathic principle is being applied whenever a sick person is treated using a method or drug that can cause similar symptoms in healthy persons. For example, conventional medicine uses radiation therapy, which causes cancer, to treat this disease. Orthodox medicine, however, does not follow other fundamental principles of homeopathy, such as the use of infinitesimal doses.

Homeopathy stimulates the defense mechanism to make it work more effectively and works on the concept of healing instead of simply treating a disease, combating illness, or suppressing symptoms. In the United States, both the Food and Drug Administration (FDA) and traditional homeopaths have been concerned about the use of homeopathic remedies to treat serious problems, such as cancer, and their use by unlicensed practitioners. In some cases, the ability to prescribe homeopathic remedies has been restricted to osteopaths, naturopaths, and medical doctors. In some cases, homeopathy does not work; the reason is unknown.

Diagnostic and Treatment Techniques

The first step in treating an illness using homeopathy is taking the case history or symptom picture (the detailed account of what is wrong with the patient as a whole). The symptoms are divided in three categories: general, mental/emotional, and physical. The homeopath then consults the *Materia Medica* (the encyclopedia of drug effects) and/or the *Repertory* (an index of symptoms from the *Materia Medica* listed in alphabetical order, used as a cross-referencing system between symptoms and remedies) to decide on the remedy to be used. The professional homeopath works with a number of *Materia Medica* texts compiled by different homeopaths. The classical homeopath will give only one remedy at a time in order to gauge its effect more efficiently.

Homeopathic remedies are always nontoxic because of the small concentrations used. They come from the plant, mineral, and animal kingdoms. Plants are the source of more than half of the remedies. They are harvested in their natural state according to strict norms by qualified specialists and are used fresh after thorough botanical inspection. Mineral remedies include natural salts and metals, always in their purest state. Animal remedies may contain venoms, poisonous insects, hormones, or physiological secretions such as musk or squid ink.

The starting remedy is made from a mixture of the substance itself, which has been steeped in alcohol for a period of time and then strained. This starting liquid is called a tincture or mother tincture. In the decimal scale, a mixture of one-tenth tincture and nine-tenths alcohol is shaken vigorously, a process known as succussion; this first dilution is called a 1X. (The number in the remedy reveals the number of times that it has been diluted and succussed; thus, 6X means diluted and succussed six times.) In the centesimal scale, the remedy is diluted using one part tincture in a hundred, and the letter C is used after the number. The number indicates the degree of the dilution, while the letter indicates the technique of preparation (decimal or centesimal). Insoluble substances are diluted by grinding them in a mortar with lactose to the desired dilution. The greater the dilution of a remedy, the greater its potency, the longer it acts, the deeper it heals, and the fewer doses are needed.

Homeopathic remedies are most commonly available in tablet form, combined with sugar from cow's milk. The tablets can be soft (so that they dissolve easily under the tongue and are easy to crush) or hard (so that they must be chewed and held in the mouth for a few seconds before being swallowed), or they can be prepared as globules (tiny round pills). The liquid remedies are dissolved in alcohol. Also available are powders that are wrapped individually in small squares of paper, wafers, suppositories, and liniments. Homeopathic tablets will keep their strength for years without deteriorating, but they must be stored in a cool, dark, and dry place with their bottle tops screwed on tightly, away from strong-smelling substances.

The prescribed quantities are the same for babies, children, adults, and older people. The size of a dose is immaterial; it is how often it is taken that counts. The strength (potency) that is needed changes with the circumstances. The greater the similarity between the symptoms and the remedy, the greater the potency to be used (that is, the more dilute the remedy).

RISKS AND BENEFITS

As with all treatments, there are some dangers associated with homeopathic cures, such as unintentional provings. These take place when, after an initial improvement, the symptoms characteristic of the remedy appear, creating a worse situation for the patient. Sometimes, this reaction takes place because the individual has been taking the remedy for too long, and it can be stopped by discontinuing the remedy or by using an antidote. In other cases, there is a confused symptom picture, the effect being that the remedy is working in a limited way or curing a restricted number of symptoms.

Homeopathy is important in the treatment of bacterial infections (where resistance to antibiotics can develop) and viral conditions. Homeopathic remedies stimulate the person's resistance to infection without the side effects of antibiotics, and they help the body without suppressing the organism's self-protective responses. The remedies used are safer than regular medicines because they exhibit minimal side effects and counterreactions between medicines can be prevented.

Homeopathic remedies are exempt from federal review in the United States. In 1938, any drug listed in the *Homeopathic Pharmacopoeia of the United States* was accepted by the FDA. Consequently, prescribed homeopathics do not have to undergo the rigorous safety and effectiveness testing the regulating agency requires of drugs used in orthodox medicine. Nonprescription homeopathics are also exempt and can be purchased in pharmacies, greengroceries, and health food stores throughout the country. The FDA requires that, as with any over-the-counter drug, a remedy can be sold only for a self-limiting condition (such as headaches, menstrual cramps, or insomnia) and that the indications be printed on the label. The ingredients and their dilution must also be listed. Nonhomeopathic active ingredients cannot be included in the preparation.

The Status of Homeopathy

The 1860's through the 1880's saw the heyday of homeopathy in the United States, with the institution of training programs, hospitals, and asylums and the training of thousands of homeopaths in the country. By the 1990's, however, only five hundred to one thousand medical doctors used homeopathics in their practices, though the number of homeopaths and osteopaths prescribing them had probably increased. Although the American Medical Association (AMA) has no official statement on homeopathy, it is no longer part of the medical school curriculum.

Homeopathy has exhibited a renaissance, and it is popular throughout the world, especially in France. Perhaps the reasons for this revived popularity include both skepticism surrounding conventional medicine and a need for alternatives in the face of challenging health problems: Homeopathy offers a safe alternative as it seeks to improve the general level of health of the whole person, emotionally as well as physically. It must not be forgotten, however, that this brand of medicine has a long way to go before its curative powers are proven.

—Maria Pacheco

See also Alternative medicine; Holistic medicine; Immunizations for children; Immunizations for the elderly; Medications and the elderly; Stress.

For Further Information:
Aubin, Michel, and Philippe Picard. *Homœopathy: A Different Way of Treating Common Ailments.* Translated by Pat Campbell and Robin Campbell. Bath, England: Ashgrove Press, 1989. An easy-to-read book which includes a

critical analysis of orthodox medicine from the perspective of an ortho-dox doctor turned homeopath, a description of homeopathy, and a section on self-treatment with homeopathy.

Castro, Miranda. *The Complete Homeopathy Handbook: A Guide to Everyday Health Care*. New York: St. Martin's Press, 1991. Examines the principles underlying the theory of homeopathy, as well as how to prescribe and learn the best use of homeopathic medicines that are available over the counter. Written for the reader who has had some experience with homeopathy. Includes a *Materia Medica* and *Repertory* for internal and external remedies, as well as some sample cases.

_____. *Homeopathic Guide to Stress*. New York: St. Martin's Griffin, 1997. An introduction to homeopathy, with a focus on stress. Suggests several homeopathic treatments for more than four dozen specific emotional states, with instructions on how to choose the most appropriate solutions.

McCabe, Vinton. *Practical Homeopathy: A Beginner's Guide*. New York: St. Martin's Press, 2000. McCabe, president of the Connecticut Homeo-pathic Association and a member of the faculty and board of the Hudson Valley School of Classical Homeopathy, joins philosophy and pharmacy in a practical way in this resource. Includes homeopathic remedies.

Ullman, Dana. *Discovering Homeopathy: Medicine for the Twenty-first Century*. Rev. ed. Berkeley, Calif.: North Atlantic Books, 1991. Includes sections on the history and research methods of homeopathy and an excellent section on sources (books, computer programs, tapes) and general infor-mation on homeopathy. Lists pharmacies, organizations, schools, and training programs in the United States. Information on how to choose a practitioner and about the use of homeopathy in specific areas is pre-sented.

✦ HORMONE REPLACEMENT THERAPY

Type of issue: Medical procedures, treatment, women's health
Definition: The use of oral or injectable forms of hormones to replace inadequate gland secretions.

Hormones are critical substances released by glands, the organs of the endocrine system. Hormone replacement therapy is needed when insuffi-cient amounts of hormones are being produced. Glands can slow or cease secretion because of destruction by tumors, infections, poor nutrition, environmental toxins, normal aging, heredity, and trauma. The most com-mon problems exist with the thyroid (hypothyroidism), pancreas (diabetes mellitus), and ovaries (the menopause). Both thyroid and pancreatic insulin hormone replacement are lifesaving therapies.

After careful testing reveals a hormone deficiency, hormones are administered as either pills or injections. While symptoms, simple blood tests, and X rays may point to a diagnosis, more sophisticated tests are often needed. A sensitive blood test called a radioimmunoassay can determine exact hormone levels. Nuclear scans, using injected radioactive materials, provide vivid images of the affected gland. Biopsies, which are samples of tissue taken from the gland through a needle or incision, can be viewed directly.

Uses of Hormone Replacement Therapy

Hormone replacement therapy reverses the symptoms of hormone deficiency diseases. Without treatment, the diabetic patient, lacking the insulin that regulates blood sugar levels, will suffer coma and death. The patient who lacks sufficient thyroid hormone to regulate the rate of metabolism will also have a fatal outcome if this condition is left untreated. Postmenopausal women, whose ovaries have ceased the production of estrogen and progesterone because of normal aging, may have uncomfortable and sometimes disabling symptoms which can be relieved by hormone replacement.

Definite risks are associated with hormone use because it is very difficult to imitate the precision with which the body normally maintains the blood concentrations of internally produced hormones. Excess dosages can have devastating consequences: Excess amounts of thyroid or insulin hormones can lead to death. Considerable controversy surrounds postmenopausal hormone replacement because of its association with breast and uterine cancer, liver disease, and blood clots. As with all drugs, the benefits and risks of hormones must be weighed and blood levels carefully monitored.

—Connie Rizzo, M.D.

See also Diabetes mellitus; Genetic engineering; Hysterectomy; Menopause; Women's health issues.

For Further Information:
Braunwald, Eugene, et al., eds. *Harrison's Principles of Internal Medicine.* 15th ed. New York: McGraw-Hill, 2000.
Dennerstein, Lorraine, and Julia Shelley, eds. *A Woman's Guide to Menopause and Hormone Replacement Therapy.* Washington, D.C.: American Psychiatric Press, 1998.
Goldstein, Steven R. *The Estrogen Alternative.* New York: Putnam, 1998.
Jacobwitz, Ruth S. *The Estrogen Answer Book: 150 Most-Asked Questions About Hormone Replacement Therapy.* Boston: Little, Brown, 1999.
Stolar, Mark. *Estrogen.* New York: Avon Books, 1997.

✧ HOSPICE

Type of issue: Ethics, mental health, social trends
Definition: A holistic approach to caring for the dying and their families by addressing their physical, emotional, and spiritual needs.

Hospice is a philosophy of care directed toward persons who are dying. Hospice care uses a family-oriented holistic approach to assist these individuals in making the transition from life to death in a manner that preserves their dignity and comfort. This approach, as Elisabeth Kübler-Ross would say, allows dying patients "to live until they die." Hospice care encourages patients to participate fully in determining the type of care that is most appropriate for their comfort. By creating a secure and caring community sensitive to the needs of the dying and their families and by providing palliative care that relieves patients of the distressing symptoms of their disease, hospice care can aid the dying in preparing mentally as well as spiritually for their impending death.

Unlike traditional health care, where the patient is viewed as the client, hospice care with its holistic emphasis treats the family unit as the client. In addition to the stress of caring for the physical needs of the dying, family members often feel tremendous pressure maintaining their own roles and responsibilities within the family itself. The conflict of caring for their own nuclear families while caring for dying relatives places a huge strain on everyone involved and can be a source of anxiety and guilt for the patient as well. Another area of stress experienced by family involves concern for themselves, that is, having to put their own lives on hold, maintaining their own health, dealing with their newly acquired time constraints, and viewing themselves as isolated from friends and family. Compounding this is the guilt that many caregivers feel over not caring for the dying relative as well or as patiently as they might, or secretly wishing for the caregiving experience to reach an end.

Due to the holistic nature of the care provided, the hospice team is actually an interdisciplinary team composed of physicians, nurses, psychological and social workers, pastoral counselors, and trained volunteers. This medically supervised team meets weekly to decide on how best to provide physical, emotional, and spiritual support for dying patients and to assist the surviving family members in the subsequent grieving process.

This type of care can be administered in three different ways. It can be home health-agency based, delivered in the patient's own home. It can be dispensed in an institution devoted solely to hospice care. It can even be administered in traditional medical facilities (such as hospitals) that allot a certain amount of space (perhaps a wing or floor, or even a certain number of beds) to this type of care. Fewer than 20 percent of hospices are totally independent and have no affiliation with one or more hospitals.

Hospice care attempts to enhance the quality of dying patients' final days by providing them with as much comfort as possible. It is predicated on the belief that death is a natural process with which humans should not interfere. The principles of hospice care, therefore, revolve around alleviating the anxieties and physical suffering that can be associated with the dying process, and not prolonging the dying process by using invasive medical techniques. Hospice care is also based on the assertion that dying patients have certain rights that must be respected. These rights include a right to absent themselves from social responsibilities and commitments, a right to be cared for, and the right to continued respect and status. The following seven principles are basic components of hospice care.

PRINCIPLES OF HOSPICE CARE

The first principle is highly personalized and holistic care of the dying, which includes treating dying patients emotionally and spiritually as well as physically. This interpersonal support, known as bonding, helps patients in their final days to live as fully and as comfortably as possible, while retaining their dignity, autonomy, and individual self-worth in a safe and secure environment. This one-on-one attention involves what can be called therapeutic communication. Knowing that someone has heard, that someone understands and is concerned, can be profoundly healing.

Another principle is treating pain aggressively. To this end, hospice care advocates the use of narcotics at a dosage that will alleviate suffering while, at the same time, enable patients to maintain a desired level of alertness. Efforts are made to employ the least invasive routes to administer these drugs (usually orally, if possible). In addition, pain medication is administered before the pain begins, thus alleviating the anxiety of patients waiting for pain to return. Since it has been shown that fear of pain often increases the pain itself, this type of aggressive pain management gives dying patients more time and energy to respond to family members and friends and to work through the emotional and spiritual stages of dying. This dispensation of pain medication before the pain actually occurs, however, has proven to be perhaps the most controversial element in hospice care, with some critics charging that the dying are being turned into drug addicts.

A third principle is the participation of families in caring for the dying. Family members are trained by hospice nurses to care for the dying patients and even to dispense pain medication. The aim is to prevent the patients from suffering isolation or feeling as if they are surrounded by strangers. Participation in care also helps to sustain the patients' and the families' sense of autonomy.

The fourth principle is familiarity of surroundings. Whenever possible, it is the goal of hospice care to keep dying patients at home. This eliminates the necessity of the dying to spend their final days in an institutionalized setting, isolated from family and friends when they need them the most. It is estimated that close to 90 percent of all hospice care days are spent in patients' own homes. When this is not possible and patients must enter institutional settings, rules are relaxed so that their rooms can be decorated or arranged in such a way as to replicate the patients' home surroundings. Visiting rules are suspended when possible, and visits by family members, children, and sometimes even pets are encouraged.

The fifth principle is emotional and spiritual support for the family caregivers. Hospice volunteers are specially trained to use listening and communicative techniques with family members and to provide them with emotional support both during and after the patient's death. In addition, because the care is holistic, the caregivers' physical needs are attended to (for example, respite is provided for exhausted caregivers), as are their emotional and spiritual needs. This spiritual support applies to people of all faith backgrounds, as impending death tends to put faith into a perspective where particular creeds and denominational structures assume less significance. In attending to this spiritual dimension, the hospice team is respectful of all religious traditions while realizing that death and bereavement have the ability to both strengthen and weaken faith.

The sixth principle is having hospice services available twenty-four hours a day, seven days a week. Because of its reliance on the assistance of trained volunteers, round-the-clock support is available to patients and their families.

The seventh principle is bereavement counseling for the survivors. At the time of death, the hospice team is available to help families take care of tasks such as planning the funeral and probating the will. In the weeks after the death, hospice volunteers offer their support to surviving family members in dealing with their loss and grief and the various phases of the bereavement process, always aware of the fact that not all bereaved need or want formal interventions.

COST

Because of hospice care's reliance on heavily trained volunteers and contributions, and because death is seen as a natural process that should not be prolonged by invasive and expensive medical techniques, hospice care is much less costly than traditional acute care facilities. Because hospice care is a philosophy of care rather than a specific facility, though, legislation to provide monetary support for hospice patients took a great deal of time to be approved. In 1982, the U.S. Congress finally added hospice care as a Medicare benefit. In 1986, it was made a permanent benefit. Medicare requires, however, that there be a prognosis of six months or less for the patient to live. Hospice care is also reimbursable by many private insurance companies.

—Mara Kelly-Zukowski

See also Death and dying; Euthanasia; Hospitalization of the elderly; Nursing and convalescent homes; Terminal illnesses.

For Further Information:

Buckingham, Robert W. *The Handbook of Hospice Care.* New York: Prometheus Books, 1996. Covers the history and philosophy of hospice care while providing practical information as to its cost, how to find hospice programs in your own community, and how to manage grief. Focuses on two target populations for hospice care: children and AIDS victims.

Byock, Ira. *Dying Well: The Prospect for Growth at the End of Life.* New York: Riverhead Books, 1997. President of the American Academy of Hospice and Palliative Medicine at the time he wrote this book, Dr. Byock uses the personal stories of his patients to show the best ways to die. Provides information for the families of the dying who wish to make their loved ones' final days as comfortable and meaningful as possible.

Corr, Charles A., and Donna M. Corr, eds. *Hospice Care: Principles and Practice.* New York: Springer, 1983. A collection of salient essays on hospice care addressing issues ranging from the needs of the dying to the stress associated with caregiving to the terminally ill. Contributors include Cicely Saunders, physicians, hospice directors, psychologists, and chaplains.

Kübler-Ross, Elisabeth. *On Death and Dying.* New York: Macmillan, 1969. Landmark work which outlines the psychological stages of dying and the deficiencies in modern medicine's ability to care for dying patients in an appropriate manner.

Lattanzi-Licht, Marcia, John J. Mahoney, and Galen W. Miller. *The Hospice Choice: In Pursuit of a Peaceful Death.* New York: Simon & Schuster, 1998. Definitive resource from the National Hospice Organization. Provides practical information such as range of hospice services, methods of payment, and so on. Intersperses stories of families who have received hospice care with a thorough explanation of its history, principles, and benefits. Provides personal accounts of hospice nurses and volunteers with discussion of psychological and emotional responses to life-threatening illnesses.

✧ Hospitalization of the Elderly

Type of issue: Economic issues, elder health, public health, treatment
Definition: The specific needs of the elderly in hospital settings, particularly pertaining to acute and long-term care.

In 1996, those aged sixty-five and over accounted for 38 percent of the admissions to nonfederal, acute care hospitals. Those aged forty-five through sixty-four accounted for 20 percent of all admissions. The average length of stay (ALOS) was 5.3 days for people forty-five through sixty-four and 6.5 days for those sixty-five and over. Although the major portion of inpatient services is provided in acute care community hospitals, elderly patients may also receive inpatient services in hospitals operated by the Department of Veterans Affairs or in proprietary facilities such as psychiatric hospitals.

Approximately 97 percent of all hospital care in the United States is financed by third parties. The vast majority of Americans over the age of sixty-five (33.4 million people in 1996) had hospital insurance through the Medicare program. According to data compiled by the Health Care Financing Administration (HCFA), the administrative agency for the Medicare program, the largest component of national health expenditure is hospital care. Inpatient hospital care for beneficiaries resulted in costs to the Medicare program of $79.9 billion in 1996.

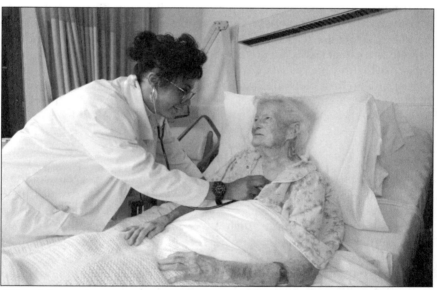

Older adults may find themselves hospitalized for acute illnesses, chronic illnesses, or injuries—all of which present higher risks for the elderly than for younger adults. (Digital Stock)

COST AND PAYMENTS

Medicare pays most short-stay hospitalization under a prospective payment system (PPS) in which hospitals are reimbursed for services according to the diagnosis-related group (DRG) to which the patient is assigned. The DRG system is used to classify patients based on their principal diagnosis and other patient data, such as comorbidity or coexisting conditions. Medicare has set a fixed, preestablished amount of payment for each DRG based on the average cost of resources needed to treat a patient with that particular diagnosis.

The PPS was instituted as a means of containing costs for hospital services by replacing the cost-plus payment system. Since the hospital is paid a fixed amount for each patient stay, the incentive is for the hospital to reduce the average length of stay per inpatient episode. The PPS has been effective in reducing the growth of short-stay hospitalization by providing financial incentives to shift services from inpatient to outpatient settings, to provide services in a more efficient manner, and to reduce the length of stay. These measures were effective in reducing the ALOS from 8.8 days in 1990 to 6.5 days in 1996 and reducing the portion of Medicare payments for inpatient services to 47.8 percent in the same year (from a high of 69.7 percent in 1974).

Approximately 7 million Medicare recipients were hospitalized in 1996, representing 23.1 percent of all people enrolled and 79.1 percent of all Medicare payments for the year. Yearly payments for Medicare enrollees who had been hospitalized averaged $18,925, which was approximately thirteen times higher than payments for nonhospitalized enrollees. One factor that accounts for the higher costs is that in the last months of life, Medicare services, including hospital usage, intensify. During 1996, 6.4 percent (1.9 million) of all Medicare enrollees died; they accounted for 20.5 percent of all yearly Medicare payments.

Diseases and Procedures

Hospitalization for an elderly individual commonly occurs because of acute illness such as pneumonia; because of the exacerbation of a chronic illness, such as an episode of pulmonary edema caused by chronic heart failure; for a major operative procedure, such as coronary artery bypass surgery; because of injury, such as a fracture; or for complex diagnostic procedures, such as an endoscopy.

The most frequent diagnostic category resulting in short-stay hospitalization for Medicare beneficiaries in 1996 was heart disease. These patients made up 20 percent of all Medicare hospitalizations—accounting for 23.7 percent of all payments—and had an ALOS of 5.6 days with an average cost of $7,893 per hospital stay. Related conditions include chest pain (angina), with an ALOS of 2.3 days; cardiac arrhythmia and conduction disorder, with an average cost per episode of $4,548; and coronary artery bypass surgery, with an average cost of $51,583 per patient.

The second most common diagnostic category was cerebrovascular disease (stroke), accounting for 5.7 percent of all hospitalizations and 4.9 percent of all payments. The ALOS for this group was 6.0 days, and payments averaged $5,945 per patient. Pneumonia was the third most frequent cause of hospitalization, accounting for 5.6 percent of discharges, resulting in 5.2

percent of all payments, and having an ALOS of 7.4 days. Malignant neo-plasms (cancers), the fourth leading cause of hospitalization, with 5.5 per-cent of all Medicare discharges affected, resulted in an ALOS of 7.9 days and accounted for 7.5 percent of all payments. The fifth-leading condition resulting in hospitalization was fractures, which accounted for 3.7 percent of all Medicare hospitalizations and 3.9 percent of all payments, with an ALOS of 6.6 days. The highest ALOS, at 14.9 days, was hospitalization for rehabilitative services.

Of all Medicare payments, 74 percent were applied to hospitalizations involving a medical procedure. The most frequent procedure in 1996 was an endoscopy of the small intestines, which may have included a tissue biopsy, performed on 330,035 patients, or 4.9 percent of all Medicare admissions. The ALOS for this procedure was 6.7 days, and the average cost was $4,648. Cardiac catheterization was the second most common medical procedure performed on hospitalized patients, involving 4.4 percent of all patients. The ALOS for this group was 4.7 days, with an average cost of $5,882 per patient. Other medical procedures commonly performed during hospitalization were computed tomography (CT) scan, diagnostic ultra-sound, and respiratory therapy.

In 1996, the rate per 1,000 population for inpatient procedures was 62.9 in the fifteen through forty-five age group, 77.2 in the forty-five through sixty-four age group, and 196.5 for the sixty-five and over age group.

ADVERSE REACTIONS

Longer and more frequent hospitalizations place the elderly patient at higher risk for iatrogenic complications (those accidentally induced by the physician), nosocomial infections (those acquired in the hospital), and falls. The most frequently encountered problem in hospitalized elderly is an adverse drug reaction. The elderly are especially prone to adverse drug reactions because of age-related changes in body composition and function, resulting in altered ability to absorb, metabolize, and excrete medications. Elderly patients frequently require a number of medications (polyphar-macy) to control multiple health problems, and additions to and changes in the medication regimen are common during hospitalization.

Functional decline of the elderly person is a common problem leading to hospitalization, and deterioration in function can be worsened during hospitalization. Factors that contribute to a decline in functional level are the disease process itself, medical procedures and treatments, and decondi-tioning caused by restricted activity. Patients most likely to experience reduced functional ability during hospitalization are those who are older, those with cognitive impairments, and those who exhibited functional losses prior to hospitalization. Early recognition and intervention can decrease the likelihood of functional losses during and after hospitalization.

Delirium or confusion develops in many hospitalized elderly. The development of delirium can have multiple causes, such as drug reactions, sepsis, or the disruption caused by hospitalization. Rapid identification and treatment of the cause is essential to prevent permanent impairment. Elderly patients are more likely to develop respiratory tract infections as a result of immobility, decreased immunity, and decreased respiratory function. They are also more susceptible to urinary tract infections caused by urinary stasis or the use of indwelling catheters. Age-related skin and circulatory changes often increase the older patient's risk of developing pressure ulcers. Pressure, or decubital, ulcers (commonly called bedsores) are more likely to develop in patients who are immobile, incontinent, febrile, or malnourished, or in those who have poor circulation. Special attention to the skin care of the hospitalized elderly is important in preventing skin breakdown.

Visitation by family members and friends plays a therapeutic role in the patient's recovery. Interacting with familiar people helps keep the patient mentally alert and oriented, decreases the sense of loneliness, and increases motivation. Because of the special needs of elderly hospitalized patients, a team approach to treatment is suggested. Involvement by physical therapists, nutritionists, pharmacists, and social workers, as well as nurses and physicians, can be beneficial in promoting rapid and maximum recovery.

ADVANCE DIRECTIVES

The federal Patient Self-Determination Act, which went into effect on December 1, 1991, dictates that all Medicare providers, including hospitals, must have policies and procedures in place that ensure that all patients receive information about advance directives at the time of admission. Advance directives, such as "do not resuscitate" orders or living wills, allow competent people to extend their right of self-determination regarding health care into the future. Such directives ensure that the patient's decisions regarding the acceptance or rejection of particular types of treatment will be respected should the patient become incompetent. At admission, patients should be asked whether they have an advance directive, and, if they do, it should be included in the medical record. Advance directives are especially important for elderly patients, since they are more prone to cognitive impairments caused by illness.

—Roberta Tierney

See also Aging; Cancer; Broken bones in the elderly; Health insurance; Heart attacks; Heart disease; Iatrogenic disorders; Illnesses among the elderly; Injuries among the elderly; Living wills; Medications and the elderly; Nursing and convalescent homes; Overmedication; Strokes; Terminal illnesses.

FOR FURTHER INFORMATION:

Graves, Edmund J., and Maria F. Owings. "1996 Summary: National Hospital Discharge Survey." In *Data: Vital and Health Statistics of the Centers for Disease Control and Prevention/National Center for Health Statistics*. Hyattsville, Md.: U.S. Department of Health and Human Services, Public Health Service, Centers for Disease Control and Prevention, National Center for Health Statistics, 1998.

Health Care Financing Administration. *Health Care Financing Review: Statistical Supplement*. Baltimore, Md.: U.S. Department of Health and Human Services, 1998.

Holmes, H. Nancy, ed. *Mastering Geriatric Care*. Springhouse, Pa.: Springhouse, 1997.

Luggen, Ann Schmidt, ed. *National Gerontological Nursing Association Core Curriculum for Gerontological Nursing*. St. Louis: Mosby, 1996.

Owings, Maria F., and Lola Jean Kozak. "Ambulatory and Inpatient Procedures in the United States, 1996." In *Data: Vital and Health Statistics of the Centers for Disease Control and Prevention/National Center for Health Statistics*. Hyattsville, Md.: U.S. Department of Health and Human Services, Public Health Service, Centers for Disease Control and Prevention, National Center for Health Statistics, 1998.

✧ HYDROCEPHALUS

Type of issue: Children's health, mental health

Definition: A collection of excessive amounts of cerebrospinal fluid (CSF) within the cranial cavity, which can cause increased pressure within the brain and skull, leading to brain tissue damage and, in infants, enlargement of the skull.

Frequently referred to as "water on the brain," hydrocephalus is a disorder most commonly seen in newborns and infants but sometimes occurring in older children and adults. The water is actually a relatively small amount (about 10 cubic centimeters for every kilogram of body weight) of cerebrospinal fluid (CSF), which surrounds and cushions the brain and spinal cord on both the inside and the outside. Within the brain are four CSF-filled spaces called ventricles. The CSF is continuously formed here and then moves down through the central canal, a tube that runs the length of the spinal cord. From the base of the spine, the fluid moves upward on the outside of the spinal cord, returning to the skull, where it covers the outer surfaces of the brain. Here it is absorbed by the brain's outer lining. If interference occurs in any part of this, CSF continues to accumulate in the brain. This usually causes increased pressure to develop within the skull.

Abnormally high pressure can lead to permanent brain damage and even death. In the infant, this accumulation also causes the skull to enlarge, since the growth regions of the skull have not yet become firm.

Excessive CSF may develop due to overproduction of fluid in the brain, a blockage of the fluid's circulation, or a blockage of fluid reabsorption on the brain's surface. Hydrocephalus can be congenital or may develop as a result of a head injury, infection, brain hemorrhage, or tumor. Congenital hydrocephalus and most hydrocephalus that begins in infancy are characterized by an enlarged head, which continues to grow at an abnormally rapid pace.

Symptoms and signs that accompany congenital hydrocephalus include lethargy, vomiting, irritability, epilepsy, rigidity of the legs, and the loss of normal reflexes. If left untreated, the condition causes drowsiness, seizures, and severe brain damage, leading to death possibly within days or weeks. Hydrocephalus is also often associated with other anomalies of the brain and nervous system, such as spina bifida.

When hydrocephalus develops in older children and adults, the head size will not increase since the growth lines in the bones of the skull have hardened. If the CSF pressure increases, resulting symptoms include headaches, vomiting, vision problems, problems with muscle coordination, and a progressive decrease in mental activity.

Treatment and Therapy

Diagnosis of hydrocephalus and related nervous system defects sometimes can be made before birth, either by fetal ultrasound or by testing for the presence of an abnormal amount of a brain-associated protein, alpha-fetoprotein, in the pregnant woman's blood. However, even with early diagnosis and surgical intervention promptly after birth, the prognosis is guarded.

Older children and adults suspected of having hydrocephalus should be examined by a neurologist. A computed tomography (CT) scan or magnetic resonance imaging (MRI) of the brain can visualize the structure of the brain and the extent of the hydrocephalus.

Surgical correction is the primary treatment for hydrocephalus. The excess pressure must be drained from within the brain or a balance between the production and elimination of CSF must be established. In some cases, a combination of surgery and medication is successful. For example, the drugs furosemide (Lasix) and acetazolamide (Diamox), when used for increased CSF pressure from brain hemorrhage, may reduce the amount of CSF fluid produced and thereby decrease the amount of swelling.

Relieving the CSF pressure within the brain is generally achieved by the surgical insertion of a tube, called a shunt, through brain tissue into one of the cerebral ventricles. A one-way valve is attached to the tube; this allows CSF to escape from the skull cavity when the pressure exceeds a certain level. The tubing is then passed beneath the skin into either the right side of the heart or the abdominal cavity, where the excessive CSF can be absorbed safely. Complications of this procedure are fairly common and include repeated infections, septicemia, peritonitis, or meningitis.

The outcome of treated patients with hydrocephalus has improved over the years, but the condition is still associated with long-term problems. A modest percentage of newborns with congenital hydrocephalus will survive and achieve normal intelligence.

—*Cynthia Beres*

See also Birth defects; Childbirth complications; Children's health issues; Meningitis; Mental retardation; Prenatal care; Spina bifida.

FOR FURTHER INFORMATION:

Clayman, Charles B., ed. *The American Medical Association Encyclopedia of Medicine.* 3d ed. New York: Random House, 1994.
Professional Guide to Diseases. 7th ed. Springhouse, Pa.: Springhouse, 2001.

✧ HYPERTENSION

Type of issue: Elder health, public health
Definition: High blood pressure, usually defined as a systolic measurement of 140 millimeters or higher, and a diastolic measurement of 90 millimeters or higher.

High blood pressure that is not controlled by medication or lifestyle can damage the body. The higher the blood pressure, the harder the heart must work to pump blood throughout the body. When the heart has to work harder, the heart muscle gets larger, or hypertrophies. An enlarged heart can work well at first, but as it gets larger, it does not function efficiently and begins to fail. Additionally, arteries get harder and less elastic with age. Having high blood pressure accelerates this process, resulting in further degradations in heart function.

A serious concern of high blood pressure is the increased potential for a stroke, which has been the leading cause of disability in the United States. A stroke occurs when a blood vessel in the brain becomes clogged or bursts. The brain tissue that gets its blood from the affected vessel is deprived of oxygen and begins to die within minutes. The death of the brain tissue can cause paralysis, loss of vision, difficulty talking or hearing, or, in extreme cases, death.

Another complication of hypertension is related to the kidneys. When systolic pressures get high, small blood vessels in the kidneys can rupture and bleed. Over time, this can destroy kidney cells, resulting in impaired function and higher blood pressure. In order to make the kidneys filter blood effectively after the damage, the body must increase the blood pressure, further complicating the health of the whole body. In the extreme cases, this process results in the need for kidney dialysis, which is very costly and a burden for the individuals involved. Blood vessel ruptures can cause complications with the eyes as well. High pressures can damage the eye's retina tissues. In many cases, it can cause blindness.

Hypertension is a major health problem by itself. When left untreated, it can complicate and contribute to many other health problems. Therefore, individuals must be screened periodically and make the necessary lifestyle modifications to minimize their risk of this disease.

Diagnosis of Hypertension

Because no symptoms are felt by individuals with hypertension, it is important to have one's blood pressure checked periodically by a qualified person. Blood pressure is measured by a sphygmomanometer (blood pressure cuff) and a stethoscope. The cuff is wrapped around the upper arm and filled with air to compress the brachial artery. The pressure is slowly released while the health practitioner listens for blood flow through the stethoscope. When the pulsating blood is first heard, the systolic blood pressure is recorded. After the pulsating sound stops, the diastolic blood pressure is recorded. All values are measured in millimeters of mercury. Systolic blood pressure indicates the pressure the blood exerts against the blood vessel walls when the heart is contracting. A value of 140 millimeters or higher would be considered high blood pressure. In general, the greater the value is over 140, the more severe the hypertension. Diastolic blood pressure is the pressure the blood exerts against the blood vessel walls when the heart is at rest (between beats). A value of 90 millimeters or higher denotes high blood pressure. As with the systolic blood pressure, the greater the value is over 90, the more severe the hypertension.

Although there are two different measures for blood pressure, only one of them has to be elevated to be diagnosed as hypertension. Diastolic and systolic blood pressures are highly correlated to one another. Additionally, both are correlated with cardiovascular disease when considered alone and when combined. Generally, the risks of complications are higher for elevated systolic blood pressure than for elevated diastolic blood pressure. An important factor to understand is that blood pressure fluctuates greatly over the course of a day. Therefore, one random reading that happens to be high should not immediately be used to diagnose hypertension. High values at rest on two or more days are required to make an accurate diagnosis.

RISK FACTORS FOR HYPERTENSION

Conditions that increase an individual's likelihood of having a disease are called risk factors. There are several risk factors for high blood pressure. Some risk factors are controllable, while others are uncontrollable. Three risk factors have been identified that cannot be controlled. Heredity is one: Individuals from families with a history of high blood pressure, strokes, or heart attacks are more likely to have high blood pressure. Age is another uncontrollable risk factor: Individuals over the age of thirty-five are more likely to have hypertension than younger individuals. Ethnic background has also been found to be an uncontrollable risk factor: African Americans, Puerto Ricans, Mexican Americans, and Cuban Americans are more likely to have high blood pressure than European Americans.

Fortunately, there are several risk factors that can be controlled. Individuals who are overweight are more likely to have high blood pressure. Also, individuals who consume more than one alcoholic drink per day are at a higher risk. Some individuals are sensitive to sodium (a major component of table salt). These individuals are more likely to have hypertension if they consume too much salt or other sodium-containing products. It has also been found that women who use some types of birth control pills are more likely to develop high blood pressure. Lack of exercise is another risk factor that can be controlled. Proper aerobic exercise has been found to decrease blood pressure.

Risk factors indicate the likelihood for health problems. Not having any risk factors is no guarantee of good health. Therefore, medical experts urge all individuals to have their blood pressure checked at least annually (and more often if risk factors are present) to be sure the "silent killer" is not present.

LIFESTYLE MANAGEMENT

Based on the risk factors identified for high blood pressure, there are several activities that can decrease the likelihood of having hypertension. It is recommended that individuals maintain a proper weight and that overweight individuals implement a reduced-calorie diet. All individuals can benefit from regular exercise. Continuous, vigorous activities are best. Besides developing a stronger cardiovascular system, they can also help people lose weight. These exercises should be done three to four days per week. Long, steady walks can be as good as running for many people.

Other controllable activities include using an alternative to birth control pills, decreasing or discontinuing the consumption of alcoholic beverages, and reducing the intake of sodium. For individuals who have been diagnosed with hypertension, strict adherence to the medication regimen is critical. High blood pressure medication works by getting rid of excess body fluids and sodium, opening up narrowed blood vessels, or preventing blood vessels from narrowing or constricting. It can lower the pressures substantially if taken as directed by a physician. A major problem exists with individuals forgetting or skipping doses and trading medicines with family and friends. It is critical that blood pressure medications be taken exactly as directed and other lifestyle modification recommendations are followed.

A lifestyle habit that indirectly affects hypertension is smoking. Although smoking contributes no known, long-term risk, it does cause immediate, short-term increases in blood pressure. This can complicate an elevated blood pressure by pushing it even higher. Additionally, smoking has been found to increase the risk of coronary artery disease and stroke. Both of these major health problems are related to and complicated by hypertension.

Hypertension can have serious negative effects on health. This disease can affect individuals at any age, but its incidence increases with age. Fortunately, proper lifestyle habits can significantly improve the chances of avoiding hypertension. It is important that people implement positive lifestyle habits early in life rather than waiting until after the problems develop later in life.

—Bradley R. A. Wilson

See also Aging; Alcoholism; Alcoholism among the elderly; Exercise; Exercise and the elderly; Heart attacks; Heart disease; Heart disease and women; Illnesses among the elderly; Nutrition and the elderly; Smoking; Strokes.

For Further Information:
American Heart Association. *About High Blood Pressure.* Dallas: Author, 1995.
_____. *Human Blood Pressure Determination by Sphygmomanometry.* Dallas: Author, 1994.
_____. *Sodium and Blood Pressure.* Dallas: Author, 1996.
Delaney, Lisa. "The Ultimate High-Blood-Pressure Prevention Plan." *Prevention* 45 (November, 1993).
Smith, Susan C. "Take Control of High Blood Pressure in Two Weeks." *Prevention* 50 (September, 1998).